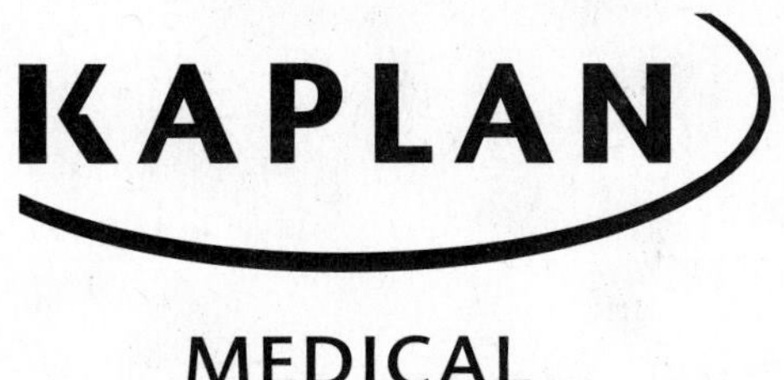

USMLE®

STEP 2 CK

Lecture Notes 2017

Obstetrics and Gynecology

Published by Kaplan Medical, a division of Kaplan, Inc.
750 Third Avenue
New York, NY 10017

10 9 8 7 6 5 4 3 2 1

Course ISBN: 978-1-5062-0804-6

Retail Kit ISBN: 978-1-5062-0815-2
This item comes as a set and should not be broken out and sold separately.

Editor

Elmar Peter Sakala, M.D., M.A., M.P.H., F.A.C.O.G.
Professor of Gynecology and Obstetrics
Division of Maternal Fetal Medicine
Department of Gynecology and Obstetrics
Loma Linda University School of Medicine
Loma Linda, CA

Contributor

Joshua P. Kesterson, M.D.
Assistant Professor
Department of Obstetrics and Gynecology, Division of Gynecologic Oncology
Penn State College of Medicine
Hershey, PA

We want to hear what you think. What do you like or not like about the Notes?
Please email us at **medfeedback@kaplan.com**.

Contents

Section I. Obstetrics

Section II. Gynecology

SECTION I

Obstetrics

Reproductive Basics 1

Learning Objectives

- ❑ Describe the basic physiology of spermatogenesis, ovulation, pregnancy, and lactation
- ❑ List the stages of fetal development and risks related to premature birth
- ❑ Answer questions about the terminology and epidemiology of perinatal statistics and genetic disorders detectable at birth

PHYSIOLOGY OF REPRODUCTION

Human Chorionic Gonadotropin (hCG)

Source—It is produced by the placental syncytiotrophoblast, first appearing in maternal blood 10 days after fertilization, peaking at 9–10 weeks, and then gradually falling to a plateau level at 20–22 weeks.

Structure—By chemical structure it is a glycoprotein with two subunits. The α-subunit is similar to luteinizing hormone (LH), follicle-stimulating hormone (FSH), and thyrotropin (TSH). The β-subunit is specific for pregnancy.

Purposes

- **Maintain corpus luteum production** of progesterone until the placenta can take over maintenance of the pregnancy.
- **Regulate steroid biosynthesis** in the placenta and fetal adrenal gland as well.
- **Stimulate testosterone production** in the fetal male testes.

If levels are excessive—**twin pregnancy**, **hydatidiform mole**, choriocarcinoma, embryonal carcinoma.

If levels are inadequate—**ectopic pregnancy**, **threatened abortion**, missed abortion.

Human Placental Lactogen

Structure—Chemically it is similar to anterior pituitary growth hormone and prolactin.

Pregnancy change—Its level parallels placental growth, rising throughout pregnancy.

OB Triad

Human Chrorionic Gonadotropin (hCG)

- Produced by syncytiotrophoblast
- Similar to LH, FSH, & TSH
- Maintains corpus luteum

OB Triad

Human Placental Lactogen (hPL)

- Produced by syncytiotrophoblast
- Similar to HGH, prolactin
- Decreases insulin sensitivity

Effect—It **antagonizes** the cellular action of insulin, decreasing insulin utilization, thereby contributing to the predisposition of pregnancy to glucose intolerance and diabetes.

If levels are low—threatened abortion, intrauterine growth restriction (IUGR).

Progesterone

Structure—This is a steroid hormone produced after ovulation by the luteal cells of the corpus luteum to induce endometrial secretory changes favorable for blastocyst implantation.

Source—It is initially produced exclusively by the corpus luteum up to 6–7 menstrual weeks. Between 7 and 9 weeks, both the corpus luteum and the placenta produce progesterone. After 9 weeks the corpus luteum declines, and progesterone production is exclusively by the placenta.

Purposes

- **In early pregnancy** it induces endometrial secretory changes favorable for blastocyst implantation.
- **In later pregnancy** its function is to induce immune tolerance for the pregnancy and prevent myometrial contractions.

OB Triad

Progesterone

- Produced by corpus luteum
- Prepares endometrium for implantation
- Decreased myometrial contractility

Estrogen

These are steroid hormones, which occur in 3 forms, each of unique significance during a woman's life.

Estradiol is the predominant moiety **during** the nonpregnant **reproductive years.** It is converted from androgens (produced from cholesterol in the follicular theca cells), which diffuse into the follicular granulosa cells containing the aromatase enzyme that completes the transformation into estradiol.

Estriol is the main estrogen **during pregnancy**. Dehydroepiandrosterone-sulfate (DHEAS) from the fetal adrenal gland is the precursor for 90% of estriol converted by sulfatase enzyme in the placenta.

Estrone is the main form **during menopause**. Postmenopausally, adrenal androstenedione is converted in peripheral adipose tissue to estrone.

Table 1-1. Estrogens Throughout a Woman's Life

Estra*di*ol	Nonpregnant reproductive years	**Follicle** Granulosa
Es*tri*ol	Pregnancy	**Placenta** from fetal adrenal DHEAS
Estr*one*	After menopause	**Adipose** from adrenal steroids

PHYSIOLOGIC CHANGES IN PREGNANCY

Skin

Striae gravidarum—"Stretch marks" that develop in genetically predisposed women on the abdomen and buttocks.

Spider angiomata and **palmer erythema**—From increased skin vascularity.

Chadwick sign—Bluish or purplish discoloration of the vagina and cervix as a result of increased vascularity.

Linea nigra—Increased pigmentation of the lower abdominal midline from the pubis to the umbilicus.

Chloasma—Blotchy pigmentation of the nose and face.

Cardiovascular

Arterial blood pressure—Systolic and diastolic values both decline early in the first trimester, reaching a nadir by 24–28 weeks, then they gradually rise toward term but never return quite to prepregnancy baseline. Diastolic falls more than systolic, as much as 15 mm Hg. **Arterial blood pressure is never normally elevated in pregnancy.**

Venous blood pressure—Central venous pressure (CVP) is **unchanged with pregnancy**, but femoral venous pressure (FVP) increases two- to threefold by 30 weeks' gestation.

Plasma volume—Plasma volume increases up to 50% with a significant increase by the first trimester. Maximum increase is by 30 weeks. This increase is even greater with multiple fetuses.

Systemic vascular resistance (SVR)—SVR equals blood pressure (BP) divided by cardiac output (CO). Because BP decreases and CO increases, SVR **declines** by 30%, reaching its nadir by 20 weeks. This enhances uteroplacental perfusion.

Cardiac output (CO)—CO **increases** up to 50% with the major increase by 20 weeks. CO is the product of heart rate (HR) and stroke volume (SV), and both increase in pregnancy. HR increases by 20 beats/min by the third trimester. SV increases by 30% by the end of the first trimester. **CO is dependent on maternal position.** CO is the lowest in the supine position because of inferior vena cava compression resulting in decreased cardiac return. CO is the highest in the left lateral position. CO increases progressively through the three stages of labor.

Murmurs—A systolic ejection murmur along the left sternal border is normal in pregnancy owing to increased CO passing through the aortic and pulmonary valves. **Diastolic murmurs are never normal in pregnancy** and must be investigated.

Table 1-2. Cardiovascular Changes

Arterial blood pressure	Systolic	↓
	Diastolic	↓↓
Venous pressure	Central	Unchanged
	Femoral	↑
Peripheral vascular resistance		↓

Hematologic

Red blood cells (RBC)—RBC mass **increases** by 30% in pregnancy; thus, oxygen-carrying capacity increases. However, because plasma volume increases by 50%, the calculated hemoglobin and hematocrit values decrease by 15%. The nadir of the hemoglobin value is at 28–30 weeks' gestation. **This is a physiologic dilutional effect, not a manifestation of anemia.**

White blood cells (WBC)—WBC count **increases** progressively during pregnancy with a mean value of up to 16,000/mm^3 in the third trimester.

Erythrocyte sedimentation rate (ESR)—ESR **increases** in pregnancy because of the increase in gamma globulins.

Platelet count—Platelet count normal reference range is **unchanged** in pregnancy.

Coagulation factors—Factors V, VII, VIII, IX, XII, and von Willebrand Factor **increase** progressively in pregnancy, leading to a hypercoagulable state.

Gastrointestinal

Stomach—Gastric motility **decreases** and emptying time **increases** from the progesterone effect on smooth muscle. This increase in stomach residual volume, along with upward displacement of intraabdominal contents by the gravid uterus, predisposes to aspiration pneumonia with general anesthesia at delivery.

Large bowel—Colonic motility **decreases** and transit time **increases** from the progesterone effect on smooth muscle. This predisposes to increased colonic fluid absorption resulting in constipation.

Pulmonary

Tidal volume (Vt)—Vt is volume of air that moves in and out of the lungs at rest. Vt **increases** with pregnancy to 40%. It is the only lung volume that does not decrease with pregnancy.

Minute ventilation ($\dot{V}e$)—$\dot{V}e$ **increases** up to 40% with the major increase by 20 weeks. $\dot{V}e$ is the product of respiratory rate (RR) and Vt. RR remains unchanged with Vt increasing steadily throughout the pregnancy into the third trimester.

Residual volume (RV)—RV is the volume of air trapped in the lungs after deepest expiration. RV decreases up to 20% by the third trimester. To a great extent this is because of the upward displacement of intraabdominal contents against the diaphragm by the gravid uterus.

Blood gases—The rise in Vt produces a **respiratory alkalosis** with a decrease in Pco_2 from 40–30 mm Hg and an increase in pH from 7.40 to 7.45. An increased renal loss of bicarbonate helps compensate, resulting in an alkalotic urine.

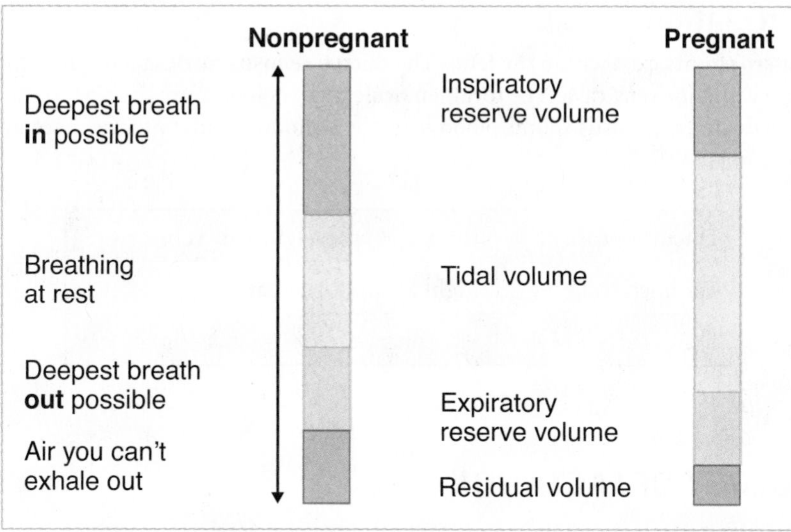

Figure I-1-1. Changes in Pulmonary System

Renal

Kidneys—The kidneys **increase** in size because of the increase in renal blood flow. This hypertrophy doesn't reverse until 3 months postpartum.

Ureters—Ureteral diameter **increases** owing to the progesterone effect on smooth muscle. The right side dilates more than the left in 90% of patients.

Glomerular filtration rate (GFR)—GFR, renal plasma flow, and creatinine clearance all **increase** by 50% as early as the end of the first trimester. This results in a 25% decrease in serum blood urea nitrogen (BUN), creatinine, and uric acid.

Glucosuria—Urine glucose normally **increases**. Glucose is freely filtered and actively reabsorbed. However, the tubal reabsorption threshold falls from 195 to 155 mg/dL.

Proteinuria—Urine protein remains **unchanged**.

Endocrine

Pituitary—Pituitary size **increases** by 100% by term from increasing vascularity. This makes it susceptible to ischemic injury (Sheehan syndrome) from postpartum hypotension.

Adrenals—Adrenal gland size is unchanged, but production of cortisol **increases** two- to threefold.

Thyroid—Thyroid size **increases** 15% from increased vascularity. Thyroid binding globulin (TBG) increases, resulting in **increased** total T_3 and T_4, although free T_3 and free T_4 remain **unchanged**.

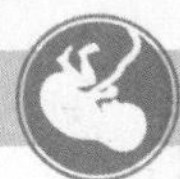

Fetal Circulation

Three **in utero shunts** exist within the fetus. The **ductus venosus** carries blood from the umbilical vein to the inferior vena cava. The **foramen ovale** carries blood from the right to the left atrium, and the **ductus arteriosus** shunts blood from the pulmonary artery to the descending aorta.

Ductus venosus	Umbilical vein → inferior vena cava
Foramen ovale	Right atrium → left atrium
Ductus arteriosus	Pulmonary artery → descending aorta

OB Triad

Fetal Circulation Shunts

- Ductus venosus (UA → IVC)
- Foramen ovale (RA → LA)
- Ductus arteriosus (PA → DA)

PHYSIOLOGY OF LACTATION

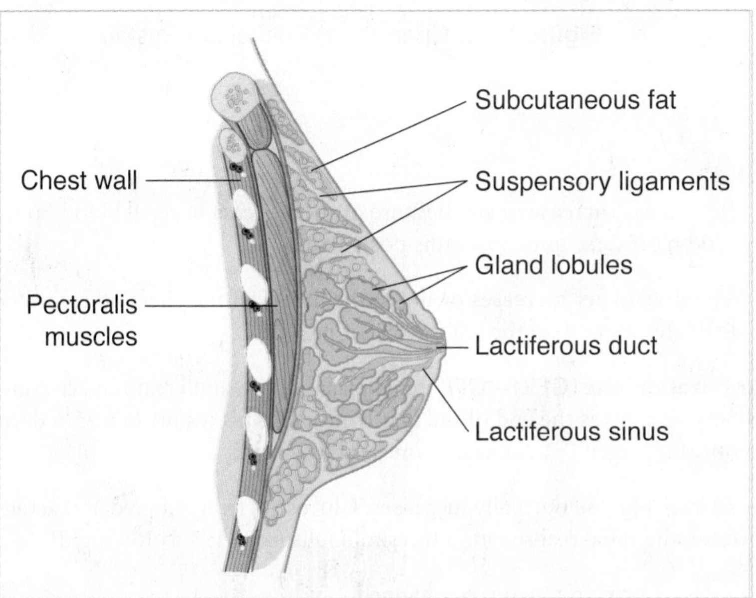

Figure I-1-2. Sagittal View of Breast

Embryology

Breasts begin developing in the embryo about 7 to 8 weeks after conception, consisting only of a thickening or ridge of tissue.

- From weeks 12 to 16, tiny groupings of cells begin to branch out, laying the foundation for future **ducts** and milk-producing **glands**. Other tissues develop into **muscle** cells that will form the nipple (the protruding point of the breast) and areola (the darkened tissue surrounding the nipple).
- In the later stages of pregnancy, maternal hormones cause breast cells to organize into branching, tubelike structures, thus forming the milk ducts. In the final 8 weeks, lobules (milk-producing glands) mature and actually begin to secrete a liquid substance called colostrum.

- In both female and male newborns, swellings underneath the nipples and areolae can easily be felt and a clear liquid discharge (colostrum) can be seen.

Puberty

From infancy to just before puberty, there is no difference between female and male breasts.

- With the beginning of female puberty, however, the release of estrogen—at first alone, and then in combination with progesterone when the ovaries functionally mature—causes the breasts to undergo dramatic changes which culminate in the fully mature form.
- This process, on average, takes 3 to 4 years and is usually complete by age 16.

Anatomy

The breast is made of lobes of glandular tissue with associated ducts for transfer of milk to the exterior and supportive fibrous and fatty tissue. On average, there are 15 to 20 lobes in each breast, arranged roughly in a wheel-spoke pattern emanating from the nipple area. The distribution of the lobes, however, is not even.

- There is a preponderance of glandular tissue in the upper outer portion of the breast. This is responsible for the tenderness in this region that many women experience prior to their menstrual cycle.
- About 80–85% of normal breast tissue is fat during the reproductive years. The 15 to 20 lobes are further divided into lobules containing alveoli (small saclike features) of secretory cells with smaller ducts that conduct milk to larger ducts and finally to a reservoir that lies just under the nipple. In the nonpregnant, nonlactating breast, the alveoli are small.
- During pregnancy, the alveoli enlarge; and during lactation, the cells secrete milk substances (proteins and lipids). With the release of oxytocin, the muscular cells surrounding the alveoli contract to express the milk during lactation.
- Ligaments called **Cooper's ligaments**, which keep the breasts in their characteristic shape and position, support breast tissue. In the elderly or during pregnancy, these ligaments become loose or stretched, respectively, and the breasts sag.
- The lymphatic system drains excess fluid from the tissues of the breast into the axillary nodes. Lymph nodes along the pathway of drainage screen for foreign bodies such as bacteria or viruses.

Hormones

Reproductive hormones are important in the development of the breast in puberty and in lactation.

- **Estrogen**, released from the ovarian follicle, promotes the growth ducts.
- **Progesterone**, released from the corpus luteum, stimulates the development of milk-producing alveolar cells.
- **Prolactin**, released from the anterior pituitary gland, stimulates milk production.
- **Oxytocin**, released from the posterior pituitary in response to suckling, causes milk ejection from the lactating breast.

Table 1-3. Effect of Hormones on Breast

Estrogen	Ducts, nipples, fat
Progesterone	Lobules, alveoli
Prolactin	Milk production
Oxytocin	Milk ejection

Lactation

The breasts become fully developed under the influence of **estrogen**, **progesterone**, and **prolactin** during pregnancy. **Prolactin** causes the production of milk, and **oxytocin** release (via the suckling reflex) causes the contraction of smooth-muscle cells in the ducts to eject the milk from the nipple.

- The first secretion of the mammary gland after delivery is colostrum. It contains more protein and less fat than subsequent milk, and contains IgA antibodies that impart some **passive immunity** to the infant. Most of the time it takes 1 to 3 days after delivery for milk production to reach appreciable levels.
- The expulsion of the placenta at delivery initiates milk production and causes the drop in circulating estrogens and progesterone. **Estrogen** antagonizes the positive effect of prolactin on milk production.
- The physical stimulation of suckling causes the release of oxytocin and stimulates prolactin secretion, causing more milk production.

EMBRYOLOGY AND FETOLOGY

Embryonic and Fetal Development

Postconception Week 1

The most significant event of week 1 is the **implantation of the blastocyst** on the endometrium. Week 1 begins with fertilization of the egg and ends with implantation of the blastocyst onto the endometrial surface. Fertilization usually occurs in the distal part of the oviduct. The egg is capable of being fertilized for 12–24 hours. The sperm is capable of fertilizing for 24–48 hours.

OB Triad

Post-Conception Week 1

- **Starts** at conception
- **Ends** with implantation
- **Yields** morula → blastula

Week 1 can be divided into 2 phases:

- The **intratubal** phase extends through the first half of the first week. It begins at conception (day 0) and ends with the entry of the morula into the uterine cavity (day 3). The conceptus is traveling down the oviduct as it passes through the 2-cell, 4-cell, and 8-cell stages.
- The **intrauterine** phase begins with entry of the morula into the uterus (day 3) and ends with implantation of the blastocyst onto the endometrial surface (day 6). During this time the morula differentiates into a hollow ball of cells. The outer layer will become the trophoblast or placenta, and the inner cell mass will become the embryo.

Postconception Week 2

The most significant event of week 2 is the development of the **bilaminar germ disk with epiblast and hypoblast layers.** These layers will eventually give rise to the 3 primordial germ layers.

Another significant event is the invasion of the maternal sinusoids by syncytiotrophoblast. Because β-human chorionic gonadotropin (β-hCG) is produced in the syncytiotrophoblast, this now allows β-hCG to enter the maternal blood stream. **β-hCG pregnancy test now can be positive for the first time.**

OB Triad

Post-Conception Week 2

- **Starts** with implantation
- **Ends** with 2-layer embryo
- **Yields** bi-laminar germ disk

Postconception Week 3

The most significant event of week 3 is the migration of cells through the primitive streak between the epiblast and hypoblast to form the **trilaminar germ disk with ectoderm, mesoderm, and endoderm layers**. These layers will give rise to the major organs and organ systems.

OB Triad

Post-Conception Week 3

- **Starts** with 2-layer embryo
- **Ends** with 3-layer embryo
- **Yields** tri-laminar germ disk

Postconception Weeks 4–8

During this time the major organs and organ systems are being formed. This is the period of major teratogenic risk.

- **Ectoderm**—central and peripheral nervous systems; sensory organs of seeing and hearing; integument layers (skin, hair, and nails).
- **Mesoderm**—muscles, cartilage, cardiovascular system, urogenital system.
- **Endoderm**—lining of the gastrointestinal and respiratory tracts.

OB Triad

Post-Conception Week 4-8

- 3 germ layers differentiating
- Greatest risk of malformations
- Folic acid prevents NTD

Paramesonephric (Müllerian) Duct

This duct is present in all early embryos and is the primordium of the female internal reproductive system. **No hormonal stimulation is required.**

- In males the Y chromosome induces gonadal secretion of müllerian inhibitory factor (MIF), which causes the müllerian duct to involute.
- In females, without MIF, development continues to form the fallopian tubes, corpus of the uterus, cervix, and proximal vagina.

Female External Genitalia

No hormonal stimulation is needed for differentiation of the external genitalia into labia majora, labia minora, clitoris, and distal vagina.

Mesonephric (Wolffian) Duct

This duct is also present in all early embryos and is the primordium of the male internal reproductive system. **Testosterone stimulation is required** for development to continue to form the vas deferens, seminal vesicles, epididymis, and efferent ducts. This is present in males from testicular sources. In females, without androgen stimulation, the Wolffian duct undergoes regression. If a genetic male has an absence of androgen receptors, the Wolffian duct will also undergo regression.

Male External Genitalia

Dihydrotestosterone (DHT) stimulation is needed for differentiation of the external genitalia into a penis and scrotum. If a genetic male has an absence of androgen receptors, external genitalia will differentiate in a female direction.

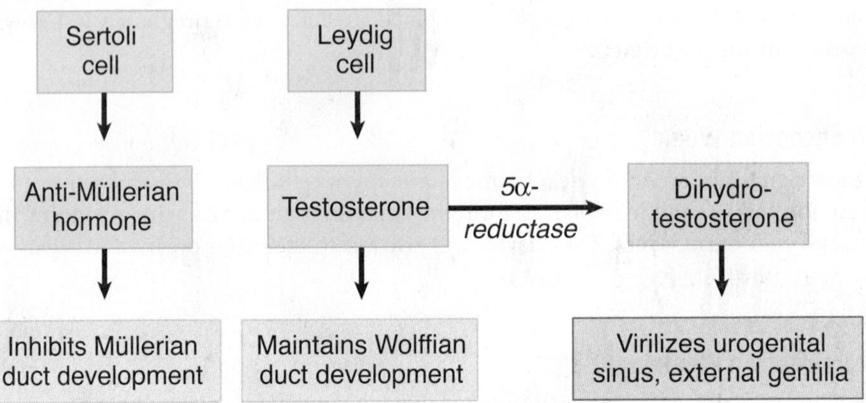

Figure 1-3. Testicular Function

Hormones Needed for Genital Development		
♀	External?	None
	Internal?	
♂	External?	Androgen
	Internal?	

Table 1-4. Embryology

Primordia	Female	Male	Major Determinant Factors
Gonadal			
Germ cells	Oogonia	Spermatogonia	Sex chromosomes
Coelomic epithelium	Granulosa cells	Sertoli cells	
Mesenchyme	Theca cells	Leydig cells	
Mesonephros	Rete ovarii	Rete testis	
Ductal			
Paramesonephric (Müllerian)	Fallopian tubes Uterus Part of vagina	Testis hydatid	Absence of Y chromosome Testosterone Müllerian-inhibiting factor
Mesonephric (Wolffian)	Gartner's duct	Vas deferens Seminal vesicles Epididymis	
Mesonephric tubules	Epoophoron Paraoophron	Efferent ducts	
External Genitalia			
Urogenital sinus	Vaginal contribution Skene's glands Bartholin's glands	Prostate Bulbourethral glands Prostatic utricle	Presence or absense of testosterone, dihydrotestosterone, and 5-alpha reductase enzyme
Genital tubercle	Clitoris	Penis	
Urogenital folds	Labia minora	Corpora spongiosa	
Genital folds	Labia majora	Scrotum	

Teratology

A 36-year-old woman underwent a barium enema for rectal bleeding on February 1 with estimated radiation dose of 4 rad. Her last menstrual period (LMP) was January 1 and she has 35-day cycles. She was not using any contraception. A urine pregnancy test was positive on March 15. She inquires about the risk to her fetus of teratogenic injury.

Definition. A teratogen is any agent that disturbs normal fetal development and affects subsequent function. The nature of the agent as well as its timing and duration after conception are critical. There are critical periods of susceptibility with each teratogenic agent and with each organ system.

Stages of Teratogenesis

- **From conception to end of second week**—The embryo will either survive intact or die because the 3 germ layers have not yet been formed.
- **Postconception weeks 3–8**—This is the period of greatest teratogenic risk from formation of the 3 germ layers to completion of organogenesis.
- **After week 9 of postconception**—During this time teratogenicity is low, but adverse effects may include diminished organ hypertrophy and hyperplasia.

Types of Agents Resulting in Teratogenesis or Adverse Outcomes

Infectious: Agents in this category include bacteria (e.g., chlamydia and gonorrhea cause neonatal eye and ear infections), viral (e.g., rubella, cytomegalovirus, herpes virus), spirochetes (e.g., syphilis), or protozoa (e.g., toxoplasmosis).

Ionizing radiation: No single diagnostic procedure results in radiation exposure to a degree that would threaten the developing pre-embryo, embryo, or fetus. No increase is seen in fetal anomalies or pregnancy losses with exposure of <5 rads. The greatest risk of exposure is between 8 and
15 weeks' gestation with the risk a nonthreshold, linear function at doses of at least 20 rads.

Chemotherapy: Risk is predominantly a first-trimester phenomenon. Second- and third-trimester fetuses are remarkably resistant to chemotherapeutic agents.

Environmental: Tobacco is associated with intrauterine growth restriction (IUGR) and preterm delivery, but no specific syndrome. Alcohol is associated with fetal alcohol syndrome: midfacial hypoplasia, microcephaly, mental retardation, and IUGR.

Recreational drugs: Cocaine is associated with placental abruption, preterm delivery, intraventricular hemorrhage, and IUGR. Marijuana is associated with preterm delivery but not with any syndrome.

Medications: These agents account for 1–2% of congenital malformations. The ability of a drug to cross the placenta to the fetus depends on molecular weight, ionic charge, lipid solubility, and protein binding. Drugs are listed by the FDA as category A, B, C, D, and X.

FDA Categories of Drugs

- **Category A—Controlled studies show no risk.** Adequate studies show no risk to the fetus in any pregnancy trimester. This includes acetaminophen, thyroxine, folic acid, and magnesium sulfate.
- **Category B—No evidence of risk in animals but human studies have not been done.** This includes penicillins, cephalosporins, methyldopa, insulin, Pepcid, Reglan, Tagamet, Vistaril, Paxil, Prozac, Benadryl, and Dramamine.
- **Category C—Risk cannot be ruled out.** Risk is present in animals but controlled studies are lacking in humans. This includes codeine, Decadron, methadone, Bactrim, Cipro, AZT, β-blockers, Prilosec, heparin, Protamine, Thorazine, Alupent, Robitussin, and Sudafed.
- **Category D—Positive evidence of risk.** Studies demonstrate fetal risk, but potential benefits of the drug may outweigh the risk. This includes aspirin, Valium, tetracycline, Dilantin, Depakote, and Lithium.
- **Category X—Contraindicated in pregnancy.** Studies demonstrate fetal risk, which outweighs any possible benefit. This includes Accutane (isotretinoin), Danocrine, Pravachol, Coumadin, and Cafergot.

Specific Syndromes

Alcohol. Fetal alcohol syndrome—IUGR, **midfacial hypoplasia**, developmental delay, short palpebral fissures, **long philtrum**, multiple joint anomalies, cardiac defects.

Diethylstilbestrol. DES syndrome—**T-shaped uterus**, **vaginal adenosis** (with predisposition to **vaginal clear cell carcinoma**), cervical hood, incompetent cervix, preterm delivery.

Dilantin. Fetal hydantoin syndrome—IUGR, **craniofacial dysmorphism** (epicanthal folds, depressed nasal bridge, oral clefts), **mental retardation, microcephaly**, nail hypoplasia, heart defects.

Isotretinoin (Accutane). Congenital deafness, microtia, CNS defects, congenital heart defects.

Lithium. Ebstein's anomaly (right heart defect).

Streptomycin. VIII nerve damage, hearing loss.

Tetracycline. After fourth month, deciduous teeth discoloration.

Thalidomide. Phocomelia, limb reduction defects, ear/nasal anomalies, cardiac defects, pyloric or duodenal stenosis.

Trimethadione. Facial dysmorphism (short upturned nose, slanted eyebrows), cardiac defects, IUGR, mental retardation.

Valproic acid (Depakote). Neural tube defects (spina bifida), cleft lip, renal defects.

Warfarin (Coumadin). Chondrodysplasia (stippled epiphysis), microcephaly, mental retardation, optic atrophy.

PERINATAL STATISTICS AND TERMINOLOGY

Table 1-5. Terminology for Perinatal Statistics

Terminology	Definition
Gravidity	Total number of pregnancies irrespective of the pregnancy duration
Nulligravida	Woman who is not currently pregnant and has never been pregnant
Primigravida	Woman who is pregnant currently for the first time
Multigravida	Woman who is pregnant currently for more than the first time
Parity	Total number of pregnancies achieving ≥20 weeks' gestation
Nullipara	Woman who has never carried a pregnancy achieving ≥20 weeks' gestation
Primipara	Woman who has carried one pregnancy achieving ≥20 weeks' gestation
Multipara	Woman who has carried more than one pregnancy to ≥20 weeks' gestation
Parturient	Woman who is in labor
Puerpera	Woman who has just given birth

Table 1-6. Terminology for Perinatal Losses

Terminology	Definition
Abortion	Pregnancy loss prior to 20 menstrual weeks
Antepartum death	Fetal death between 20 menstrual weeks and onset of labor
Intrapartum death	Fetal death from onset of labor to birth
Fetal death	Fetal death between 20 menstrual weeks and birth
Perinatal death	Fetal/neonatal death from 20 menstrual weeks to 28 days after birth
Neonatal death	Newborn death between birth and the first 28 days of life
Infant death	Infant death between birth and first year of life
Maternal death	A woman who died during pregnancy or within 90 days of birth

Table 1-7. Terminology for Mortality Rates

Terminology	Definition
Birth rate	Number of live births per 1,000 total population
Fertility rate	Number of live births per 1,000 women ages 15–45 years
Fetal mortality rate	Number of fetal deaths per 1,000 total births
Neonatal mortality rate	Number of neonatal deaths per 1,000 live births
Perinatal mortality rate	Number of fetal + neonatal deaths per 1,000 total births
Infant mortality rate	Number of infant deaths per 1,000 live births
Maternal mortality ratio	Number of maternal deaths per 100,000 live births

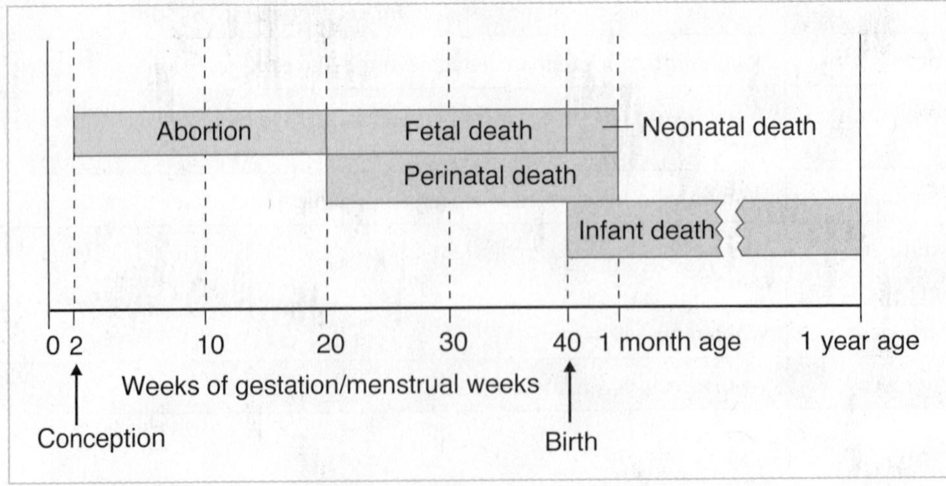

Figure I-1-4. Perinatal Mortality Terminology

GENETIC DISORDERS

Human Genetics and Indications for Genetic Counseling

A 37-year-old G5 P0 Ab4 comes for prenatal care at 7 weeks' gestation. She has experienced 4 previous spontaneous first-trimester abortions. She is concerned about the likelihood of her next pregnancy being successful.

- **Advanced maternal age:** women ≥35 years of age at increased risk of fetal nondisjunction trisomies (e.g., trisomies 21 and 18)
- **Incidence of chromosomal abnormalities by maternal age:**

Age	Down Syndrome	Total Risk
20	1 in 1,670	1:525
25	1 in 1,250	1:475
30	1 in 885	1:385
35	1 in 365	1:180
40	1 in 110	1:63
45	1 in 32	1:18
49	1 in 12	1:7

- **Multiple fetal losses**
- **Previous child:** neonatal death, mental retardation, aneuploidy, known genetic disorder
- **Pregnancy or fetal losses:** stillborn with birth defect, multiple pregnancy or fetal losses
- **Family history:** genetic diseases, birth defects, mental retardation
- **Abnormal prenatal tests:** triple marker screen, sonogram
- **Parental aneuploidy**

Chromosomal Aberration

Aneuploidy

This refers to **numeric chromosome abnormalities** in which cells do not contain 2 complete sets of 23 chromosomes. This usually occurs because of **nondisjunction**. The **most common** aneuploidy is **trisomy**, the presence of an extra chromosome. Most autosomal trisomies result in spontaneous abortions. The **most common** trisomy in first-trimester losses is trisomy 16. The **most common** trisomy at term is trisomy 21.

Polyploidy

This refers to numeric chromosome abnormalities in which cells contain complete **sets of extra chromosomes**. The most common polyploidy is **triploidy** with 69 chromosomes, followed by **tetraploidy** with 92 chromosomes. An example of triploidy is **incomplete molar** pregnancies, which occurs from fertilization of an egg by two sperm.

Structural alterations

This refers to conditions in which chromosomal material is deleted, gained, or rearranged. It can involve single or multiple chromosomes. An example of a chromosomal deletion is del (5p) or cri du chat syndrome, which is a deletion of the short arm of chromosome 5.

Mosaicism

This refers to the presence of ≥2 cytogenetically distinct cell lines in the same individual. Mosaicism can involve the placenta, the fetus, or both. Gonadal mosaicism can result in premature ovarian failure and predispose the gonad to malignancy.

Common aneuploidies are as follows:

Trisomy	Extra single	47,XX+21
Monosomy	Missing single	45,X
Polyploidy	Extra set	69,XXY

Translocations

Reciprocal

This involves any two or more nonhomologous chromosomes, and occurs when there is a **breakage and reunion** of portions of the involved chromosomes to yield new products. Carriers of **balanced reciprocal translocations** have 46 chromosomes, with both derivative chromosomes present. The offspring may also have 46 chromosomes but have only one of the derivative chromosomes present.

Robertsonian

This always involves the **acrocentric chromosomes**, and is caused by centric fusion after loss of the satellite region of the short arms of the original acrosomic chromosome. The karyotype of a balanced Robertsonian translocation will appear to have only 45 chromosomes; however, the full complement of genetic material is present, and there are no clinical effects. The offspring may have 46 chromosomes but have double the genetic material of a particular chromosome.

Genetics of Pregnancy Loss

Miscarriage

At least 50% of first-trimester abortuses have abnormal chromosomes. The 2 **most common** aneuploidies in miscarriages are trisomy 16 and monosomy X. Fifty percent of these abnormalities are autosomal trisomies, with trisomy 16 being the most common.

Turner Syndrome (45,X)

Also known as **gonadal dysgenesis** or **monosomy X**, Turner syndrome is seen in 1 in 2,000 births. In most cases it is the result of loss of the paternal X chromosome. Ninety-eight percent of these conceptions abort spontaneously. Obstetric ultrasound shows the characteristic nuchal skin-fold thickening and cystic hygroma. Those fetuses that survive to term have absence of secondary sexual development, short stature, streak gonads, primary amenorrhea, primary infertility, broad chest, and neck webbing. Urinary tract anomalies, bicuspid aortic valve, and aortic coarctation are commonly seen. Intelligence is usually normal. Mosaic patterns can occur with ovarian follicles present.

Klinefelter Syndrome (47,XXY)

Klinefelter syndrome is seen in 1 in 1,000 births. Diagnosis is seldom made before puberty. Physical findings include tall stature, testicular atrophy, azoospermia, gynecomastia, and truncal obesity. Learning disorders, autoimmune diseases, and low IQ are common.

Down Syndrome

Trisomy 21 is seen in 1 in 800 births and accounts for 50% of all cytogenetic diseases at term. IUGR and polyhydramnios are common. T21 incidence increases with advancing maternal age. The syndrome is characterized by mental retardation, short stature, muscular hypotonia, brachycephaly, and short neck. The typical facial appearance is oblique orbital fissures, flat nasal bridge, small ears, nystagmus, and protruding tongue. Congenital heart disease (endocardial cushion defects) is more common along with duodenal atresia.

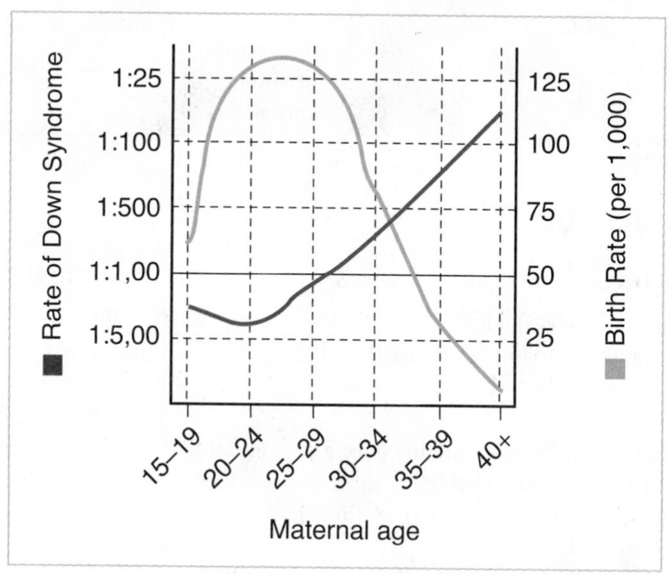

Figure I-1-5. Birth Rate and Rate of Down Syndrome versus Maternal Age

OB Triad

Turner Syndrome

- Primary amenorrhea
- Web neck
- Streak gonads

OB Triad

Klinefelter Syndrome

- Testicular atrophy
- Gynecomastia
- Azoospermia

OB Triad

Down Syndrome

- Short stature
- Mental retardation
- Endocardial cushion cardiac defects

Edward syndrome

Trisomy 18 is seen in 1 in 5,000 births and is more frequent with advancing maternal age. IUGR is common. It is associated with profound mental retardation. Unique findings are rocker-bottom feet and clenched fists. Eighty percent of cases occur in females. Survival to 1 year of age is <10%. Mean survival is 14 days.

Patau syndrome

Trisomy 13 is also seen more frequently with advancing maternal age. It is associated with profound mental retardation. Associated findings include IUGR, cyclopia, proboscis, holoprosencephaly, and severe cleft lip with palate. Survival to 1 year of age is rare, with mean survival 2 days.

Table 1-8. Genetic Syndromes

<table>
<tr><th>Name</th><th>Karyotype</th><th colspan="2">Stature IQ</th><th>Unique finding</th></tr>
<tr><td>Klinefelter</td><td>47,XXY</td><td>TALL</td><td>↓ IQ</td><td>Microgenitals, infertility</td></tr>
<tr><td>Turner</td><td>45,X</td><td rowspan="4">SHORT</td><td>Normal IQ</td><td>Web neck, coarctation aorta</td></tr>
<tr><td>Down</td><td>T21</td><td rowspan="3">Functional MR
↓
Severe MR
↓
Profound mental retardation</td><td>Duodenal atresia, AV canal defect</td></tr>
<tr><td>Edward</td><td>T18</td><td>Abnormal feet, fist</td></tr>
<tr><td>Patau</td><td>T13</td><td>Holoprosencephaly
Cyclops</td></tr>
</table>

Mendelian Genetics

A 23-year-old black primigravida is seen at 12 weeks' gestation. She has been diagnosed with sickle cell trait (AS). Her husband and father of the baby is also AS. She inquires as to the risk of her baby having sickle cell disease (SS).

Prevalence. About 1% of liveborn infants have a congenital Mendelian disorder. **15%** of all birth defects are attributable to Mendelian disorders. Of these, **70%** are autosomal dominant. The remainder are autosomal recessive or X-linked.

Autosomal dominant genetics

Transmission occurs equally to males and females, and serial generations are affected. **Gross anatomic abnormalities are the most common findings.** Age of onset is usually delayed, with variability in clinical expression. Each affected individual has an affected parent (unless this is a new mutation). Affected individuals will transmit the disease to 50% of their offspring. Unaffected individuals will bear unaffected children (if penetrance is complete). **There are no carrier states.**

OB Triad

Autosomal Recessive

- Transmitted by both sexes
- Often skips generations
- Male and female carriers

Autosomal dominant examples:

Polydactyly	Marfan syndrome	Polycystic kidneys
Huntington chorea	Myotonic dystrophy	Neurofibromatosis
Achondroplasia		Osteogenesis imperfecta

Autosomal recessive

Transmission occurs equally to males and females, but the disease often skips generations. Enzyme deficiencies are most common findings. Age of onset is usually earlier with consistency in clinical expression. If both parents are heterozygous for the gene, 25% of offspring are affected, 50% are carriers, and 25% are normal. If one parent is homozygous and one is heterozygous, 50% of offspring will be affected, and 50% will be carriers. If both parents are homozygous, 100% of children will be affected. **Carrier states are common.**

Autosomal recessive examples:

Deafness	Albinism	Phenylketonuria (PKU)
Cystic fibrosis (CF)	Sickle cell anemia	Congenital adrenal hyperplasia (CAH)
Thalassemia	Tay-Sachs (TS) disease	Wilson disease

X-linked recessive

These conditions are functionally dominant in men, but may be dominant or recessive in women. There is no male-to-male transmission (because the father gives only his Y chromosome to his son), but transmission is 100% male to female. The usual transmission is from heterozygous females to male offspring in an autosomally dominant pattern. The disease is expressed in all males who carry the gene. Family history reveals the disorder is only found in male relatives, and commonly in maternal uncles.

X-linked recessive examples:

Hemophilia A	Diabetes insipidus	G-6-PD deficiency
Color blindness	Hydrocephalus	Duchenne muscular dystrophy
Complete androgen insensitivity		

OB Triad

X-Linked Recessive

- No male–male transmission
- Expressed only in males
- Female carriers

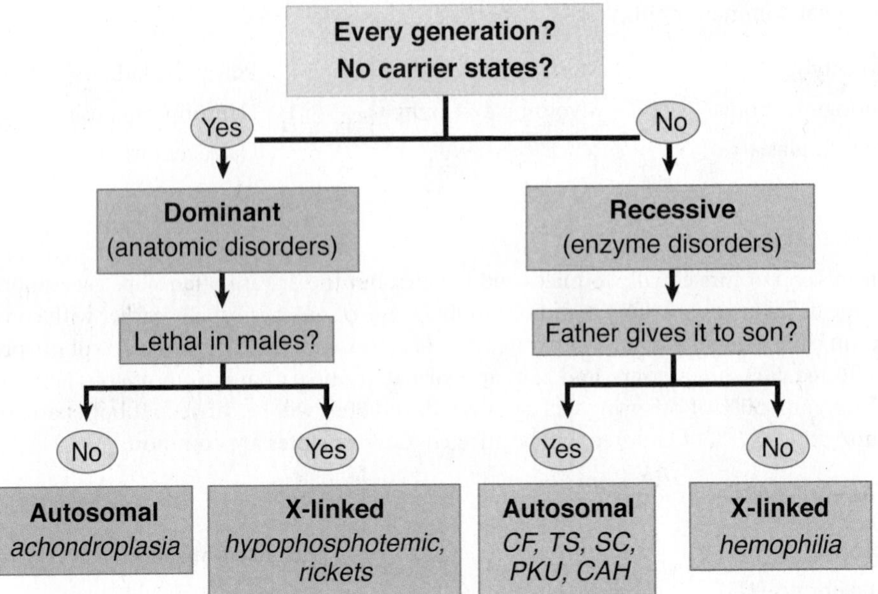

Figure I-1-6. Mendelian Genetics

X-linked dominant

These conditions may show up as two types of disorders: (1) manifested in female heterozygotes as well as carrier males (hemizygotes). Example is hypophosphatemic rickets. (2) manifested in female heterozygotes but lethal in males. The increased spontaneous abortion rate represents male fetuses. Examples are incontinentia pigmenti, focal dermal hypoplasia, and orofaciodigital syndrome.

	A	S
A		
A		

	A	S
A		
S		

	S	S
A		
S		

Calculations of Autosomal Recessive Risk

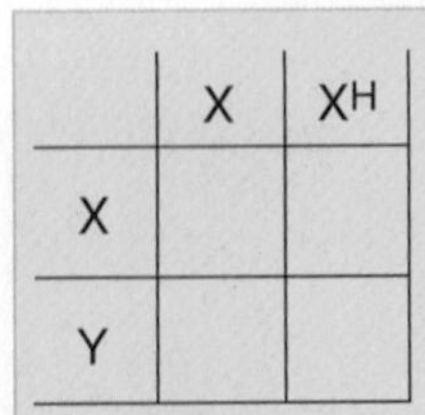

Figure I-1-7. Calculations of X-linked Risk (Hemophilia)

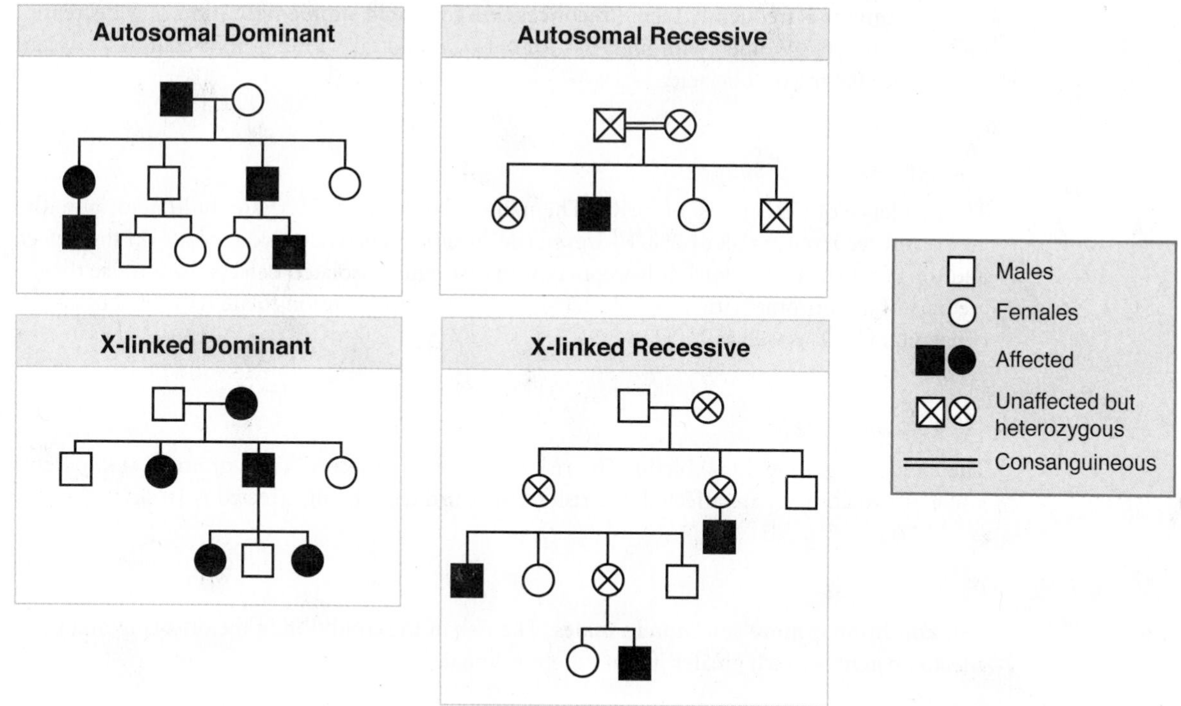

Figure 1-8. Familial Transmission Patterns of Inheritance

Multifactorial Inheritance

A 32-year-old woman with corrected tetralogy of Fallot is pregnant at 18 weeks' gestation with a male fetus. She inquires as to the chance that her son has congenital heart disease.

Prevalence. The majority of birth defects (70%) are multifactorial or polygenic in origin, which means there is an interaction of multiple genes with environmental factors. Characteristic Mendelian patterns are not found, but there is an increased frequency of the disorder or phenotype in families. **The overall recurrence rate is 2–3%.**

- As the number of genes for a multifactorial trait increases, the liability for the disease increases.
- The more severe the malformation, the higher the risk for recurrence.
- Examples of multifactorial inheritance include neural tube defects, congenital heart disease, cleft lip and palate, and pyloric stenosis.

Neural tube defects (NTD)

The incidence of NTD is 1–2 per 1,000 births. These anomalies result from failure of neural tube closure by **day 22–28 postconception**. The spectrum ranges from anencephaly to very slight vertebral defects. Anencephaly and spina bifida occur with equal frequency.

Polyhydramnios is frequently seen. **Preconception folic acid supplementation** may decrease incidence of NTD. Women with high risk for NTD should take **4 mg** of folic acid. All women should take **0.4 mg** of folic acid.

Congenital heart disease (CHD)

The incidence of CHD is 1% of births. The majority of isolated CHD are multifactorial **with an overall recurrence risk of 2%**. However, the specific recurrence risk depends on the defect and the family history details. It is important to distinguish isolated defects from those that are part of a syndrome with a higher recurrence risk. Preconception folate reduces the risk of congenital CHD, as well as NTD.

Cleft lip and palate

The incidence is 1 per 1,000 births. The risk of cleft lip in a second child of unaffected parents is 4%. If two children are affected, the risk of the third child being affected is 10%.

Pyloric stenosis

This condition is more common in males. The risk of the condition in the offspring of an affected parent is much greater if that parent is female.

Failed Pregnancy 2

Learning Objectives

- ❑ Describe the detection and risks of ectopic pregnancy
- ❑ List the approaches to induced abortion at different stages of fetal development
- ❑ Describe the epidemiology and management of early pregnancy bleeding and fetal demise

INDUCED ABORTION

Nearly half of all pregnancies among American women are unintended, and 4 in 10 of these are terminated by abortion. A quarter of all pregnancies (excluding miscarriages) end in abortion.

- Early first-trimester abortions pose virtually no long-term risk of infertility, ectopic pregnancy, spontaneous abortion (miscarriage), or congenital malformation (birth defect), and little or no risk of preterm or low birth-weight deliveries. <0.3% of abortion patients experience a complication that requires hospitalization.
- Numerous epidemiologic studies have shown no association between abortion and breast cancer or any other type of cancer.
- The risk of maternal death associated with abortion increases with advancing gestational age. The maternal mortality associated with childbirth is about 12 times as high as that associated with early first-trimester abortion.

First-Trimester Methods

Vacuum curettage—dilation and curettage (D&C)

- This is the **most common** abortion procedure in the United States (90%), and is performed before 13 weeks' gestation.
- Prophylactic antibiotics are given to reduce the infection rate, and conscious sedation and paracervical block local anesthetic are administered for pain relief.
- The cervical canal is dilated with tapered metal cervical dilators or hygroscopic/osmotic dilators such as **laminaria.**
- Complications are rare but include endometritis, treated with outpatient antibiotics; and retained products of conception (POC), treated by repeat curettage.
- Maternal mortality ratio: **1 per 100,000** women.

Medical abortion

- Mifepristone has been marketed over the past decade as an alternative to surgical abortion.
- Medical induction of abortion can be induced using oral mifepristone (Mifeprex; a **progesterone antagonist**) and oral misoprostol (Cytotec; prostaglandin E1). Use is limited to the first 63 days of amenorrhea.
- Approximately 85% of patients will abort within 3 days. The earlier the gestational age, the higher the success rate. About 2% of patients abort incompletely and require vacuum curettage.
- Rare cases of ***Clostridium sordellii*** sepsis have been reported.

Second-Trimester Methods

The more advanced the gestation, the higher the rate of complications.

Dilation and evacuation (D&E)

- This is the most common second-trimester abortion procedure.
- Cervical dilation is performed by inserting osmotic laminaria dilators 24 hours prior to the procedure. The cervical dilation in millimeters equals the number of weeks of gestation (e.g., at 18 weeks, the cervix should be dilated 18 mm).
- Early second-trimester abortions (13–14 weeks) can be performed by vacuum aspiration. After 14 weeks, the fetus is morcellated and removed in pieces. Ultrasound guidance can ensure complete evacuation of pregnancy tissues. A D&E is difficult to perform after 20 weeks due to toughness of fetal tissues.
- An **intact D&E** involves more advanced pregnancies, with 2 or more days of laminaria treatment to obtain wide cervical dilation allowing assisted breech delivery of the fetus under ultrasound guidance and decompression of the calvaria, with the fetus otherwise delivered intact. In lay terminology, this has been called a "partial birth" abortion. An intact D&E can be performed up to 24 weeks.
- Pain relief is achieved through local, intravenous, or spinal anesthesia.
- Immediate complications may include uterine perforation, retained tissue, hemorrhage, infection, and, rarely, disseminated intravascular coagulation.
- Delayed complications may include cervical trauma with resulting cervical insufficiency.
- Maternal mortality ratio: **4 per 100,000** women.

Labor induction methods

Stimulation of **uterine contractions** to dilate the cervix can be achieved with any of the following: **prostaglandins** (intra-amniotic $PGF_{2\alpha}$), vaginal PGE_2 (dinoprostone [Cervidil®]), IM 15-methyl $PGF_{2\alpha}$ (carboprost tromethamine [Hemabate®]), PGE_1 (misoprostol [Cytotec®]). Interval from induction to delivery may be up to 24 hours.

Delivery of a live fetus may occur with use of prostaglandin (PG) analogs; feticidal agents used include intracardiac injection of KCl or digoxin.

Immediate complications include retained placenta (the most common problem with all PG abortions), hemorrhage, and infection. **Delayed complications** include cervical trauma with resulting cervical insufficiency.

Maternal mortality ratio: **8 per 100,000** women.

Table 2-1. Methods of Induced Abortion

Trimester	Method	Procedure	Maternity-Mortality Ratio
First Trimester	Surgical	Suction dilation & curettage (D&C)	1
	Medical	Mifepristone (progesterone antagonist)	1
Second Trimester	Surgical	Dilation & evacuation (D&E)	4
	PGE_1	Induction of labor contractions	8
Any Trimester	Major surgery	Hysterotomy, hysterectomy	25

EARLY PREGNANCY BLEEDING

A 40-year-old woman (G3 P1 Ab1) at 9 weeks' gestation comes to the office complaining of vaginal bleeding. A urine pregnancy test was positive 3 weeks ago. She initially experienced breast tenderness; however, it has now disappeared. She denies passage of any tissue vaginally.

Note

For more discussion about antiphospholipid syndrome, refer to the thrombophilias section in chapter 10.

Definition. Bleeding that occurs before 12 weeks' gestation. The most common cause of early pregnancy loss is fetal in origin.

Etiology

- **Cytogenetic etiology.** The majority of early pregnancy losses are caused by gross chromosomal abnormalities of the embryo or fetus.
- **Mendelian etiology.** Other losses may be caused by autosomal or X-linked dominant or recessive diseases.
- **Antiphospholipid syndrome.** An uncommon cause of early pregnancy loss. Some women with SLE produce antibodies against their own vascular system and fetoplacental tissues. Treatment is subcutaneous heparin.

Clinical Presentation: Speculum examination is essential to rule out vaginal or cervical lesions that are causing bleeding.

- **RhoGAM** should be administered to all Rh-negative gravidas who undergo dilatation and curettage (D&C).
- Molar and ectopic pregnancy should be ruled out in all patients with early pregnancy bleeding.

Clinical Entities

The following diagnoses represent findings along a continuum from the beginnings of losing the pregnancy to complete expulsion of the products of conception (POC).

Missed abortion

Sonogram finding of a nonviable pregnancy without vaginal bleeding, uterine cramping, or cervical dilation. **Management:** Scheduled suction D&C, conservative management awaiting a spontaneous completed abortion, or induce contractions with misoprostol (Cytotec®) (PGE 1).

Threatened abortion

Sonogram finding of a viable pregnancy with vaginal bleeding but no cervical dilation. Half of these pregnancies will continue to term successfully. **Management:** Often the cause is implantation bleeding. Observation. No intervention is generally indicated or effective.

Inevitable abortion

Vaginal bleeding and uterine cramping leading to cervical dilation, but no POC has yet been passed. **Management:** Emergency suction D&C if bleeding is heavy to prevent further blood loss and anemia. Otherwise conservative management awaiting a spontaneous completed abortion or induce contractions with misoprostol (Cytotec®) PGE 1.

Incomplete abortion

Vaginal bleeding and uterine cramping leading to cervical dilation, with some, but not all, POC having been passed. **Management:** Emergency suction D&C if bleeding is heavy to prevent further blood loss and anemia. Otherwise conservative management awaiting a spontaneous completed abortion or induce contractions with misoprostol (Cytotec(R)) PGE1.

Completed abortion

Vaginal bleeding and uterine cramping have led to all POC being passed. This is confirmed by a sonogram showing no intrauterine contents or debris. **Management:** Conservative if an intrauterine pregnancy had been previously confirmed. Otherwise, serial β-human chorionic gonadotropin (β-hCG) titers should be obtained weekly until negative to ensure an ectopic pregnancy has not been missed.

FETAL DEMISE

A 28-year-old multigravida at 33 weeks' gestation comes to the office stating she has not felt her baby move for 24 hours. A previous 18-week sonogram showed a single fetus with grossly normal anatomy. You are unable to find fetal heart tones by auscultation with a Doppler stethoscope.

Definition. From a medical viewpoint, the term applies to any death after the embryo period (**≥10 menstrual weeks**). From a perinatal statistics viewpoint, the term applies to in utero death of a fetus after 20 weeks' gestation before birth. **Antenatal demise** occurs before labor. **Intrapartum demise** is the term if death occurs after the onset of labor.

Significance

- Disseminated intravascular coagulation (DIC) is the most serious consequence with prolonged fetal demise (>2 weeks) resulting from release of tissue thromboplastin from deteriorating fetal organs.
- Grief resolution may be prolonged if psychosocial issues are not appropriately addressed.

Risk Factors. Fetal demise is most commonly idiopathic. When a cause is identified, risk factors include antiphospholipid syndrome, overt maternal diabetes, maternal trauma, severe maternal isoimmunization, fetal aneuploidy, and fetal infection.

Presentation

- Before 20 weeks' gestation, the most common finding is uterine **fundus less than dates**.
- After 20 weeks' gestation, the most common symptom is maternal report of **absence of fetal movements**.

Diagnosis. Ultrasound demonstration of lack of fetal cardiac activity.

Management

- **DIC present.** DIC is usually not seen until 4 weeks after demise. Coagulopathy should be ruled out with appropriate laboratory testing: platelet count, d-dimer, fibrinogen, prothrombin time, partial thromboplastin time. If DIC is identified, immediate delivery is necessary with selective blood product transfusion as clinically indicated.
- **No DIC present.** Delivery may best be deferred for a number of days to allow for an appropriate grief response to begin. Or if the patient wishes conservative management, follow weekly serial DIC laboratory tests. Ninety percent of patients start spontaneous labor after 2 weeks.
- **Mode of delivery.** A dilatation and evacuation (D&E) procedure may be appropriate in pregnancies of <23 weeks' gestation if no fetal autopsy is indicated. Induction of labor with vaginal prostaglandin is appropriate in pregnancies of ≥23 weeks or if a fetal autopsy is indicated. Cesarean delivery is almost never appropriate for dead fetus.
- **Psychosocial issues.** Acceptance of the reality of the loss may be enhanced by allowing the patient and her family to see the fetus, hold the fetus, name the fetus, and have a burial. Encouraging expression of feelings and tears may speed grief resolution.
- **Identify cause.** Workup may include cervical and placental cultures for suspected infection, **autopsy** for suspected lethal anatomic syndrome, **karyotype** for suspected aneuploidy, **total body x-ray** for suspected osteochondrodysplasia, maternal blood for **Kleihauer-Betke** (peripheral smear for suspected fetomaternal bleed). Amniocentesis can yield living fetal amniocyte cells although the fetus is demised. Up to 10% of the karyotypes show aneuploidy.

ECTOPIC PREGNANCY

A 28-year-old patient visits the emergency department complaining of unilateral left-sided abdominal pain and vaginal spotting of 3 days' duration. Her last menstrual period was 8 weeks ago, and before this episode she had menses every 28 days. Her only previous pregnancy was an uncomplicated term spontaneous vaginal delivery. She had used intrauterine contraception for 3 years in the past. On pelvic examination the uterus is slightly enlarged and there is left adnexal tenderness but no palpable mass. A quantitative serum β-hCG value is 2,600 mIU.

GYN Triad

Ectopic Pregnancy

- **Secondary** amenorrhea
- **Unilateral** abdominal/pelvic pain
- Vaginal bleeding

Definition. This is a pregnancy in which implantation has occurred outside of the uterine cavity. The most common location of ectopic pregnancies is an oviduct. The **most common** location within the oviduct is the distal ampulla.

Differential Diagnosis. With a positive pregnancy test, the differential diagnosis consists of a threatened abortion, incomplete abortion, ectopic pregnancy, and hydatidiform mole. In a reproductive age woman with abnormal vaginal bleeding, the possibility of pregnancy or complication of pregnancy should always be considered.

Risk Factors. The **most common** predisposing cause is previous pelvic inflammatory disease (PID). Ectopic pregnancy risk is increased from any obstruction of normal zygote migration to the uterine cavity from tubal scarring or adhesions from any origin: infectious (PID, IUD), postsurgical (tubal ligation, tubal surgery), or congenital (diethylstilbestrol [DES] exposure). One percent of pregnancies are ectopic pregnancies, and if the patient has had one ectopic pregnancy, the incidence becomes 15%.

Table 2-2. Risk Factors for Ectopic Pregnancy

Scarring or Adhesions Obstructing Normal Zygote Migration	
Infectious	Pelvic inflammatory disease
Postsurgical	Tuboplasty/ligation
Congenital	Diethylstilbestrol
Idiopathic	No risk factors

Clinical Findings

- **Symptoms.** The **classic triad** with an unruptured ectopic pregnancy is amenorrhea, vaginal bleeding, and unilateral pelvic-abdominal pain. With a ruptured ectopic pregnancy, the symptoms will vary with the extent of intraperitoneal bleeding and irritation. Pain usually occurs after 6–8 menstrual weeks.
- **Signs.** The classic findings with an unruptured ectopic pregnancy are unilateral adnexal and cervical motion tenderness. Uterine enlargement and fever are usually absent. With a ruptured ectopic pregnancy, the findings reflect peritoneal irritation and the degree of hypovolemia. Hypotension and tachycardia indicate significant blood loss. This results in abdominal guarding and rigidity.
- **Investigative findings.** A β-hCG test will be positive. Sonography may or may not reveal an adnexal mass, but most significantly no intrauterine pregnancy (IUP) will be seen.

Diagnosis. The diagnosis of an unruptured ectopic pregnancy rests on the results of a quantitative serum β-hCG titer combined with the results of a vaginal sonogram. It is based on the assumption that when a normal intrauterine pregnancy has progressed to where it can be seen on vaginal sonogram at 5 weeks' gestation, the serum β-hCG titer will exceed 1,500 mIU. With the lower resolution of abdominal sonography, an IUP will not consistently be seen until 6 weeks' gestation. The β-hCG discriminatory threshold for an abdominal ultrasound to detect an intrauterine gestation is 6,500 mIU compared with 1,500 mIU for vaginal ultrasound.

Specific criteria. Failure to see a normal intrauterine gestational sac when the serum β-hCG titer is >1,500 mIU is presumptive diagnosis of an ectopic pregnancy.

Diagnosis of unruptured ectopic pregnancy is presumed when:

β-hCG titer >1,500 mIU
No intrauterine pregnancy is seen with vaginal sonogram

Management

- **Ruptured ectopic.** The diagnosis of ruptured ectopic pregnancy is presumed with a history of amenorrhea, vaginal bleeding, and abdominal pain in the presence of a hemodynamically unstable patient. Immediate surgical intervention to stop the bleeding is vital, usually by laparotomy.
- **Intrauterine pregnancy.** If the sonogram reveals an IUP, management will be based on the findings. If the diagnosis is hydatidiform mole, the patient should be treated with a suction curettage and followed up on a weekly basis with β-hCG.
- **Possible ectopic.** If the sonogram does not reveal an IUP, but the quantitative β-hCG is <1,500 mIU, it is impossible to differentiate a normal IUP from an ectopic pregnancy. Because β-hCG levels in a normal IUP double every 58 hours, the appropriate management will be to repeat the quantitative β-hCG and vaginal sonogram every 2–3 days until the β-hCG level exceeds 1,500 mIU. With that information an ectopic pregnancy can be distinguished from an IUP.
- **Unruptured ectopic.** Management can be medical with methotrexate or surgical with laparoscopy. Medical treatment is preferable because of the lower cost, with otherwise similar outcomes.
  - **Methotrexate.** This **folate antagonist** attacks rapidly proliferating tissues including trophoblastic villi. Criteria for methotrexate include pregnancy mass <3.5 cm diameter, absence of fetal heart motion, β-hCG level <6,000 mIU, and no history of folic supplementation. Single dose 1 mg/kg is 90% successful. Patients with an ectopic pregnancy should be advised of the somewhat increased incidence of recurrent ectopic pregnancies. Follow-up with **serial β-hCG levels** is crucial to ensure pregnancy resolution. Rh-negative women should be administered **RhoGAM**.
  - **Laparoscopy.** If criteria for methotrexate are not met, surgical evaluation is performed through a laparoscopy or through a laparotomy incision. The preferred procedure for an unruptured ampullary tubal pregnancy is a **salpingostomy**, in which the trophoblastic villi are dissected free preserving the oviduct. Isthmic tubal pregnancies are managed with a **segmental resection**, in which the tubal segment containing the pregnancy is resected.

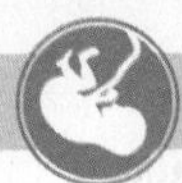

- **Salpingectomy** is reserved for the patient with a ruptured ectopic pregnancy or those with no desire for further fertility. After a salpingostomy β-hCG titers should be obtained on a weekly basis to make sure that there is resolution of the pregnancy. Rh-negative women should be administered **RhoGAM.**

Follow-Up. Patients who are treated with methotrexate or salpingostomy should be followed up with β-hCG titers to assure there has been complete destruction of the ectopic trophoblastic villi.

Obstetric Procedures 3

Learning Objectives

- ❑ Describe routine and high risk prenatal diagnostic testing
- ❑ Describe the appropriate use of obstetrical monitoring procedures including U/S, chorionic villus sampling, amniocentesis, percutaneous umbilical blood sampling, and fetoscopy

OBSTETRIC ULTRASOUND

This imaging modality uses low-energy, high-frequency sound waves.

MODALITIES

- **Transvaginal sonogram:** used in first trimester, producing high-resolution images that are not influenced by maternal BMI. Dating accuracy of first trimester sonogram is +/- 5–7 days.
- **Transabdominal sonogram:** used any time during the pregnancy, but image quality may be limited by maternal obesity. No adverse fetal effects have been noted during decades of research studies. Dating accuracy of early second trimester sonogram is +/- 7-10 days.
- **Doppler** ultrasound studies: used to assess umbilical artery (UA) and middle cerebral artery (MCA) blood flow. This modality assesses fetal well-being in **IUGR** pregnancies as well as fetal anemia in alloimmunized pregnancies.

Indications for obstetrical ultrasound include:

- Pregnancy location & viability, gestational age dating
- Multiple gestation (zygosity, chorionicity, amnionicity)
- Amniotic fluid volume (oligohydramnios, polyhydramnios)
- Fetal growth (IUGR, macrosomia)
- Fetal anomalies, fetal well-being
- Pregnancy bleeding, fetal anemia

Note

Accuracy of Sonogram Dating

Crown-Rump Length (CRL)

+/- 5 days	<9 weeks
+/- 7 days	9-14 weeks

BPD, HC, AC, FL

+/- 7 days	14-16 weeks
+/- 10 days	16-22 weeks
+/- 14 days	22-28 weeks
+/- 21 days	28+ weeks

Genetic sonogram, ideally performed at 18-20 weeks, looks for anatomic markers of fetal aneuploidy which includes:

- **Generic:** any structural abnormalities
- **Specific:** nuchal skin fold thickness (strongest predictor), short long bones, pyelectasis, echogenic intracardiac focus, hyperechoic bowel.

Nuchal translucency (NT) **measurement** is a screening test, performed between 10-14 weeks, measuring the fetal fluid collection behind the neck.

- A thickened NT increases the likelihood of aneuploidy and cardiac disease.
- It is combined with two maternal blood tests (free β-hCG & PAPP-A) in first-trimester screening to increase the sensitivity and specificity for aneuploidy screening.

CHORIONIC VILLUS SAMPLING (CVS)

CVS is a diagnostic outpatient office procedure performed under ultrasound guidance without anesthesia. Procedure-related pregnancy loss rate is 0.7%.

- The catheter is placed directly into the placental tissue without entering the amniotic cavity. Chorionic villi, which are placental precursors, are aspirated from a pregnant uterus between 10 and 12 weeks' gestation.
- The tissue is sent to the laboratory for karyotyping. The chromosomes of the villi are almost always identical to those of the embryo.
- The procedure can be performed either **transcervically** or **transabdominally**. Since the fetus and chorionic villi are both derived from a common origin (the zygote), their karyotype is identical more than 99% of the time.

AMNIOCENTESIS

Amniocentesis is a diagnostic, outpatient office procedure performed **after 15 weeks** under ultrasound guidance without anesthesia. Pregnancy loss rate is 0.5%

- A needle is placed into a pocket of amniotic fluid under direct ultrasound guidance, aspirating amniotic fluid containing desquamated living fetal cells **(amniocytes)**.
- Fetal karyotyping is performed on amniocytes. NTD (neural tube defect) screening is performed on amniotic fluid with biochemical analysis (**AFP and acetylcholinesterase**).

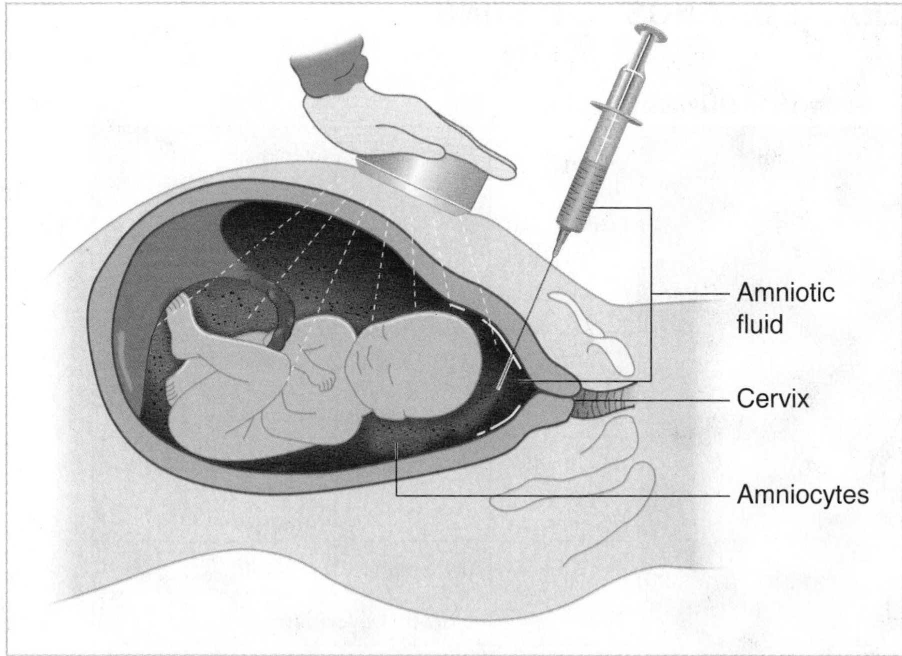

Figure I-3-1. Amniocentesis

PERCUTANEOUS UMBILICAL BLOOD SAMPLE (PUBS)

This transabdominal procedure, performed under ultrasound guidance, aspirates fetal blood from the umbilical vein after 20 weeks' gestation.

- The procedure can be **diagnostic** (e.g., blood gases, karyotype, IgG and IgM antibodies) as well as **therapeutic** (e.g., intrauterine transfusion with fetal anemia).
- Procedure-related pregnancy loss rate is **1–2%.**

FETOSCOPY

A fetoscopy is a **transabdominal** procedure performed with a fiberoptic scope in the operating room **after 20 weeks** under regional or general anesthesia.

- Indications for fetoscopy include **intrauterine surgery** or **fetal skin biopsy**.
- Laser is used for coagulating placental vessels in twin–twin transfusion syndrome (TTTS). Skin biopsy may be performed for suspected fetal ichthyosis.
- **Risks** are bleeding, infection, membrane rupture, fetal loss.
- The pregnancy loss rate is **2–5%.**

PRENATAL DIAGNOSTIC TESTING

Table 3-1. Prenatal Diagnostic Testing

CVS	10-12 wks	0.7% pregnancy loss rate
		Placental precursor
First Trimester	10-14 wks	0% pregnancy loss rate
		Nuchal T, PAPP-A
Amniocentesis	≥15 wks	0.5% pregnancy loss rate
		Amniocytes; amniotic fluid AFP
Expanded X-AFP	15-20 wks	0% pregnancy loss rate
		MS-AFP, β-hCG, estriol, inhibin
Sonogram	18-20 wks	0% pregnancy loss rate
		Non-invasive anatomy scan
Fetoscopy	18-20 wks	3-5% pregnancy loss rate
		Laser in TTTS, fetal biopsy
PUBS	≥20 wks	1-2% pregnancy loss rate
		Umbilical vein blood

Prenatal Management of the Normal Pregnancy 4

Learning Objectives

- ❑ Describe methods for diagnosing pregnancy, establishing gestational age, and identifying risk factors
- ❑ List normal pregnancy events and complaints
- ❑ Differentiate between safe and unsafe immunizations in pregnancy

DIAGNOSIS OF PREGNANCY

Presumptive signs of pregnancy include amenorrhea, breast tenderness, nausea and vomiting, increased skin pigmentation, and skin striae.

Probable signs of pregnancy include **enlargement of the uterus**, maternal sensation of uterine contractions or fetal movement, Hegar sign (softening of the junction between the corpus and cervix), and positive urine or **serum β-human chorionic gonadotropin** (β-hCG) testing.

Positive signs of pregnancy include hearing **fetal heart tones, sonographic visualization of a fetus**, perception of fetal movements by an external examiner, and x-ray showing a fetal skeleton.

Table 4-1. Signs of Pregnancy

Presumptive	Unrelated to uterus or fetus	Amenorrhea
Probable	Related to uterus or mother's feelings	↑ uterine size β-hCG
Definitive	Related to the fetus	Sonogram of fetus Heard FHT

ESTABLISHING GESTATIONAL AGE

Conception Dating

Normal pregnancy duration postconception is 266 days or 38 weeks. However, most women can't identify conception date accurately.

Menstrual Dating

Because the last menstrual period (LMP) is more easily identified than conception, pregnancy duration in most cases is determined to be 280 days or 40 weeks from the LMP. We assume a 28-day menstrual cycle in which ovulation occurs on day 14 after the beginning of the LMP. Yet only 10% of women have a 28-day cycle. A normal cycle length can vary from 21 to 35 days.

Naegele's Rule

Assuming 28-day cycles, a due date can be estimated as the LMP minus 3 months + 7 days.

Table 4-2. Pregnancy Dating

Duration of pregnancy using:	Conceptional dating	266 days or 38 weeks
Duration of pregnancy using:	Menstrual dating	280 days or 40 weeks
Assumed cycle length		28 days
Calculate due date	Naegele's rule	LMP–3 months + 7 days

Definition of abbreviations: LMP, last menstrual period.

Basal Body Temperature (BBT)

The rise in BBT is assumed to be caused by the thermogenic effect of progesterone produced by the corpus luteum that formed after ovulation. The accuracy of BBT is ±1 week.

Menstrual History

Menstrual dating assumes ovulation occurred on day 14 after the first day of the LMP. However, normal menstrual cycles can vary from 21 to 35 days, making ovulation possible on day 7 to day 21. Because most women's cycles are more or less than 28 days, adjustment of the due date may be necessary. Accuracy of menstrual dating is variable depending on the patient's memory and record keeping. The accuracy of menstrual history is ±1 week.

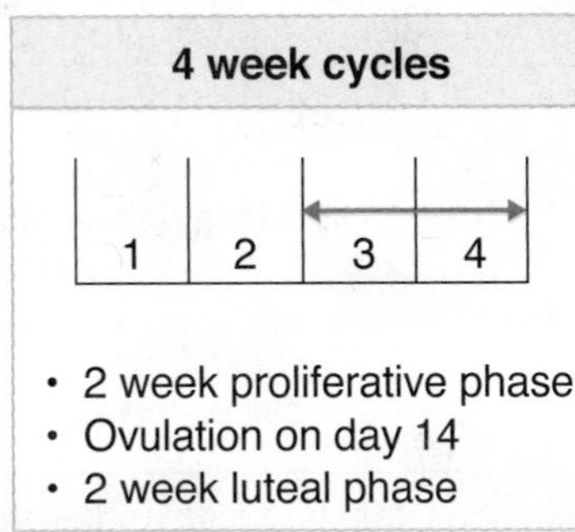

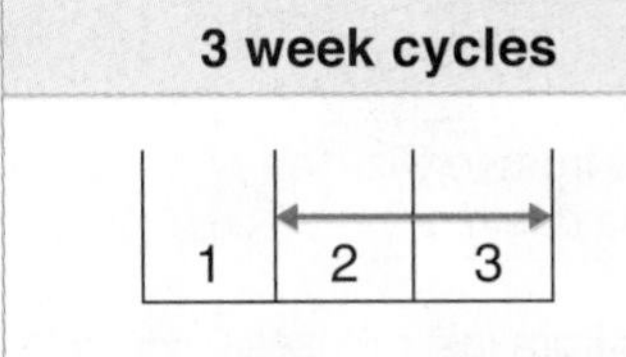

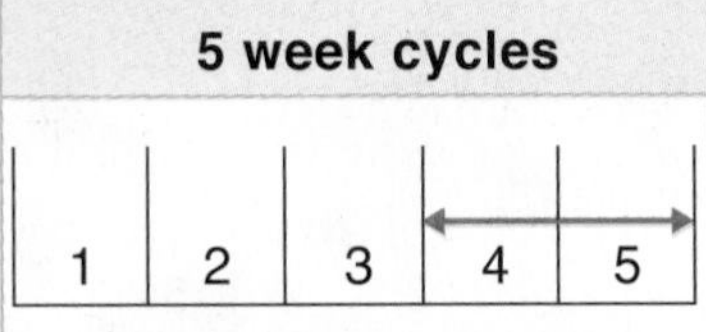

Figure I-4-1. Variations in Menstrual Cycle

OB Triad

Precise Day of Ovulation

- **21-day cycle:** day 7
- **28-day cycle:** day 14
- **35-day cycle:** day 21

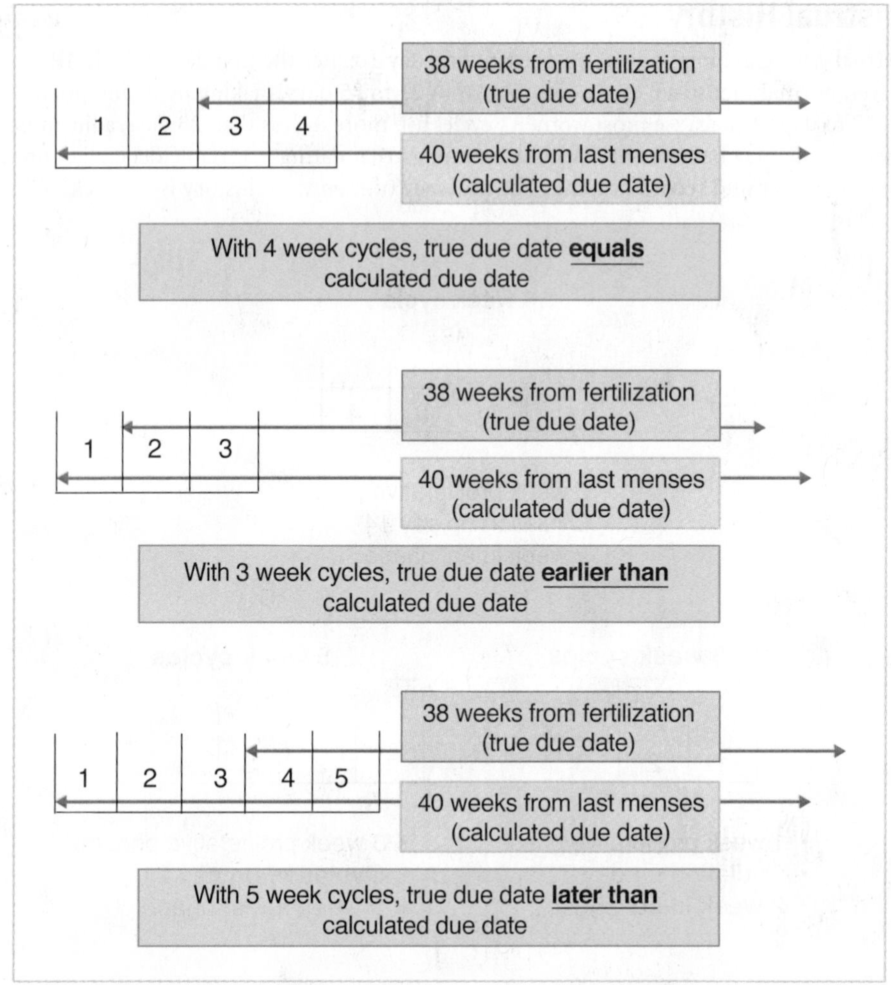

Figure I-4-2. Effect of Cycle Length on Calculated Due Date

IDENTIFICATION OF RISK FACTORS

Obstetrical history—number of pregnancies, pregnancy duration, complications, mode of delivery, perinatal outcome

Medical and surgical history—diabetes mellitus, hypertension, cardiac, thyroid, seizure disorder, anemia

Social history—educational level, marital status, social support, abusive relationships

Family history—inherited diseases, mental retardation, birth defects, perinatal deaths

Sexual history—age of first intercourse, current partners, lifetime sexual partners, previous sexual abuse

Lifestyle—alcohol, tobacco, recreational drugs, poor nutrition, eating disorders

Teratogenic exposure—x-radiation, toxins, chemicals, prescription medications

NORMAL PREGNANCY EVENTS

First Trimester

Assuming a 40 menstrual week pregnancy, the first trimester is assumed to extend from conception through to 13 weeks.

- Normal symptoms seen in the majority of pregnancies include nausea, vomiting, fatigue, breast tenderness, and frequent urination.
- **Spotting and bleeding** occur in 20% of pregnancies, 50% of which will continue successfully.
- Average weight gain is 5–8 pounds.
- Complications—spontaneous abortion.

Second Trimester

Assuming a 40 menstrual week pregnancy, the second trimester is assumed to extend from 13 to 26 weeks.

- Normal symptoms are an improved feeling of general well-being.
- Round ligament pain is common.
- **Braxton-Hicks** contractions are painless, low-intensity, long-duration contractions that can be palpated as early as 14 weeks.
- **Quickening** (maternal awareness of fetal movement) is detected at 18–20 weeks by primigravidas and 16–20 weeks by multigravidas.
- Average weight gain is 1 pound per week after 20 weeks.
- Complications include incompetent cervix (painless cervical dilation leading to delivery of a nonviable fetus); premature membrane rupture, and premature labor.

Third Trimester

Assuming a 40 menstrual week pregnancy, the third trimester is assumed to extend from 26 to 40 weeks.

- Normal symptoms include decreased libido, lower back and leg pain, urinary frequency, and Braxton-Hicks contractions.
- **Lightening** describes descent of the fetal head into the pelvis resulting in easier maternal breathing, pelvic pressure.
- **Bloody show** describes vaginal passage of bloody endocervical mucus, the result of cervical dilation before labor.
- Average weight gain is 1 pound per week after 20 weeks.
- Complications include premature membrane rupture, premature labor, preeclampsia, urinary tract infection, anemia, and gestational diabetes.

NORMAL PREGNANCY COMPLAINTS

- **Backache** is very common, especially in the latter part of pregnancy because of the change in center of gravity with the enlarging uterus. Muscles and ligaments are now used that otherwise would not be. **Management** is encouragement of correct posture.

- **Bleeding gums** is caused by the increase of blood flow to the gums with pregnancy. If it is associated with clinical swelling, it is known as epulis. **Management** is conservative.
- **Breast enlargement.** Each breast increases in size by 400 grams and may result in an increase of one to two cup sizes. **Management** is a support bra.
- **Carpal tunnel.** As many as 50% of pregnant women will experience numbness, tingling, burning, or pain in at least two of the three digits supplied by the median nerve. **Management** is fitting with a wrist splint (most cases will spontaneously resolve after delivery).
- **Complexion changes**. Some women develop brownish or yellowish patches called chloasma, or the "mask of pregnancy," on their faces. Others may develop a linea nigra on the lower abdominal midline, as well as hyperpigmentation of the nipples and external genitalia. **Management** is conservative.
- **Dizziness.** BP normally decreases in pregnancy, which may lead to postural hypotension. **Management** is avoiding rapid postural changes, such as standing up quickly.
- **Fatigue** is very common in pregnancy, probably because of rapid hormonal changes. **Management** is adequate resting and the avoidance of excessive activity.
- **Fluid retention.** Increased circulating steroid levels and decreased serum albumin results in edema in over half of pregnant women. Edema is not a criterion for preeclampsia. **Management** is elevating legs and using support hose.
- **Hair and nails.** Hair shedding decreases in pregnancy. **Telogen effluvium** is the excessive shedding of hair occurring 1–5 months after pregnancy. Telogen effluvium occurs in 40–50% of women. Nails may become more brittle. **Management** is conservative.
- **Headaches.** Muscle contraction and migraine headaches are more common in pregnancy probably because of increased estrogen levels. **Management** is physical therapy (e.g., ice packs, massage) with medication only as a last resort.
- **Leg cramps.** Lower extremity muscle cramps are frequent in pregnancy. **Management** is hydration, stretching exercises, and calcium supplementation.
- **Morning sickness.** Nausea and vomiting are common in early pregnancy and are probably mediated by elevated hCG levels. **Management** is eating small meals emphasizing crackers and carbohydrates.
- **Nosebleeds.** Vasodilation and increased vascular supply results in more frequent nosebleeds. **Management** is saline drops and the avoidance of nasal sprays.
- **Stretch marks.** Genetic predisposition and pregnancy can result in striae gravidarum. Women with stretch marks have increased risk of delivery lacerations. **Management** is conservative.
- **Stress incontinence.** Pressure on the bladder with an enlarging uterus frequently results in an involuntary loss of urine. **Management** is strengthening the pelvic diaphragm with Kegel exercises.
- **Varicose veins.** Increased blood volume, the relaxing effect of progesterone on smooth muscle, and an increased lower-extremity venous pressure often result in lower-extremity varicosities. **Management** is discouraging prolonged standing and sitting.

Table 4-3. Pregnancy Danger Signs

Complaint	Possible Diagnosis
Vaginal bleeding	Early (spontaneous abortion) Later (abruption, previa)
Vaginal fluid leakage	Rupture of membrane (ROM) Urinary incontinence
Epigastric pain	Severe preeclampsia
Uterine cramping	Preterm labor Preterm contractions
↓ fetal movement	Fetal compromise
Persistent vomiting	Hyperemesis (early) Hepatitis Pyelonephritis
Headache, visual changes	Severe preeclampsia
Pain with urination	Cystitis Pyelonephritis
Chills and fever	Pyelonephritis Chorioamnionitis

SAFE AND UNSAFE IMMUNIZATIONS

Safe

Safe immunizations include antigens from killed or inactivated organisms:

- Influenza (all pregnant women in flu season)
- Hepatitis B (pre- and postexposure)
- Hepatitis A (pre- and postexposure)
- Pneumococcus (only high-risk women)
- Meningococcus (in unusual outbreaks)
- Typhoid (not routinely recommended)

Unsafe

Unsafe immunizations include antigens from live attenuated organisms:

- Measles
- Mumps
- Polio
- Rubella
- Yellow fever
- Varicella

Prenatal Laboratory Testing 5

Learning Objectives

- ❑ Use knowledge of first trimester laboratory tests
- ❑ Use knowledge of second trimester laboratory tests
- ❑ Explain information related to third-trimester laboratory tests

FIRST TRIMESTER LABORATORY TESTS

A 21-year-old primigravida G1 PO presents for her first prenatal visit at 11 weeks' gestation, which is confirmed by obstetric sonogram. She has no risk factors. What laboratory tests should be ordered on her?

Complete Blood Count

Hemoglobin and hematocrit

Normal pregnancy hemoglobin reference range is 10–12 g/dL. Although nonpregnant female hemoglobin reference range is 12–14 g/dL, normal values in pregnancy will reflect the dilutional effect of greater plasma volume increase than red blood cell (RBC) mass.

Mean corpuscular volume (MCV)

Because hemoglobin and hematocrit reflect pregnancy dilution, MCV may be the most reliable predictor of true anemia. A low hemoglobin and low MCV (<80 μm^3) most commonly suggests iron deficiency, but may also be caused by thalassemia. A low hemoglobin and high MCV (>100) suggests folate deficiency or, rarely, vitamin B12 deficiency.

Platelet count

A low platelet count (<150,000/mm^3) is most likely indicative of gestational (pregnancy-induced) thrombocytopenia. Preeclampsia with severe features and idiopathic thrombocytopenic purpura (ITP) are uncommon causes of low platelets. Disseminated intravascular coagulation is rare.

Leukocyte count

White blood cell count in pregnancy is normally up to 16,000/mm^3. Leukopenia suggests immune suppression or leukemia.

Rubella IgG Antibody

Immunity

The presence of rubella antibodies rules out a primary infection during the pregnancy. Antibodies derived from a natural, wild infection lead to lifelong immunity. Antibodies from a live-attenuated virus are not as durable.

Susceptibility

An absence of antibodies leaves the woman at risk for a primary rubella infection in pregnancy that can have devastating fetal effects, particularly in the first trimester. Rubella immunization is contraindicated in pregnancy because it is made from a live virus but is recommended after delivery.

Hepatitis B Virus (HBV)

Surface antibody

HBV surface antibodies are expected from a successful vaccination.

Surface antigen

The presence of HBV surface antigen represents either a previous or current infection. HBV surface antigen indicates **high risk for vertical transmission** of HBV from the mother to the fetus or neonate. This is the only specific hepatitis test obtained routinely on the prenatal laboratory panel.

E antigen

The presence of HBV E antigen signifies a highly infectious state.

Type, Rh, and Antibody Screening

Direct Coombs test

The patient's blood type and Rh is determined with the **direct Coombs test**. If the patient is Rh negative, she is at risk for anti-D isoimmunization.

Indirect Coombs test or atypical antibody test (AAT)

The presence of atypical RBC antibodies is determined with the indirect Coombs test. Isoimmunization is identified if atypical antibodies are present. Follow-up testing is necessary to identify whether the fetus is at risk.

STD Screening

Cervical cultures

Screening cultures for **chlamydia** and **gonorrhea** will identify whether the fetus is at risk from delivery through an infected birth canal.

Syphilis

Nonspecific screening tests (**veneral disease research laboratory** [VDRL] or **rapid plasma reagin** [RPR]) are performed on all pregnant women. Positive screening tests must be followed up with treponema-specific tests (microhemagglutination assay for antibodies to *T. pallidum* [**MHA-TP**] or **fluorescent treponema antibody absorption** [FTA]). **Treatment** of syphilis in pregnancy requires penicillin to ensure adequate fetal treatment.

Hepatitis B

Maternal hepatitis-B surface antigen (HBsAg) screening assesses if the mother could have active hepatitis, as well as if she could transmit HBV to her newborn at the time of delivery.

Table 5-1. Initial Prenatal Labs STDs

<table>
<tr><td>Chlamydia/Gonorrhea (GC)</td><td>Screening</td><td>DNA probes</td></tr>
<tr><td>Hepatitis B virus</td><td>Screening</td><td>HBsAg</td></tr>
<tr><td rowspan="2">Syphilis</td><td>Screening</td><td>VDRL/RPR</td></tr>
<tr><td>Definitive</td><td>MHA/FTA</td></tr>
<tr><td rowspan="2">HIV</td><td>Screening</td><td>ELISA</td></tr>
<tr><td>Definitive</td><td>Western Blot</td></tr>
</table>

Definition of abbreviations: FTA, fluorescent treponema antibody absorption; HBsAg, hepatitis B surface antigen; ELISA, enzyme-linked, immunosorbant assay; MHA, microhemagglutination assay; RPR, rapid plasma reagin.

Urine Screening

Urinalysis

Assessment of proteinuria, ketones, glucose, leukocytes, and bacteria is important to screen for **underlying renal disease**, diabetes, and infection.

Culture

Screening for **asymptomatic bacteriuria** (ASB) is essential. Eight percent of pregnant women have ASB. Left untreated, 30% of ASB progresses to pyelonephritis, which is associated with septic shock, pulmonary edema, and adult respiratory distress syndrome.

Tuberculosis (TB) Screening

PPD or Tine test

This screening skin test determines **previous exposure to TB**. A positive test is induration, not erythema. If the screening test is negative, no further follow-up is necessary. TB screening is not done routinely and performed only on high-risk populations.

Chest x-ray

A chest x-ray is performed to rule out active disease only if the screening skin test is positive. If the chest x-ray is negative, isoniazid (INH) (and vitamin B_6) is given for 9 months. If the chest x-ray is positive, induced sputum is cultured and triple medications begun until cultures define the organisms involved. Antituberculosis drugs are not contraindicated in pregnancy.

HIV Screening

Screening

HIV screening is recommended for all pregnant women as part of the initial lab testing. The CDC recommends **Informed Refusal** (or "**Opt Out**," where a patient is tested unless she refuses), rather than **Informed Consent** (or "**Opt In**," where a patient must specifically consent). Retesting should take place in the third trimester in areas of high HIV prevalence or an at-risk patient. Rapid HIV testing in labor is recommended if the patient's HIV status is not known.

ELISA test

This **screening test** assesses presence of detectable HIV antibodies. A 3-month lag exists between HIV infection and a positive ELISA test. All babies born to HIV-positive women will be HIV antibody positive from passive maternal antibodies.

Western blot test

This **definitive test** identifies the presence of HIV core and envelope antigens. Triple antiviral therapy is recommended for all HIV-positive women starting at 14 weeks and continuing through delivery. With cesarean delivery and triple antiviral therapy, transmission rates are as low as 1%.

Cervical Pap Smear

Cervical cytologic screening can identify if the mother has cervical dysplasia or malignancy.

SECOND TRIMESTER LABORATORY TESTS

A 23-year-old woman (G3 P1 Ab1) is seen at 16 weeks' gestation. Her previous pregnancy resulted in an anencephalic fetus that did not survive. She took 4 mg of folate preconception before this pregnancy but wants to know whether this fetus is affected.

Maternal Serum α-Fetoprotein (MS-AFP)

AFP

This is the **major serum glycoprotein** of the embryo. The concentration peaks at 12 weeks in the fetus and amniotic fluid (AF), then rises until 30 weeks in the maternal serum. Fetal structural defects (open neural tube defect [NTD] and ventral wall defects) result in increased spillage into the amniotic fluid and maternal serum. Other causes include twin pregnancy, placental bleeding, fetal renal disease, and sacrococcygeal teratoma.

Table 5-2. Alpha-Fetoprotein

Major Serum Glycoprotein of the Embryo		
Normal AFP changes	Fetal serum	Peaks at **12** weeks
	Amniotic fluid	Peaks at **12** weeks
	Maternal serum	Peaks at **30** weeks

MS-AFP

MS-AFP is reported in multiples of the median (MoM) and is always performed as part of multiple marker screenings. Maternal serum testing is performed within a gestational window of **15–20 weeks**. Because reference ranges are specific to gestational age, accurate pregnancy dating is imperative.

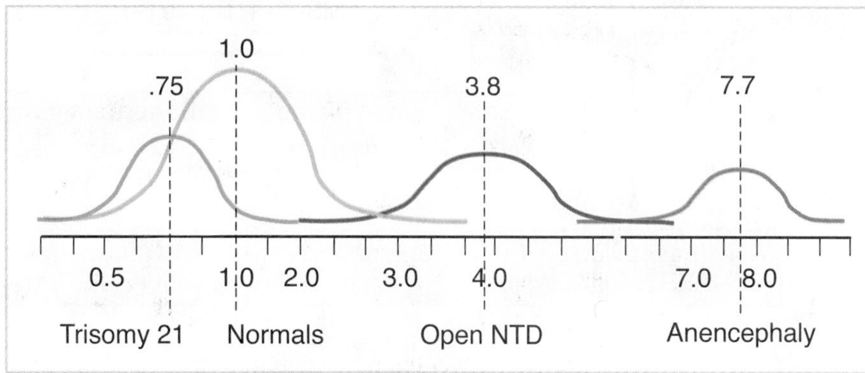

Figure I-5-1. Midpoints of MSAFP

Elevated MS-AFP

A positive high value is >2.5 MoM. The next step in management is to obtain an obstetric ultrasound to confirm gestational dating. The most common cause of an elevated MS-AFP is **dating error**.

- If the true gestational age is more advanced than the assumed gestational age, it would explain the positive high value. In cases of dating error, repeat the MS-AFP if the pregnancy is still within the 15- to 20-week window. A normal MS-AFP will be reassuring.

- If the dates are correct and no explanation is seen on sonogram, perform amniocentesis for AF-AFP determination and acetylcholinesterase activity. Elevated levels of **AF acetylcholinesterase** activity are specific to open NTD.
- With unexplained elevated MS-AFP but normal AF-AFP, the pregnancy is statistically at risk for intrauterine growth restriction (IUGR), stillbirth, and preeclampsia.

Low MS-AFP

A positive low value is **<0.85 MoM**. The sensitivity of MS-AFP alone for trisomy 21 is only 20%. The next step in management is to obtain an obstetric ultrasound to confirm gestational dating. The most common cause of a low MS-AFP is **dating error**.

- If the true gestational age is less than the assumed gestational age, it would explain the positive low value. In cases of dating error, repeat the MS-AFP if the pregnancy is still within the window. A normal MS-AFP will be reassuring.
- If the dates are correct and no explanation is seen on sonogram, perform amniocentesis for **karyotype**.

This is an elective prenatal test, not a routine one.

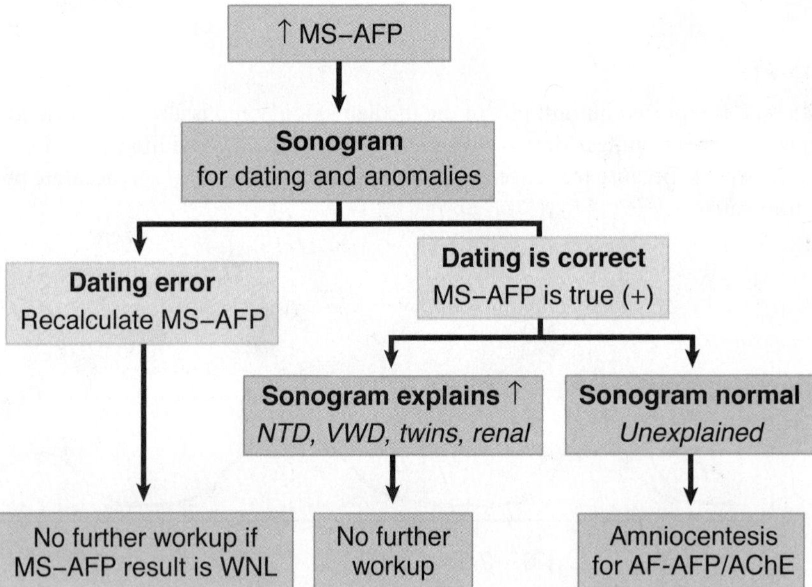

Figure I-5-2. Midtrimester Labs

Quadruple Marker Screen

Trisomy screening

The sensitivity for trisomy 21 detection can be increased to 80% by performing maternal serum screen for not only **MS-AFP**, but also **hCG**, **estriol**, and **inhibin-A**. The window for testing is also **15–20 weeks**. Because reference values are gestational age specific, accurate dating is important.

Trisomy 21

With Down syndrome, levels for MS-AFP and estriol are decreased, but **hCG and inhibin-A are, increased.** Perform an amniocentesis for **karyotype.**

Trisomy 18

With Edward syndrome, levels for **all 4 markers** (MS-AFP, estriol, inhibin-A, and hCG) **are decreased.** Perform an amniocentesis for **karyotype.**

THIRD-TRIMESTER LABORATORY TESTS

A 33-year-old woman (G4 P3) is at 25 weeks' gestation. Her height is 63 inches and weight 250 pounds. She has gained 30 pounds thus far this pregnancy. With her last pregnancy she gained 60 pounds, was diagnosed with gestational diabetes, and delivered a 4,300-g female neonate by cesarean section. She wants to know whether she has diabetes with this pregnancy.

Diabetic Testing

1-h 50-g oral glucose tolerance test (OGTT)

This **screening** test is administered to all pregnant women between 24 and 28 weeks' gestation. No fasting state is needed. A 50-g glucose load is given, and serum glucose is measured 1 h later. A **normal value** is <140 mg/dL. Fifteen percent of pregnant women will have an abnormal screening test, which is ≥140 mg/dL. **Management** is a 3-h 100-g OGTT.

3-h 100-g OGTT

This is the **definitive** test for glucose intolerance in pregnancy. Fifteen percent of women with an abnormal screening test will be found to have gestational diabetes mellitus. After an overnight fast, a fasting blood sugar (FBS) is drawn. An FBS >125 mg/dL indicates overt diabetes mellitus, and no further testing is performed. If the FBS is <126 mg/dL, administer a 100-g glucose load, followed by glucose levels at 1, 2, and 3 h. Normal values are FBS <95 mg/dL, 1 h <180 mg/dL, 2 h <155 mg/dL, and 3 h <140 mg/dL. Gestational diabetes is diagnosed if ≥2 values are abnormal. Impaired glucose intolerance is diagnosed if only 1 value is abnormal.

Complete Blood Count

Anemia

A complete blood count (CBC) should be performed between 24 and 28 weeks' gestation in all women. With the increasing diversion of iron to the fetus in the second and third trimester, iron deficiency, which was not present early in pregnancy, may develop. This is particularly so in the woman who is not taking iron supplementation. A hemoglobin <10 g/dL is considered anemia. The most common cause is **iron deficiency**, which occurs only after bone marrow iron stores are completely depleted.

Platelet count

Reassessment of pregnancy-induced thrombocytopenia can be also be done with the CBC.

Atypical Antibody Screen

Before giving prophylactic RhoGAM to an Rh-negative woman, an indirect Coombs test is performed at 28 weeks. This is obtained to ensure she has not become isoimmunized since her previous negative AAT earlier in pregnancy. Two-tenths of a percent of Rh-negative women will become isoimmunized from spontaneous feto-maternal bleeding before 28 weeks. If it is discovered that the patient already has anti-D antibodies, administration of RhoGAM is futile.

Late Pregnancy Bleeding 6

Learning Objectives

- ❑ Differentiate between placenta disorders and late pregnancy bleeding, including abruptio placenta, placenta previa, vasa previa, placenta accreta, placenta increta, and placenta precreta
- ❑ Describe the risk factors for and prognosis of uterine rupture

DIFFERENTIAL DIAGNOSIS OF LATE PREGNANCY BLEEDING

Definition. Vaginal bleeding occurring after 20 weeks' gestation. Prevalence is <5%, but when it does occur, prematurity and perinatal mortality quadruple.

Etiology

- **Cervical** causes include erosion, polyps, and, rarely, carcinoma.
- **Vaginal** causes include varicosities and lacerations.
- **Placental** causes include abruptio placenta, placenta previa, and vasa previa.

Initial Evaluation. What are patient's vital signs? Are fetal heart tones present? What is fetal status? What is the nature and duration of the bleeding? Is there pain or contractions? What is the location of placental implantation?

Initial Investigation. Complete blood count, disseminated intravascular coagulation (DIC) workup (platelets, prothrombin time, partial thromboplastin time, fibrinogen, **D-dimer**), type and cross-match, and sonogram for placental location. **Never perform a digital or speculum examination until ultrasound study rules out placenta previa.**

Initial Management. Start an IV line with a large-bore needle; if maternal vital signs are unstable, run isotonic fluids without dextrose wide open and place a urinary catheter to monitor urine output. If fetal jeopardy is present or gestational age is ±36 weeks, the goal is delivery.

OB Triad

Abruptio Placenta

- Late trimester **painful** bleeding
- Normal placental implantation
- Disseminated intravascular coagulopathy (DIC)

ABRUPTIO PLACENTA

A 32-year-old multigravida at 31 weeks' gestation is admitted to the birthing unit after a motor-vehicle accident. She complains of sudden onset of moderate vaginal bleeding for the past hour. She has intense, constant uterine pain and frequent contractions. Fetal heart tones are regular at 145 beats/min. On inspection her perineum is grossly bloody.

Etiology/Pathophysiology

- A normally implanted placenta (not in the lower uterine segment) separates from the uterine wall before delivery of the fetus. Separation can be partial or complete.
- Most commonly bleeding is **overt and external**. In this situation blood dissects between placental membranes exiting out the vagina.
- Less commonly, if bleeding remains **concealed or internal**, the retroplacental hematoma remains within the uterus, resulting in an increase in fundal height over time.

Diagnosis. This is based on the presence of painful late-trimester vaginal bleeding with a normal fundal or lateral uterine wall **placental implantation** not over the lower uterine segment.

Clinical Presentation. Abruptio placenta is the most common cause of late-trimester bleeding, occurring in 1% of pregnancies at term. It is the most common cause of painful late-trimester bleeding.

Classification

- With **mild abruption**, vaginal bleeding is minimal with no fetal monitor abnormality. Localized uterine pain and tenderness is noted, with incomplete relaxation between contractions.
- With **moderate abruption**, symptoms of uterine pain and moderate vaginal bleeding can be gradual or abrupt in onset. From 25 to 50% of placental surface is separated. Fetal monitoring may show tachycardia, decreased variability, or mild late decelerations.
- With **severe abruption**, symptoms are usually abrupt with a continuous knifelike uterine pain. Greater than 50% of placental separation occurs. Fetal monitor shows severe late decelerations, bradycardia, or even fetal death. Severe disseminated intravascular coagulation (DIC) may occur.
- Ultrasound visualization of a retroplacental hematoma may be seen.

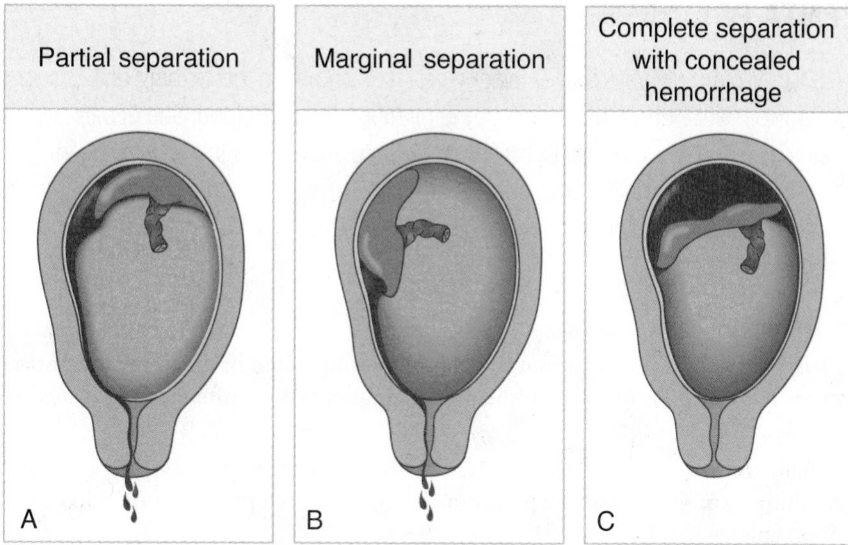

Figure I-6-1. Abruptio Placenta

Risk Factors. Abruptio placenta is seen more commonly with **previous abruption**, **hypertension**, and **maternal blunt trauma**. Other risk factors are smoking, maternal cocaine abuse and premature membrane rupture.

Management. Management is variable:

- **Emergency cesarean delivery**—This is performed if maternal or fetal jeopardy is present as soon as the mother is stabilized.
- **Vaginal delivery**—This is performed if bleeding is heavy but controlled or pregnancy is >36 weeks. Perform amniotomy and induce labor. Place external monitors to assess fetal heart rate pattern and contractions. Avoid cesarean delivery if the fetus is dead.
- **Conservative in-hospital observation**—This is performed if mother and fetus are stable and remote from term, bleeding is minimal or decreasing, and contractions are subsiding. Confirm normal placental implantation with sonogram and replace blood loss with crystalloid and blood products as needed.

Complications. Severe abruption can result in hemorrhagic shock with **acute tubular necrosis** from profound hypotension, and **DIC** from release of tissue thromboplastin into the general circulation from the disrupted placenta. **Couvelaire uterus** refers to blood extravasating between the myometrial fibers, appearing like bruises on the serosal surface.

PLACENTA PREVIA

A 34-year-old multigravida at 31 weeks' gestation comes to the birthing unit stating she woke up in the middle of the night in a pool of blood. She denies pain or uterine contractions. Examination of the uterus shows the fetus to be in transverse lie. Fetal heart tones are regular at 145 beats/min. On inspection her perineum is grossly bloody.

OB Triad

Placenta Previa

- Late trimester bleeding
- Lower segment placental implantation
- No pain

Etiology/Pathophysiology

- Placenta previa is present when the placenta is implanted in the **lower uterine segment**. This is common early in the pregnancy, but is most often not associated with bleeding.
- Usually the lower implanted placenta atrophies and the upper placenta hypertrophies, resulting in **migration of the placenta**. At term placenta previa is found in only 0.5% of pregnancies.
- Symptomatic placenta previa occurs when painless vaginal bleeding develops through avulsion of the anchoring villi of an **abnormally implanted** placenta as lower uterine segment stretching occurs in the latter part of pregnancy.

Diagnosis. This is based on the presence of **painless** late-trimester vaginal bleeding with an obstetric ultrasound showing placental implantation over the **lower uterine segment**.

Classification

- **Total, complete, or central previa** is found when the placenta completely covers the internal cervical os. This is the most dangerous location because of its potential for hemorrhage.
- **Partial previa** exists when the placenta partially covers the internal os.
- **Marginal or low-lying previa** exists when the placental edge is near but not over the internal os.

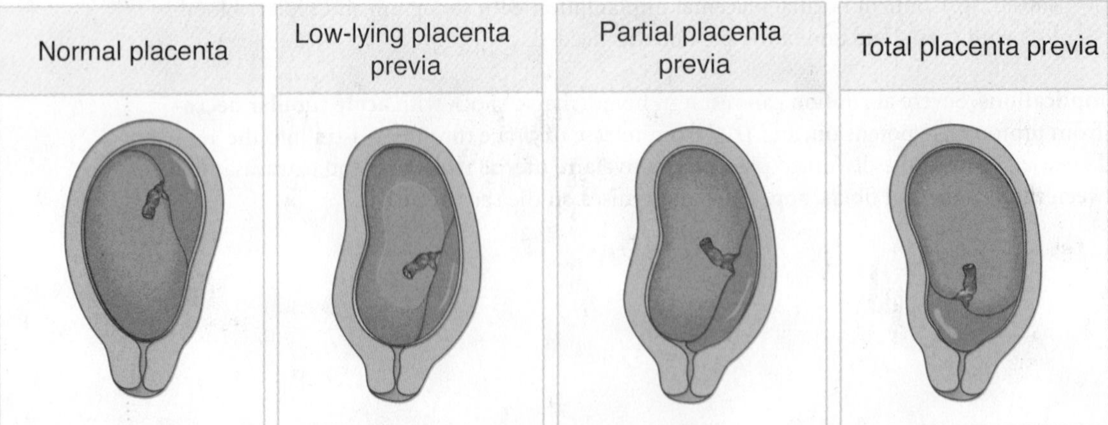

Figure I-6-2. Placenta Previa

Clinical Presentation. The classic picture is **painless** late-pregnancy bleeding, which can occur during rest or activity, suddenly and without warning. It may be preceded by trauma, coitus, or pelvic examination. The uterus is nontender and nonirritable.

Risk Factors. Placenta previa is seen more commonly with **previous placenta previa** and **multiple gestation**. Other risk factors are multiparity and advanced maternal age.

Management. Management is variable:

- **Emergency cesarean delivery**—This is performed if maternal or fetal jeopardy is present after stabilization of the mother.
- **Conservative in-hospital observation**—Conservative management of bed rest is performed in preterm gestations if mother and fetus are stable and remote from term. The initial bleed is rarely severe. Confirm abnormal placental implantation with sonogram and replace blood loss with crystalloid and blood products as needed.
- **Vaginal delivery**—This may be attempted if the lower placental edge is >2 cm from the internal cervical os.
- **Scheduled cesarean delivery**—This is performed if the mother has been stable after fetal lung maturity has been confirmed by amniocentesis, usually at 36 weeks' gestation.

Complications. If placenta previa occurs over a previous uterine scar, the villi may invade into the deeper layers of the decidua basalis and myometrium. This can result in intractable bleeding requiring **cesarean hysterectomy**. Profound hypotension can cause anterior pituitary necrosis (**Sheehan syndrome**) or **acute tubular necrosis**.

PLACENTA ACCRETA/INCRETA/PERCRETA

- Placental villi normally invade only the superficial layers of the endometrial decidua basalis. When the villi invade too deeply into the wall of the uterus, the condition is known as placenta accreta, placenta increta, or placenta percreta, depending the depth of the invasion. Approximately 1 in 2,500 pregnancies experience placenta accreta, increta, or percreta.
- **Placenta accreta** occurs when the villi invade the deeper layers of the endometrial deciduus basalis but do not penetrate the myometrium. Placenta accreta is the most common, accounting for approximately 80% of all cases.
- **Placenta increta** occurs when the villi invade the myometrium but do not reach the uterine serosal surface or the bladder. It accounts for approximately 15% of all cases.
- **Placenta percreta** occurs when the villi invade all the way to the uterine serosa or into the bladder. Placenta percreta is the least common of the 3 conditions, accounting for approximately 5% of all cases.

OB Triad

Abnormal Placental Invasion

- **Accreta:** deeper layers decidua basalis
- **Increta:** myometrium not complete
- **Percreta:** uterine serosa or bladder

VASA PREVIA

A 21-year-old primigravida at 38 weeks' gestation is admitted to the birthing unit at 6-cm dilation with contractions occurring every 3 min. Amniotomy (artificial rupture of membranes) is performed, resulting in sudden onset of bright red vaginal bleeding. The electronic fetal monitor tracing, which had showed a baseline fetal heart rate (FHR) of 135 beats/min with accelerations, now shows a bradycardia at 70 beats/min. The mother's vital signs are stable with normal blood pressure and pulse.

OB Triad

Vasa Previa

- Amniotomy–AROM
- Painless vaginal bleeding
- Fetal bradycardia

Etiology/Pathophysiology. Vasa previa is present when fetal vessels traverse the fetal membranes over the internal cervical os. These vessels may be from either a velamentous insertion of the umbilical cord or may be joining an accessory (succenturiate) placental lobe to the main disk of the placenta. If these fetal vessels rupture the bleeding is from the fetoplacental circulation, and fetal exsanguination will rapidly occur, leading to fetal death.

Diagnosis. This is rarely confirmed before delivery but may be suspected when antenatal sonogram with color-flow Doppler reveals a vessel crossing the membranes over the internal cervical os. The diagnosis is usually confirmed after delivery on examination of the placenta and fetal membranes.

Clinical Presentation. The **classic triad** is rupture of membranes and **painless** vaginal bleeding, followed by fetal bradycardia.

Risk Factors. Vasa previa is seen more commonly with **velamentous insertion** of the umbilical cord, **accessory placental lobes**, and multiple gestation.

Management. Immediate cesarean delivery of the fetus is essential or the fetus will die from hypovolemia.

OB Triad

Uterine Rupture

- Late trimester painful bleeding
- Previous uterine incision
- High perinatal mortality

UTERINE RUPTURE

A 27-year-old G2 P1 woman comes to the maternity unit for evaluation for regular uterine contractions at 34 weeks' gestation. Her previous delivery was an emergency cesarean section at 32 weeks because of hemorrhage from placenta previa. A classical uterine incision was used because of lower uterine segment varicosities. Pelvic exam shows the cervix to be closed and long. As she is being evaluated, she experiences sudden abdominal pain, profuse vaginal bleeding, and fetal bradycardia. Uterine contractions cannot be detected. The fetal head, which was at –1 station, now is floating.

Definition. Uterine rupture is **complete separation** of the wall of the pregnant uterus with or without expulsion of the fetus that endangers the life of the mother or the fetus, or both. The rupture may be **incomplete** (not including the peritoneum) or **complete** (including the visceral peritoneum).

Clinical Presentation. The most common findings are vaginal bleeding, loss of electronic fetal heart rate signal, abdominal pain, and loss of station of fetal head. Rupture may occur both before labor as well as during labor.

Diagnosis. Confirmation of the diagnosis is made by **surgical exploration** of the uterus and identifying the tear.

Risk Factors. The most common risk factors are previous **classic uterine incision, myomectomy**, and excessive oxytocin stimulation. Other risk factors are grand multiparity and marked uterine distention.

Significance. A vertical fundal uterine scar is 20 times more likely to rupture than a low segment incision. Maternal and perinatal mortality is also much higher with the vertical incision rupture.

Management. Treatment is surgical. **Immediate delivery** of the fetus is imperative. Uterine repair is indicated in a stable young woman to conserve fertility. Hysterectomy is performed in the unstable patient or one who does not desire further childbearing.

Perinatal Infections

7

Learning Objectives

- ❏ Describe the route of transmission and common complications of perinatal infections including group B beta-hemolytic streptococci, toxoplasmosis, varicella zoster, rubella, cytomegalovirus, HSV, HIV, syphilis, and hepatitis B

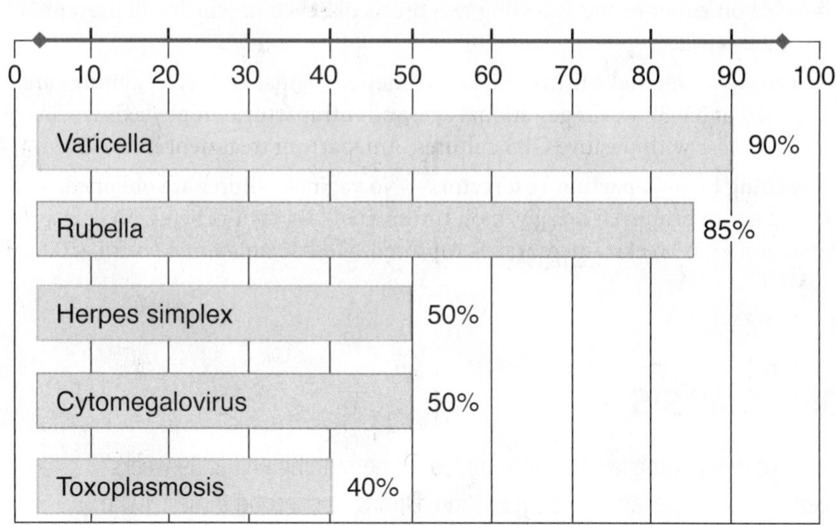

Figure I-7-1. Prevalence of IgG Seropositivity in Pregnant Women

GROUP B β-HEMOLYTIC STREPTOCOCCI (GBS)

A 20-year-old woman G2 P1 is admitted to the birthing unit at 35 weeks' gestation in active labor at 6-cm dilation. Her prenatal course was unremarkable with the exception of a positive first-trimester urine culture for GBS. Her first baby was hospitalized for 10 days after delivery for GBS pneumonia.

OB Triad

GBS Neonatal Sepsis

- Newborn sepsis
- Within hours of birth
- Bilateral diffuse pneumonia

Pathophysiology. GBS is a bacterium commonly found in normal GI tract flora. Thirty percent of women have asymptomatic **vaginal colonization** with GBS, with the majority having intermittent or transient carrier status. Most neonates delivered to colonized mothers will be culture positive.

Significance. One in 500 neonates will develop serious clinical infections or sepsis.

- **Early onset** infection is the most common finding, occurring within a few hours to days of birth, and is characterized by fulminant **pneumonia and sepsis.** This is usually vertical transmission from mother to neonate with a 30% mortality rate at or before 33 weeks but less than 5% at term.
- **Late-onset** infection is less common, occurring after the first week of life, and is characterized by meningitis. This is usually hospital acquired, with a 5% mortality rate.

Prevention. The purpose is to decrease early-onset infection only. Intrapartum antibiotic prophylaxis of neonatal GBS sepsis is given with IV penicillin G. If the patient is penicillin allergic, use clindamycin or vancomycin. Candidates for antibiotic prophylaxis are selected as follows:

- **No screening**—All women with a positive GBS urine culture or a previous baby with GBS sepsis will receive intrapartum prophylaxis. Prophylaxis of other women is based on either of the following two protocols, each of which will prevent 70% of neonatal sepsis.
- **Screening by vaginal culture**—Third-trimester vaginal and rectal cultures are obtained at 35–37 weeks gestational age, and intrapartum prophylaxis is administered only to those with positive GBS cultures. Antepartum treatment is not given.
- **Screening by intrapartum risk factors**—No vaginal cultures are obtained. Intrapartum prophylaxis is given on the basis of risk factors being present: preterm gestation (<37 weeks), membranes ruptured >18 h, or maternal fever (≥100.4°F) (38°C).

TOXOPLASMOSIS

OB Triad

Congenital *Toxoplasma*

- Chorioretinitis
- Intracranial calcifications
- Symmetrical IUGR

A 26-year-old primigravida was admitted to the birthing unit at 39 weeks' gestation in active labor at 6-cm dilation. During her second trimester she experienced a mononucleosis-like syndrome. Uterine fundal growth lagged behind that expected on the basis of a first-trimester sonogram. Serial sonograms showed symmetrical intrauterine growth retardation (IUGR). She delivered a 2,250-g male neonate who was diagnosed with microcephaly, intracranial calcifications, and chorioretinitis.

Note

Remember to distinguish between *intracranial* calcifications with *Toxoplasma* and *periventricular* calcifications with CMV.

Pathophysiology. Toxoplasmosis is caused by a **parasite** (*Toxoplasma gondii*) transmitted most commonly in the United States from exposure to infected **cat feces.** Infections can also occur from drinking raw goat milk or eating raw or undercooked infected meat.

- **Vertical transmission** from mother to fetus or neonate can only occur during the parasitemia of a primary infection because the result is residual lifelong immunity.
- Up to 40% of pregnant women are toxoplasmosis IgG seropositive.
- First-trimester infection risk is **low** (15%), but infections are **most serious**, even lethal.
- Third-trimester infection risk is **high** (50%), but infections are **mostly asymptomatic.**

Significance

- **Fetal infection**—Manifestations may include symmetric IUGR, nonimmune fetal hydrops, microcephaly, and **intracranial calcifications**.
- **Neonatal findings**—Manifestations may include **chorioretinitis**, seizures, hepatosplenomegaly, and thrombocytopenia.

Prevention. Avoid infected cat feces, raw goat milk, and undercooked meat.

Treatment. Pyrimethamine and sulfadiazine are used to treat a known infection. Spiramycin is used to prevent vertical transmission from the mother to the fetus.

VARICELLA (VZV)

A 29-year-old woman (G2 P1) is at 34 weeks' gestation. She complains of uterine contractions every 5 min. During the last few days she has developed diffuse pruritic vesicles on her neck that appear to be also developing on her chest and breasts. She has a fever and complains of malaise.

OB Triad

Congenital Varicella

- "Zig-zag" skin lesions
- Microphthalmia
- Extremity hypoplasia

Pathophysiology. Varicella zoster is a DNA virus that is the causative agent of chicken pox and herpes zoster. It is spread by **respiratory droplets**, but is less contagious than rubeola or rubella. More than 90% of women are immune by adulthood.

Significance

- **Fetal infection**—Transplacental infection rate is as low as 2% with 25% mortality.
- **Neonatal findings**—Congenital varicella syndrome is characterized by "zigzag" skin lesions, mulberry skin spots, optic atrophy, cataracts, chorioretinitis, extremity hypoplasia, and motor and sensory defects. The greatest neonatal risk is if maternal rash appears between 5 days antepartum and 2 days postpartum. No passive IgG antibodies are present.
- **Maternal infection**—10% of patients with varicella will develop **varicella pneumonia**, which has a high maternal morbidity and mortality. Communicability begins 1–2 days before vesicles appear and lasts until all vesicles are crusted over. Pruritic vesicles begin on the head and neck, progressing to the trunk. The infection can trigger labor.

Prevention. Administer **VZIG** (varicella zoster immune globulin) to a susceptible gravida within 96 h of exposure. Live-attenuated varicella virus (Varivax III) can be administered to nonpregnant or postpartum to varicella IgG-antibody–negative women.

Treatment. Administer IV antiviral treatment with **acyclovir** for varicella pneumonia, encephalitis, or the immunocompromised.

RUBELLA

An 18-year-old primigravida is at 30 weeks' gestation and is employed in a childcare center. One of the children had a rash that was diagnosed as rubella. The patient's rubella IgG titer is negative. She is concerned about the possibility of her fetus getting infected with rubella.

OB Triad

Congenital Rubella

- Congenital deafness
- Congenital cataracts
- Congenital heart disease

Pathophysiology. Rubella is a highly contagious RNA virus that is spread by **respiratory droplets**. Up to 85% of pregnant women are rubella IgG seropositive.

- **Vertical transmission** from mother to fetus or neonate can only occur during the viremia of a primary infection because the result is residual lifelong immunity.

Significance

- **Fetal infection**—Transplacental infection rate is >90% in the first 10 weeks of pregnancy, but 5% in the third trimester. Manifestations may include symmetric IUGR, microcephaly, or ventriculoseptal defect (VSD).
- **Neonatal infection**—Congenital rubella syndrome is characterized by **congenital deafness** (**most common** sequelae), **congenital heart disease**, **cataracts**, mental retardation, hepatosplenomegaly, thrombocytopenia, and "blueberry muffin" rash.
- **Maternal infection**—Rubella infection during pregnancy is generally a mild, low-morbidity condition.

Prevention. All pregnant women should undergo rubella IgG antibody screening. Rubella-susceptible women should avoid known rubella cases, then receive active immunization after delivery. Because rubella vaccine is made using a live attenuated virus, pregnancy should be avoided for 1 month after immunization.

Treatment. No specific treatment. Rubella has been eradicated from the United States; no cases have been reported here since 2004.

CYTOMEGALOVIRUS (CMV)

A 31-year-old neonatal intensive care unit nurse has just undergone an uncomplicated term spontaneous vaginal delivery of a 2,300-g female neonate with a diffuse petechial rash. At 12 weeks' gestation she experienced a flulike syndrome with right upper quadrant pain. Obstetric sonograms showed fetal growth was only at the fifth percentile.

OB Triad

Cytomegalovirus (CMV)

- Most common congenital viral syndrome
- Most common cause of deafness in children
- Neonatal thrombocytopenia and petechiae

Pathophysiology. CMV is a DNA herpes virus that is spread by infected body secretions. Up to 50% of pregnant women are CMV IgG seropositive.

Vertical transmission from mother to fetus or neonate occurs mainly during the viremia of a primary infection. However, because the result of primary infection is predisposition to a residual lifelong latency, fetal infection can occur with reactivation.

Significance

- **Fetal infection**—Transplacental infection rate is 50% with maternal primary infections regardless of the pregnancy trimester, but <1% with recurrent infections. Manifestations may include nonimmune hydrops, symmetric IUGR, microcephaly, and cerebral calcifications in a periventricular distribution.
- **Neonatal infection**—From 1 to 2% of newborns have evidence of in utero exposure to CMV. Congenital CMV syndrome is the **most common** congenital viral syndrome in the United States. CMV is the **most common** cause of sensorineural deafness in children. Only 10% of infected infants have clinical disease, which includes **petechiae**, mulberry skin spots, meningoencephalitis, periventricular calcifications, hepatosplenomegaly, thrombocytopenia, and jaundice.

- **Maternal infection**—CMV infection during pregnancy is generally a mild, low-morbidity condition appearing as a mononucleosis-like syndrome with hepatitis.

Prevention. Follow universal precautions with all body fluids. Avoid transfusion with CMV-positive blood.

Treatment. Antiviral therapy with ganciclovir.

HERPES SIMPLEX VIRUS (HSV)

A 21-year-old multipara was admitted to the birthing unit at 39 weeks' gestation in active labor at 6-cm dilation. The bag of water is intact. She has a history of genital herpes preceeding the pregnancy. Her last outbreak was 8 weeks ago. She now complains of pain and pruritis. On examination she had localized, painful, ulcerative lesions on her right vaginal wall.

Pathophysiology. HSV is a DNA herpes virus that is spread by intimate **mucocutaneous contact.** Up to 50% of pregnant women are HSV IgG seropositive.

- Most genital herpes results from HSV II, but can also occur with HSV I.
- Transplacental transmission from mother to fetus can occur with viremia during the primary infection but is rare. HSV infection predisposes to a residual lifelong latency with periodic recurrent attacks. The most common route of fetal infection is contact with **maternal genital lesions** during a recurrent HSV episode.

Diagnosis. The definitive diagnosis is a positive HSV culture from fluid obtained from a ruptured vesicle or debrided ulcer, but there is a 20% false-negative rate. PCR is 2–4x more sensitive and is best to detect viral shedding.

Significance

- **Fetal infection**—The transplacental infection rate is 50% with maternal primary infections. Manifestations may include spontaneous abortions, symmetric IUGR, microcephaly, and cerebral calcifications.
- **Neonatal infection**—With passage through an HSV-infected birth canal, the neonatal attack rate is 50% with a primary infection, but <5% with a recurrent infection. Neonatal mortality rate is 50%. Those who survive have severe sequelae: meningoencephalitis, mental retardation, pneumonia, hepatosplenomegaly, jaundice, and petechiae.
- **Maternal infection** (2 types):
  - **Primary herpes** results from a viremia and has systemic manifestations: fever, malaise, adenopathy, and diffuse genital lesions (vagina, cervix, vulva, and urethra). Transplacental fetal infection is possible. However, in 2/3 of cases, the infection is mild or subclinical.
  - **Recurrent herpes** results from migration of the virus from the dorsal root ganglion but is localized and less severe with no systemic manifestations. Fetal infection results only from passing through a birth canal with lesions present.

Prevention. A cesarean section should be performed in the presence of genital HSV lesions at the time of labor. If membranes have been ruptured >8–12 h, the virus may already have infected the fetus and cesarean delivery would be of no value.

Treatment. Acyclovir.

HUMAN IMMUNODEFICIENCY VIRUS (HIV)

A 22-year-old multigravida is a former IV drug user. She was diagnosed as HIV positive 12 months ago during her previous pregnancy. She underwent vaginal delivery of an infant who is also HIV positive. She is now pregnant again at 15 weeks' gestation.

Pathophysiology. HIV is an RNA retrovirus that is spread by infected body secretions. Sharing contaminated needles, having sexual intercourse with an infected partner, and perinatal transmission are the most common ways of transmission.

The infected patient develops acquired immunodeficiency syndrome (**AIDS**). The clinical course from HIV to AIDS is a gradual but relentless immunosuppression during a period of years, resulting in death caused by overwhelming infection from opportunistic diseases.

Significance

- **Fetal infection**—Transplacental infection occurs, but the major route of vertical transmission is contact with infected genital secretions at the time of vaginal delivery. Without maternal azidothymidine (AZT) prophylaxis, the vertical transmission rate is 30%, but with AZT the infection rate is lowered to 10% with vaginal delivery. With elective cesarean section without labor and before membrane rupture, the perinatal infection rate may be <5%. The greatest benefit to the fetus of cesarean delivery is probably in women with low CD4 counts and high RNA viral loads, making infection through a vaginal delivery much more likely.
- **Neonatal infection**—At birth neonates of HIV-positive women will have positive HIV tests from transplacental passive IgG passage. HIV-infected breast milk can potentially transmit the disease to the newborn. Progression from HIV to AIDS in infants is more rapid than in adults.
- **Maternal infection**—Pregnancy in an HIV-positive woman does not enhance progression to AIDS.

Prevention

- **Antiviral prophylaxis**—The U.S. Public Health Service recommends that HIV-infected pregnant women be offered combination treatment with HIV-fighting drugs to help protect their health and prevent passing the infection on to their babies. Infected pregnant women should take triple-drug therapy including the drug zidovudine (ZDV) as part of their drug regimen, starting at 14 weeks and continuing throughout pregnancy, intrapartum, and after delivery.
- **Mode of delivery**—Vaginal delivery should be planned at 39 weeks. The guidelines for vaginal delivery are 1) to avoid amniotomy as long as possible, 2) do not use scalp electrodes in labor, 3) avoid forceps or vacuum extractor operative delivery, and 4) use gentle neonatal resuscitation. Cesarean section is offered at 38 weeks without amniocentesis if viral load is ≥ 1,000 copies/mL.

- **Breast feeding**—This is probably best avoided in HIV-positive women.
- **Universal precautions**—Pay careful attention to handling of all body fluids.

Treatment. All HIV-positive pregnant women should be on combination triple anti-viral HAART therapy. This includes 2 nucelotide reverse transcriptase inhibitors (NRTIs) with either an NNRTI or a protease inhibitor. An example would be zidovudine, lamivudine, or ritonavir.

SYPHILIS

A 34-year-old multigravida presents for prenatal care in the second trimester. She admits to a past history of substance abuse but states she has been clean for 6 months. With her second pregnancy she experienced a preterm delivery at 34 weeks' gestation of a male neonate who died within the first day of life. She states that at delivery the baby was swollen with skin lesions and that the placenta was very large. She was treated with antibiotics but she does not remember the name or other details. On a routine prenatal panel with this current pregnancy she is found to have a positive VDRL (Venereal Disease Research Laboratory) test.

Pathophysiology. Syphilis is caused by *Treponema pallidum*, a motile anaerobic spirochete that cannot be cultured. Syphilis does not result in either a state of immunity or latency. The infection can be eradicated by appropriate treatment, but reinfection can occur over and over again. It is spread as a sexually transmitted disease by intimate contact between moist mucous membranes or congenitally through the placenta to a fetus from an infected mother.

Significance

- **Fetal infection**—Transplacental infection is common with vertical transmission rates of 60% in primary and secondary syphilis. The rate of fetal infection with latent or tertiary syphilis is lower. Without treatment, manifestations of early congenital syphilis include nonimmune hydrops, macerated skin, anemia, thrombocytopenia, and hepatosplenomegaly. Fetal death rates are high, with perinatal mortality rates approaching 50%. The placenta is typically large and edematous.
- **Neonatal infection**—Late congenital syphilis is diagnosed after age 2 years and includes "Hutchinson" teeth, "mulberry" molars, "saber" shins, "saddle" nose, and 8th nerve deafness.
- **Maternal infection** (4 types):
  - **Primary syphilis** is the first stage after infection. Papules become painless ulcers with rolled edges (chancres) which appear 2–3 weeks after contact at the site of infection, most commonly the vulva, vagina, or cervix. Darkfield microscopy of lesion exudate is positive for the spirochete, but the nonspecific serologic tests VDRL or rapid plasma reagin [**RPR**] test) are not yet positive. Without treatment the chancre spontaneously disappears.
  - **Secondary syphilis** is characterized by systemic spirochetemia. Two to three months after contact, fever, malaise, general adenopathy, and a maculopapular skin rash ("money spots") are seen. Broad exophytic excrescences (**condyloma lata**) appear on the vulva. These physical findings also spontaneously disappear without treatment. Darkfield microscopy of condyloma exudate is positive for treponema. The VDRL or RPR test will be positive, but a diagnosis of syphilis must be confirmed with a

treponema-specific test, such as the fluorescent titer antibody absorption (FTA-ABS) or microhemagglutination assay for antibodies to *T. pallidum* (MHA-TP). The treponema-specific tests do not correlate with disease activity and remain positive in spite of treatment.

– **Latent syphilis** is characterized by absence of symptoms or physical findings. One third of cases proceed to tertiary disease. The nonspecific and treponema-specific tests remain positive.
– **Tertiary syphilis** is a symptomatic stage with symptoms dependent on which organ system is affected by the classic necrotic, ulcerative nodules (**gummas**). Lesion location may include the cardiovascular system (aortitis, saccular aneurysms), CNS (meningitis, tabes dorsalis, dementia, ataxia), or bone (osteitis). Not only are the blood tests positive, but also the cerebrospinal fluid will be positive with CNS involvement.

Table 7-1. Syphilis in Pregnancy

Characteristic	Primary	Secondary
Classic lesion	Chancre	Condyloma lata ("money spots")
Extent of disease	Localized	Systemic
Lab tests (VDRL, Darkfield, FTA-ABS)	VDRL (–) Darkfield (+) FTA-ABS (+)	VDRL (+) Darkfield (+) FTA-ABS (+)
Fetal infection rate	60%	60%
Treatment of choice	Penicillin	Penicillin

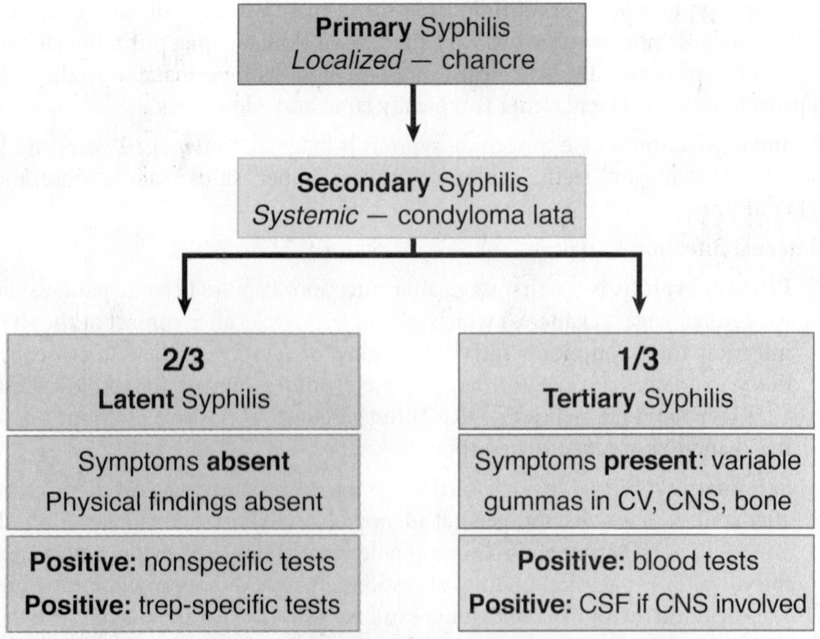

Figure I-7-2. Maternal Syphilis

Prevention

- Vaginal delivery is appropriate with cesarean section only for obstetric indications.
- Follow the principles of avoiding multiple sexual partners, and promote use of barrier contraceptives.

Management. Benzathine penicillin 2.4 million units IM × 1 is given in pregnancy to ensure adequate antibiotic levels in the fetus. Other antibiotics do not cross the placenta well. Even if the gravida is penicillin-allergic, she should still be given a full penicillin dose using an oral desensitization regimen under controlled conditions.

Follow serology titers at 1, 3, 6, 12, and 24 months. Titers should be decreased fourfold by 6 months, and should be negative in 12-24 months.

The Jarisch-Herxheimer reaction is associated with treatment and occurs in half of pregnant women. It starts in 1-2 hours, peaks in 8 hours, and resolves in 24-48 hours. It is associated with acute fever, headache, myalgias, hypotension, and uterine contractions. Management is supportive care.

HEPATITIS B (HBV)

A 29-year-old multigravida was found on routine prenatal laboratory testing to be positive for hepatitis B surface antigen. She is an intensive care unit nurse. She received 2 units of packed red blood cells 2 years ago after experiencing postpartum hemorrhage with her last pregnancy.

Pathophysiology. Hepatitis B is a DNA virus that is spread by infected body secretions. Sharing contaminated needles, having sexual intercourse with an infected partner, and perinatal transmission are the most common ways of transmission. Vertical transmission accounts for 40% of all chronic HBV infections. Most HBV infections are asymptomatic.

Significance

- **Fetal infection**—Transplacental infection is rare, occurring mostly in the third trimester. The main route of fetal or neonatal infection arises from exposure to or ingestion of infected genital secretions at the time of vaginal delivery. There is no perinatal transmission risk if the mother is positive for HBV surface antibodies but negative for HBV surface antigen.
- **Neonatal infection**—Neonatal HBV develops in only 10% of mothers positive for HBsAg but in 80% of those positive for both HBsAg and HBeAg. Of those neonates who get infected, 80% will develop chronic hepatitis, compared with only 10% of infected adults.
- **Maternal infection** (3 types):
  - **Asymptomatic HBV.** The majority of all infected patients fall into this category with no impact on maternal health. Hepatitis B surface antigen (HBsAg) is the screening test used for identifying existing infection and is obtained on all pregnant women. A positive HBsAg test is followed up with a complete hepatitis panel and liver enzymes assessing for active or chronic hepatitis.
  - **Acute hepatitis.** Acute and chronic HBV infections can result in right upper quadrant pain and lethargy varying according to the severity of the infection. Laboratory studies show elevated bilirubin and high liver enzymes. The majority of patients with acute hepatitis will recover normal liver function.

- **Chronic hepatitis.** Cirrhosis and hepatocellular carcinoma are the most serious consequences of chronic hepatitis.

Prevention

- Vaginal delivery is indicated with cesarean section only for obstetric indications.
- Avoid scalp electrodes in labor as well as scalp needles in the nursery. Neonates of HBsAg-positive mothers should receive passive immunization with hepatitis B immunoglobulin (HBIg) and active immunization with hepatitis B vaccine. Breast feeding is acceptable after the neonate has received the active immunization and HBIG.
- HBsAg-negative mothers at high risk for hepatitis B should receive HBIg passive immunization. Active immunization is safe in pregnancy because the agent is a killed virus.

Management. There is no specific therapy for acute hepatitis. Chronic HBV can be treated with interferon or lamivudine.

<table>
<tr><th></th><th>Lifelong</th><th colspan="2">Treatment/Delivery</th></tr>
<tr><td>Group β beta streptococcus</td><td>Colonization</td><td>Penicillin G</td><td rowspan="3">Vaginal Delivery</td></tr>
<tr><td>Toxoplasmosis</td><td rowspan="2">Immunity</td><td>Pyrimethamine Sulfadiazine</td></tr>
<tr><td>Rubella</td><td>None</td></tr>
<tr><td>Cytomegalovirus</td><td rowspan="3">Latency</td><td>Ganciclovir</td><td rowspan="3">Cesarean Section if active HSV or few HIV</td></tr>
<tr><td>Varicella/HSV</td><td>Acyclovir</td></tr>
<tr><td>HIV</td><td>Triple Rx antivirals</td></tr>
</table>

	Findings	Findings
Toxoplasmosis*+	Intracranial calcifications	Chorioretinitis
Varicella+	Zig zag lesions	Small eyes
Rubella*+	Deafness	Congenital heart disease
Cytomegalovirus*+	Petechiae	↑ liver, spleen
Syphilis+	Hydrops	Macerated skin
HSV, HIV, HBVΔ	None	

*Associated with IUGR
+Transplacental vertical transmission
ΔVaginal delivery vertical transmission

Obstetric Complications 8

Learning Objectives

- ❑ Describe the management of cervical insufficiency and multiple gestation
- ❑ Answer questions about alloimmunization
- ❑ List the management steps for preterm labor, premature rupture of membranes, and post-term pregnancy

CERVICAL INSUFFICIENCY

A 32-year-old primigravida at 18 weeks' gestation comes to the maternity unit complaining of pelvic pressure and increasing vaginal mucus discharge. She denies any uterine contractions. On pelvic examination the fetal membranes are seen bulging into the vagina, and no cervix can be palpated. Fetal feet can be felt through the membranes. Two years ago she underwent a cervical conization for cervical intraepithelial neoplasia.

The terms "cervical insufficiency" and "cervical incompetency" have been used to describe the inability of the uterine cervix to retain a pregnancy to viability in the absence of contractions or labor. A diagnosis was made in the past on the basis of a history of painless cervical dilation after the first trimester with expulsion of a previable living fetus.

Recent studies using ultrasound to examine cervical length suggest that cervical function is not an all-or-none phenomenon, but may be a continuous variable with a range of degrees of competency that may be expressed differently in subsequent pregnancies.

Etiology. Causes may include trauma from rapid forceful cervical dilation associated with second trimester abortion procedures, cervical laceration from rapid delivery, injury from deep cervical conization, or congenital weakness from diethylstilbestrol (DES) exposure.

Diagnosis

- Studies show the benefit of elective cervical cerclage with a history of 1 or more unexplained second-trimester pregnancy losses. The benefit of cervical cerclage placement is unclear in the following situations: sonographic findings of a short cervix or funneling, history of cervical surgery, DES exposure.
- Serial transvaginal ultrasound evaluations of the cervix after 16–20 weeks may be helpful.

OB Triad

Cervical Insufficiency

- Pregnant 18–22 weeks
- Painless cervical dilation
- Delivery of previable fetus

Management

- Elective cerclage placement at 13–14 weeks' gestation is appropriate after sonographic demonstration for fetal normality.
- Emergency or urgent cerclage may be considered with sonographic evidence of cervical insufficiency after ruling out labor and chorioamnionitis.
- Cerclage should be considered if cervical length is <25 mm by vaginal sonography prior to 24 weeks and prior preterm birth at <34 weeks gestation.
- McDonald cerclage places a removable suture in the cervix. The benefit is that vaginal delivery can be allowed to take place, avoiding a cesarean.
- Cerclage removal should take place at 36–37 weeks, after fetal lung maturity has taken place but before the usual onset of spontaneous labor that could result in avulsion of the suture.
- Shirodkar cerclage utilizes a submucosal placement of the suture that is buried beneath the mucosa and left in place. Cesarean delivery is performed at term.

MULTIPLE GESTATION

A 21-year-old primigravida at 15 weeks' gestation is seen for a routine prenatal visit. At her last visit 4 weeks ago, her uterus was appropriate for size and dates. Today, her uterine fundus is palpable at the umbilicus.

Definition. This is a pregnancy in which more than one fetus is present. The fetuses may arise from one or more zygotes and are usually separate, but may rarely be conjoined.

Risk Factors

- **Dizygotic twins** are most common. **Identifiable risk factors** include by race, geography, family history, or ovulation induction. Risk of twinning is up to 10% with clomiphene citrate and up to 30% with human menopausal gonadotropin.
- **Monozygotic twins** have **no identifiable risk factors**.

Diagnosis. Obstetric sonogram demonstration of more than one intrauterine fetus.

Complications for all twin pregnancies include nutritional anemias (iron and folate), preeclampsia, preterm labor (50%), malpresentation (50%), cesarean delivery (50%), and postpartum hemorrhage.

OB Triad

Di–Di Di or Mono–Di–Di Twins
- Twin pregnancy
- Gender same or unknown
- Two placentas seen

Mono–Mono–Di Twins
- Twin pregnancy
- Gender always same
- *One* placenta but *two* sacs

Mono–Mono–Mono Twins
- Twin pregnancy
- Gender always same
- *One* placenta and *one* sac

Table 8-1. Complications of Twin Pregnancies

ANTEpartum	Anemia ↑ 3x (iron & folate)
	Preeclampsia ↑ 3x
	Gestational diabetes ↑ 2x
	Thromboembolism ↑ 4x
INTRApartum	Preterm labor (50%)
	Malpresentation (50%)
	Cesarean delivery (50%)
POSTpartum	Hemorrhage ↑ 5x

Dizygotic twins arise from multiple ovulation with 2 zygotes. They are always dichorionic, diamnionic.

Monozygotic twins arise from one zygote. Chorionicity and amnionicity vary according to the duration of time from fertilization to cleavage.

- **Up to 72 hours** (separation up to the morula stage), the twins are **dichorionic, diamnionic**. There are 2 placentas and 2 sacs. This is the **lowest** risk of all monozygotic twins.
- **Between 4 and 8 days** (separation at the blastocyst stage), the twins are monochorionic, diamnionic. There is 1 placenta and 2 sacs. A specific additional complication is **twin–twin transfusion**, which develops in 15% of mono-di twins. The twins share a single placenta but do so unequally. The donor twin gets less blood supply, resulting in growth restriction, **oligohydramnios**, and anemia. However, neonatal outcome is usually better. The **recipient twin** gets more blood supply, resulting in excessive growth, **polyhydramnios**, and polycythemia. Intrauterine fetal surgery is indicated to laser the vascular connections on the placental surface between the 2 fetuses. Neonatal course is often complicated.

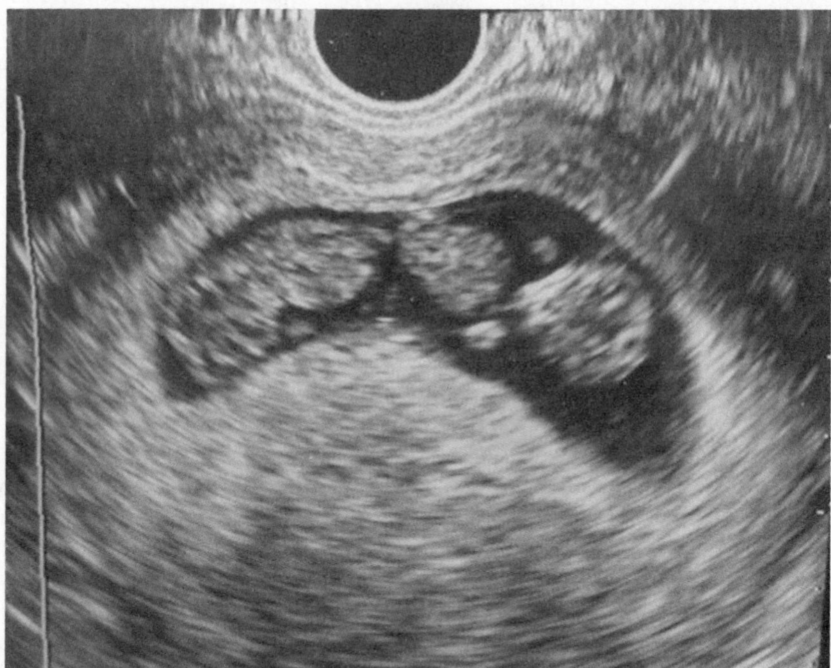

Medical Education Division of the Brookside Associates, brooksidepress.org

Figure I-8-1. Monochorionic, Diamniotic Twin Gestation

- **Between 9 and 12 days** (splitting of the embryonic disk), the twins are **monochorionic, monoamnionic.** There is only 1 placenta and 1 sac. Specific additional risks are twin–twin transfusion but particularly **umbilical cord entanglement** which can result in fetal death. This is the highest risk of all monozygotic twins.
- **After 12 days**, conjoined twins result. Most often this condition is **lethal**.

Table 8-2. Postconception Days to Identical Twin Cleavage

Dichorionic–diamnionic	0–3 days Morula
Monochorionic–diamnionic	4–8 days Blastocyst
Monochorionic–monoamnionic	9–12 days Embryonic disk
Conjoined	>12 days Embryo

Clinical Findings. Hyperemesis gravidarum is more common from high levels of β-hCG. Uterus is larger than dates. Maternal serum α-**fetoprotein** is excessively higher than with one fetus.

Management

- **Antepartum:** Give mother iron and folate supplementation to prevent anemia, monitor BP to detect preeclampsia, educate mother regarding preterm labor symptoms and signs, and perform serial ultrasound examinations looking for twin–twin transfusion (amniotic fluid discordance).
- **Intrapartum:** Route of delivery is based on presentation in labor—vaginal delivery if both are cephalic presentation (50%); cesarean delivery if first twin in noncephalic presentation; route of delivery is controversial if first twin is cephalic and second twin is noncephalic.
- **Postpartum:** Watch for postpartum hemorrhage from uterine atony owing to an overdistended uterus.

ALLOIMMUNIZATION

A 32-year-old woman, G2 P1, was seen for her first prenatal visit at 12 weeks' gestation. Her prenatal laboratory panel reveals a blood type of O negative. Her atypical antibody screen (indirect Coombs test) is positive. She has been married to the same husband for 10 years and states he is the father of both her pregnancies. She did not receive RhoGAM during her last pregnancy.

Definition. A pregnant woman has developed **antibodies to foreign red blood cells** (RBCs), most commonly against those of her current or previous fetus(es), but also caused by transfusion of mismatched blood.

Pathophysiology

- The most common RBC antigens are of the Rh system (C, c, D, E, e), with the **most common being big D**.
- Antibodies to RBC antigens are detected by **indirect Coombs test** (atypical antibody test [ATT]). The concentration of antibodies is reported in dilutional titers with the lowest level being 1:1, and titers increasing by doubling (e.g., 1:1, 1:2, 1:4, 1:8, 1:16, 1:32…1:1,024, etc.).
- **Hemolytic disease of the newborn** (HDN) is a continuum ranging from hyperbilirubinemia to erythroblastosis fetalis. HDN is caused by maternal antibodies crossing into the fetal circulation and targeting antigen-positive fetal RBCs, resulting in hemolysis. When severe, this can result in anemia, fetal hydrops, and even death.

Risk Factors. Alloimmunization most commonly occurs when **fetal RBCs enter** the mother's circulation transplacentally at delivery. It can also occur if a woman is transfused with mismatched RBCs. Other pregnancy-related risk factors are amniocentesis, ectopic pregnancy, D&C, abruptio placenta, and placenta previa.

Protective Factors. ABO incompatibility decreases the risk of maternal alloimmunization from foreign RBCs. Naturally occurring anti-A and anti-B antibodies rapidly lyse foreign RBCs before maternal lymphocytes are stimulated to produce active antibodies.

Requirements (all must be present).

- Mother must be antigen negative.
- Fetus must be antigen positive, which means the father of the pregnancy must also be antigen positive.
- Adequate fetal RBCs must cross over into the maternal circulation to stimulate her lymphocytes to produce antibodies to the fetal RBC antigens.
- Antibodies must be associated with HDN.
- A significant titer of maternal antibodies must be present to cross over into the fetal circulation and lead to fetal RBC hemolysis.

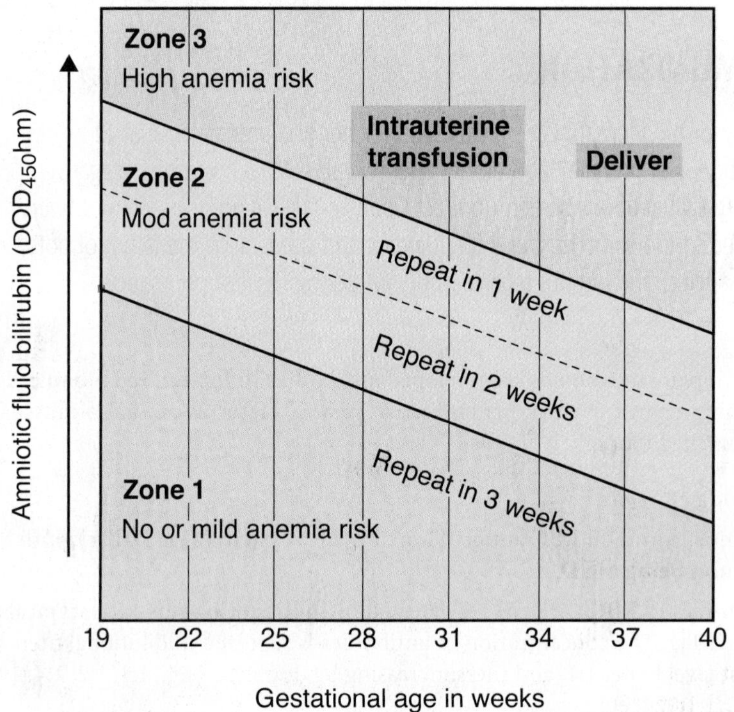

Figure I-8-2. Liley Graph

Management.

Determine whether there is any fetal risk.

- **Fetal risk is present only** if (1) atypical antibodies are detected in the mother's circulation, (2) antibodies are associated with HDN, (3) antibodies are present at a significant titer (>1:8), and (4) the father of the baby (FOB) is RBC antigen positive. Fetal blood type may be determined by amniocentesis or percutaneous umbilical blood sampling (PUBS). If the fetus is RBC antigen negative, there is no fetal risk.
- **No fetal risk is present** if (1) the AAT is negative, (2) antibodies are present but are NOT associated with HDN, (3) antibody titer is ≤1:8, or (4) the FOB is RBC antigen negative.
- **If the atypical antibody titer** is ≤1:8, management is conservative. Repeat the titer monthly as long as it remains ≤1:8.

Assess the degree of fetal if the fetus is RBC antigen positive or if fetal blood typing is impossible. This can be done by serial amniocentesis, PUBS, or ultrasound Doppler.

- **Amniotic fluid bilirubin** indirectly indicates fetal hemolysis because bilirubin accumulates as a byproduct of RBC lysis. The bilirubin is plotted on a **Liley graph.**
- **PUBS** directly measures fetal hematocrit and degree of anemia.
- **Ultrasound Doppler**—measurement of peak flow velocity of blood through the fetal middle cerebral artery (MCA). As fetal anemia worsens, the peak systolic velocity rises.

  Doppler MCA ultrasound is the **procedure of choice since it is non-invasive and has a high correlation with fetal anemia.**

Intervene if there is severe anemia. This is diagnosed when amniotic fluid bilirubin is in Liley zone III or PUBS shows fetal hematocrit to be ≤25% or MCA flow is elevated.

- Intrauterine intravascular transfusion is performed if gestational age is <34 weeks.
- Delivery is performed if gestational age is ≥34 weeks.

Prevention. RhoGAM is pooled anti-D IgG passive antibodies that are given IM to a pregnant woman when there is significant risk of fetal RBCs passing into her circulation. The passive IgG antibodies attach to the foreign RBC antigens, causing lysis to occur before the maternal lymphocytes become stimulated.

RhoGAM is routinely given to Rh(D)-negative mothers at 28 weeks, and within 72 h of chorionic villus sampling (CVS), amniocentesis, or D&C. It is also given within 72 h of delivery of an Rh(D)-positive infant. 300 mcg of RhoGAM will neutralize 15 ml of fetal RBCs or 30 mL of fetal whole blood.

Rosette test is a qualitative screening test for detecting significant feto-maternal hemorrhage (≥10 mL).

Kleihauer-Betke test quantitates the volume of fetal RBCs in the maternal circulation by differential staining of fetal and maternal RBCs on a peripheral smear. This can assess whether more than one vial of RhoGAM needs to be given when large volumes of fetal–maternal bleed may occur (e.g., abruptio placenta).

OB Triad

Preterm Contractions

- Pregnancy 20–36 weeks
- ≥3 contractions in 30 min
- Dilated <2 cm and no change

OB Triad

Magnesium Toxicity

- Preterm labor tocolysis
- Respiratory depression
- Muscle weakness

PRETERM LABOR

A 24-year-old woman, G2 P1, at 28 weeks' gestation by dates comes to the birthing unit complaining of regular uterine contractions every 7–10 min. She is a smoker with chronic hypertension. She has had no prenatal care. On examination her fundal height is 35 cm. Her previous pregnancy ended with spontaneous vaginal delivery at 30 weeks' gestation.

Preterm delivery is the most common cause of perinatal morbidity and mortality. Overall, 12% of pregnancies deliver prematurely. Many patients will have preterm contractions but not be in preterm labor. Three criteria need to be met:

- **Gestational age**—pregnancy duration ≥20 weeks, but <37 weeks
- **Uterine contractions**—at least 3 contractions in 30 min
- **Cervical change**—serial examinations show a change in dilation or effacement, or a single examination shows cervical dilation of ≥2 cm

OB Triad

Preterm Labor

- Pregnancy 20–36 weeks
- ≥3 contractions in 30 min
- Dilated ≥2 cm or changing

Preterm Delivery Categories:

- Extreme preterm: <28 weeks
- Very preterm: <32 weeks
- Moderate preterm: 32–34 weeks
- Late preterm: 34–36 6/7 weeks

Risk Factors:

- **Most common**: prior preterm birth (PTB), short transvaginal (TV) cervical length (<25 mm), PROM, multiple gestation, uterine anomaly
- Others: low maternal pre-pregnancy weight, smoking, substance abuse, and short inter-pregnancy interval (<18 months)

All gravidas should be screened:

- **History:** previous PTB
- **Sonographic cervical length:** prior to 24 weeks

Interventions to prevent preterm delivery:

- **Singleton** pregnancy:
  - Weekly IM 17-hydroxy progesterone caproate (17-0H-P) if cervical length ≥25 mm with prior spontaneous PTB
  - Weekly IM 17 -OH-P plus cervical cerclage placement if cervical length <25 mm before 24 weeks with prior PTB
  - Daily vaginal progesterone if cervical length <20 mm before 24 weeks but no prior PTB
- **Twin pregnancy:** no interventions shown to have any benefit

Symptoms. Lower abdominal pain or pressure, lower back pain, increased vaginal discharge, or bloody show. Particularly in primigravidas, the symptoms may be present for a number of hours to days but are not recognized as contractions by the patient.

Fetal Fibronectin (fFN):

fFN is a protein matrix produced by fetal cells that acts as a biological glue binding the trophoblast to the maternal decidua. It "leaks" into the vagina if PTB is likely and can be measured with a rapid test using a vaginal swab.

- Prerequisites for testing: gestation **22-35 weeks**, cervical dilation <3 cm, and membranes intact.
- Interpretation: main value of the test is a negative, since the chance of PTB in the next 2 weeks is <1%. With a positive result, the likelihood of PTB is 50%.

Intravenous Magnesium Sulfate for Fetal Neuroprotection:

Matemal IV $MgSo_4$ may reduce the severity and risk of cerebral palsy in surviving very preterm neonates.

- Start infusion if PTB is anticipated <**32 weeks** gestation regardless of the anticipated route of delivery.
- It takes 4 hours of infusion to achieve steady state of Mg in the fetus.

Antenatal Corticosteroid Therapy:

- A single course of corticosteroids is recommended for pregnant women with gestational age **23–34 weeks** of gestation who are at risk of preterm delivery within 7 days.
- A complete course is two IM 12-mg doses of betamethasone given 24 hours apart OR four IM 6-mg doses of dexamethasone given 12 hours apart.
- Neonates whose mothers receive antenatal corticosteroids have significantly lower severity, frequency, or both of respiratory distress syndrome, intracranial hemorrhage, necrotizing enterocolitis and death.

Tocolytic Contraindications. These are conditions under which stopping labor is either dangerous for mother and baby or futile (makes no difference in outcome). Examples include the following:

- **Obstetric conditions**—severe abruptio placenta, ruptured membranes, chorioamnionitis.
- **Fetal conditions**—lethal anomaly (anencephaly, renal agenesis), fetal demise or jeopardy (repetitive late decelerations).
- **Maternal conditions**—eclampsia, severe preeclampsia, advanced cervical dilation.

Tocolytic Agents. Parenteral agents may prolong pregnancy but for no more than 72 h. This does provide a window of time for (1) administration of **maternal IM betamethasone** to enhance fetal pulmonary surfactant and (2) **transportation of mother and fetus in utero** to a facility with neonatal intensive care. Oral tocolytic agents are no more effective than placebo.

- **Magnesium sulfate** is a competitive inhibitor of calcium. Clinical monitoring is based on decreasing but maintaining detectable deep tendon reflexes.
  - Side effects include muscle weakness, respiratory depression, and pulmonary edema. Magnesium overdose is treated with IV calcium gluconate.
  - Contraindications include renal insufficiency and myasthenia gravis.
- **β-Adrenergic agonists include terbutaline.** Tocolytic effect depends on the β_2-adrenergic receptor myometrial activity.
  - Cardiovascular side effects (hypertension, tachycardia) are from β_1 receptor cardiovascular activity. Other side effects are hyperglycemia, hypokalemia, and pulmonary edema.
  - Contraindications include cardiac disease, diabetes mellitus, uncontrolled hyperthyroidism.
- **Calcium-channel blockers** decrease intracellular calcium (e.g., nifedipine).
  - Side effects include tachycardia, hypotension, and myocardial depression.
  - Contraindications include hypotension.
- **Prostaglandin synthetase inhibitors** decrease smooth muscle contractility by decreasing prostaglandin production (e.g., indomethacin).
  - Side effects include oligohydramnios, in utero ductus arteriosus closure, and neonatal necrotizing enterocolitis.
  - Contraindications include gestational age >**32 weeks**.

OB Triad

Beta Agonists

- Preterm labor tocolysis
- Hypokalemia
- Hyperglycemia

OB Triad

Calcium Channel Blocker

- Preterm labor tocolysis
- Hypotension
- Myocardial depression

OB Triad

Indomethacin
- Preterm labor tocolysis
- Oligohydramnios
- PDA closure in utero

Management:
- Confirm labor using the 3 criteria listed earlier.
- Rule out contraindications to tocolysis using criteria listed above.
- Initiate IV hydration with isotonic fluids.
- Start IV $MgSo_4$ for fetal neuroprotection (if <32 weeks) at least 4 hours before anticipated birth.
- Start tocolytic therapy with terbutaline, nifedipine or indomethacin (if <32 weeks) for no longer than 48 hours to allow for antenatal steroid effect.
- Obtain cervical and urine cultures before giving IV penicillin G (or erythromycin) for group B b Streptococcus sepsis prophylaxis.
- Administer maternal IM betamethasone to stimulate fetal type II pneumocyte surfactant production if gestational age is <34 weeks.

Prevention. Weekly intramuscular injections of 17α-OH progesterone caproate starting at 20 weeks' gestation has been shown to decrease preterm deliveries in women with a history of previous idiopathic preterm deliveries.

PREMATURE RUPTURE OF MEMBRANES (PROM)

OB Triad

Ruptured Membranes
- Posterior fornix **pooling**
- Fluid is Nitrazine (phenaphthazine) (+)
- Glass slide drying: fern (+)

A 22-year-old primigravida at 33 weeks' gestation comes to the birthing unit stating that 2 h ago she had a gush of fluid from her vagina. She denies vaginal bleeding or uterine contractions. Her perineum appears moist to gross inspection. On examination her temperature is 102°F.

Definition. Rupture of the fetal membranes before the onset of labor, whether at term or preterm.

Risk Factors. Ascending infection from the lower genital tract is the most common risk factor for PROM. Other risk factors are local membrane defects and cigarette smoking.

Clinical Presentation. Typical history is a sudden gush of copious vaginal fluid. On external examination, clear fluid is flowing out of the vagina. Oligohydramnios is seen on ultrasound examination.

Diagnosis.
PROM is diagnosed by **sterile speculum examination** meeting the following criteria:
- **Pooling positive**—clear, watery amniotic fluid is seen in the posterior vaginal fornix
- **Nitrazine positive**—the fluid turns pH-sensitive paper blue
- **Fern positive**—the fluid displays a ferning pattern when allowed to air dry on a microscope glass slide

Chorioamnionitis is diagnosed **clinically** with all the following criteria needed:
- Maternal fever and uterine tenderness in the presence of confirmed PROM in the absence of a URI or UTI

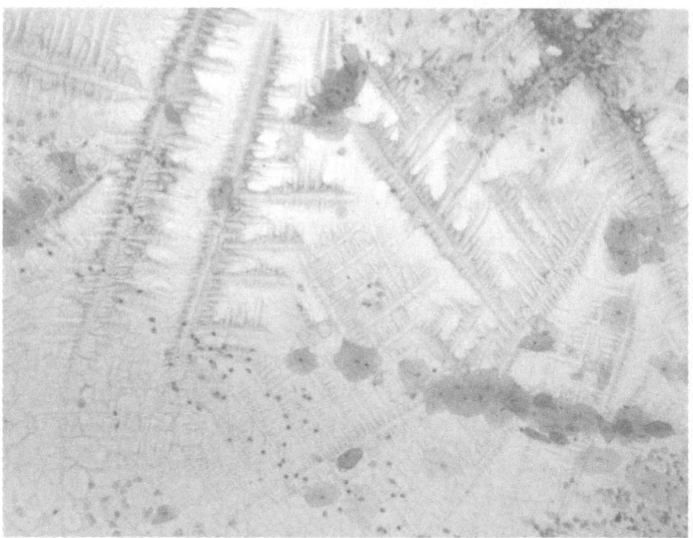
With permission, Australian Society of Cytology Inc., cytology-asc.com

Figure I-8-3. Ferning Pattern of Amniotic Fluid

Management

- If **uterine contractions** occur, tocolysis is contraindicated.
- If **chorioamnionitis** is present, obtain cervical cultures, start broad-spectrum therapeutic IV antibiotics, and initiate prompt delivery.
- If **no infection** is present, management will be based on gestational age as follows:
  - **Before viability** (<23 weeks), outcome is dismal. Either induce labor or manage patient with bed rest at home. Risk of fetal pulmonary hypoplasia is high.
  - **With preterm viability** (23 0/7–33 6/7 weeks), conservative management. Hospitalize the patient at bed rest, administer IM betamethasone to enhance fetal lung maturity if <34 weeks, obtain cervical cultures, and start a 7-day course of prophylactic ampicillin and erythromycin.
  - **At term** (≥34 weeks), initiate prompt delivery. If vaginal delivery is expected, use oxytocin or prostaglandins as indicated. Otherwise, perform cesarean delivery.

OB Triad

Chorioamnionitis
- Ruptured membranes
- Maternal fever
- No UTI or URI

Table 8-3. Hazards Associated with PROM

If Fetus Remains In Utero	If Preterm Delivery Occurs
Neonatal conditions	**Neonatal conditions**
• Infection and sepsis • Deformations • Umbilical cord compression • Pulmonary hypoplasia	• Respiratory distress syndrome (most common) • Patent ductus arteriosus • Intraventricular hemorrhage • Necrotizing enterocolitis • Retinopathy of prematurity • Bronchopulmonary dysplasia • Cerebral palsy
Maternal conditions	
• Chorioamnionitis, sepsis • Deep venous thrombosis (DVT) • Psychosocial separation	

POSTTERM PREGNANCY

A 21-year-old primigravida at 42 weeks' gestation by dates comes to the outpatient prenatal clinic. She has been seen for prenatal care since 12 weeks' gestation, confirmed by an early sonogram. She states that fetal movements have been decreasing. Fundal height measurement is 42 cm. Her cervix is long, closed, posterior, and firm. Nonstress test is reactive, but amniotic fluid index is 4 cm.

Definition

- **Academic.** The most precise definition is a pregnancy that continues for ≥40 weeks or ≥280 days postconception. This includes 6% of all pregnancies.
- **Practical.** Because most of the time the date of conception is not known, a practical definition is a pregnancy that continues ≥42 weeks or ≥294 days after the first day of the last menstrual period.
- **Statistics.** Generally, 50% of patients deliver by 40 weeks, 75% by 41 weeks, and 90% by 42 weeks. These statistics assume ovulation occurred on day 14 of a 28-day menstrual cycle. These figures probably overstate the actual number because up to half of these patients had cycles longer than 28 days.

Etiology. The most common cause of true postdates cases are idiopathic (no known cause). It does occur more commonly in young primigravidas and rarely with placental sulfatase deficiency. Pregnancies with anencephalic fetuses are the longest pregnancies reported.

Significance. Perinatal mortality is increased two- to threefold. This is a direct result of changes on placental function over time.

- **Macrosomia syndrome.** In most patients, **placental function continues** providing nutritional substrates and gas exchange to the fetus, resulting in a healthy but large fetus. **Cesarean rate is increased** owing to prolonged or arrested labor. Shoulder dystocia is more common with risks of fetal hypoxemia and brachial plexus injury.
- **Dysmaturity syndrome.** In a minority of patients, **placental function declines** as infarction and aging lead to placental scarring and loss of subcutaneous tissue. This reduction of metabolic and respiratory support to the fetus can lead to the asphyxia that is responsible for the increased perinatal morbidity and mortality. **Cesarean rate is increased** owing to nonreassuring fetal heart rate patterns. Oligohydramnios results in umbilical cord compression. Hypoxia results in acidosis and in utero meconium passage.

Management. Management is based on 2 factors.

- **Confidence in dates.** Identify how much confidence can be placed on the gestational age being truly >42 weeks.
- **Favorableness of the cervix.** Assess the likelihood of successful induction of labor by assessing cervical dilation, effacement, position, consistency, and station. The Bishop score is a numerical expression of how favorable the cervix is and the likelihood of successful labia induction.
  - Favorable cervix is dilated, effaced, soft, and anterior to mid position. Bishop score is ≥8.
  - Unfavorable cervix is closed, not effaced, long, firm, and posterior. Bishop score is ≤5.

Bishop Scoring Method

Parameter\Score	0	1	2	3
Position	Posterior	Intermediate	Anterior	-
Consistency	Firm	Intermediate	Soft	-
Effacement	0–30%	31–50%	51–80%	>80%
Dilation	0 cm	1–2 cm	3-4 cm	>5 cm
Fetal station	-3	-2	-1, 0	+1,+2

Patients can be classified into 3 groups.

- **Dates sure, favorable cervix.** Management is aggressive. There is no benefit to the fetus or mother in continuing the pregnancy. Induce labor with IV oxytocin and artificial rupture of membranes.
- **Dates sure, unfavorable cervix.** Management is controversial. Management could be aggressive, with cervical ripening initiated with vaginal or cervical prostaglandin E_2 followed by IV oxytocin. Or management could be conservative with twice weekly NSTs and AFIs awaiting spontaneous labor.
- **Dates unsure.** Management is conservative. Perform twice weekly NSTs and AFIs to ensure fetal well-being and await spontaneous labor. If fetal jeopardy is identified, delivery should be expedited.

Table 8-4. Placental Function in Post-term Pregnancy

Maintained	Deteriorates
Macrosomia (80%)	Dysmaturity (20%)
Difficult labor and delivery	Placental insufficiency
↑ C section (forceps, vacuum extractor, shoulder dystocia, birth trauma)	↑ C section (acidosis, meconium aspiration, oxygen deprivation)

Management of Meconium. Previous recommendations to prevent meconium aspiration syndrome (MAS) included:

- **In labor**, amnioinfusion (with saline infused through an intrauterine catheter) to dilute meconium and provide a fluid cushion to prevent umbilical cord compression.
- **After the head is delivered**, suction the fetal nose and pharynx to remove any upper airway meconium.
- **After the body is delivered**, visualize the vocal cords with a laryngoscope to remove meconium below the vocal cords.

Newer recommendations (American Heart Association, American Academy of Pediatrics):

- **Amnioinfusion** may be helpful to prevent umbilical cord compression; okay to perform it.
- **Suctioning of fetal nose and pharynx** makes no difference in preventing MAS; do not routinely perform.
- **Laryngoscopic visualization** of vocal cords is only indicated if the neonate is depressed; perform selectively.

Hypertensive Complications 9

Learning Objectives

- ❑ Differentiate between gestational hypertension, preeclampsia, eclampsia, and chronic hypertension with or without superimposed preeclampsia
- ❑ Describe the diagnosis, management, and complications of hypertensive syndromes in pregnancy
- ❑ Answer questions about HELLP syndrome

HYPERTENSION IN PREGNANCY

Systolic and diastolic BP both decline early in the first trimester, reaching a nadir by 24–28 weeks; then they gradually rise toward term but never return quite to prepregnancy baseline. Diastolic falls more than systolic, as much as 15 mm Hg. **Arterial BP is never normally elevated in pregnancy.**

Note

Refer to Physiologic Changes in Pregnancy in chapter 1 for a review of normal BP during pregnancy.

GESTATIONAL HYPERTENSION

A 19-year-old primigravida is seen in the outpatient prenatal clinic for routine visit. She is at 32 weeks' gestation, confirmed by first trimester sonogram. She has no complaints. She denies headache, epigastric pain, or visual disturbances. She has gained 2 pounds since her last visit 2 weeks ago. On examination her blood pressure is 155/95 mm Hg, which is persistent on repeat check 10 minutes later. She has only trace pedal edema. A spot urine dipstick is negative.

Definition. Gestational hypertension is diagnosed with **sustained** elevation of BP ≥ 140/90 mm Hg after 20 weeks of pregnancy **without** proteinuria. BP returns to normal baseline postpartum.

Symptoms. No symptoms of preeclampsia are seen, e.g., headache, epigastric pain, visual disturbances. Physical findings are unremarkable for pregnancy.

Laboratory Abnormalities. Laboratory tests are unremarkable for pregnancy. Proteinuria is absent.

Diagnostic Tests. The key finding is sustained elevation of BP >140/90 mm Hg without proteinuria.

OB Triad

Gestational Hypertension

- Pregnancy >20 wk
- Sustained HTN
- No proteinuria

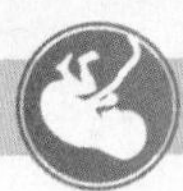

Management. Conservative outpatient management is appropriate. Close observation is prudent since 30% of patients will develop preeclampsia. Appropriate laboratory testing should be performed to rule out preeclampsia, e.g., urine protein, hemoconcentration assessment. Deliver by 40 weeks.

Differential Diagnosis. Preeclampsia should always be ruled out.

PREECLAMPSIA

A 21-year-old primigravida without severe features is seen in the outpatient prenatal clinic for routine visit. She is at 32 weeks' gestation, confirmed by first trimester sonogram. She denies headache, epigastric pain, or visual disturbances. She has gained 10 pounds since her last visit 2 weeks ago. On examination her BP is 155/95, and remains unchanged on repeat check in 15 min. She has 2+ pedal edema, and her fingers appear swollen. A spot urine dipstick shows 2+ protein.

OB Triad

Preeclampsia

- Pregnancy >20 wk
- Sustained HTN (>140/90 mm Hg)
- Proteinuria (≥300 mg/24 h)

Definition. Preeclampsia is **sustained BP** elevation in pregnancy **after 20 weeks'** gestation in the absence of preexisting hypertension.

Diagnostic Criteria. There are no pathognomic tests. The diagnostic dyad includes the following:

- **Sustained BP elevation** of ≥140/90 mm Hg.
- **Proteinuria** of ≥300 mg on a 24-h urine collection or protein/creatinine ratio of ≥0.3.

Risk Factors. Preeclampsia is found 8 times more frequently in **primiparas.** Other risk factors are multiple gestation, hydatidiform mole, diabetes mellitus, age extremes, chronic hypertension, and chronic renal disease.

Etiology/Pathophysiology. Pathophysiology involves **diffuse vasospasm** caused by (1) loss of the normal pregnancy-related refractoriness to vasoactive substances such as angiotensin; and (2) relative or absolute changes in the following **prostaglandin** substances: increases in the vasoconstrictor thromboxane along with decreases in the potent vasodilator **prostacyclin.** This vasospasm contributes to intravascular volume constriction and decreased perfusion of most organs including uteroplacental unit, kidneys, liver, brain, and heart. Decreased renal blood flow leads to decreased clearance of body metabolic wastes. Capillary injury leads to loss of intravascular volume into the interstitial space and subsequent edema.

Presenting Symptoms and Physical Examination. With preeclampsia without severe features the symptoms and physical findings, if present, are generally related to excess weight gain and fluid retention. Presence of new onset of persistent headache, epigastric pain, or visual disturbances would move the diagnosis from preeclampsia without severe features to preeclampsia with severe features.

Laboratory Abnormalities. Evidence of **hemoconcentration** is shown by elevation of hemoglobin, hematocrit, blood urea nitrogen (BUN), serum creatinine, and serum uric acid. **Proteinuria** is present (described under diagnostic criteria). Evidence of disseminated intravascular coagulation (**DIC**) or liver enzyme elevation would move the diagnosis from preeclampsia without severe features to preeclampsia with severe features.

Management. The only definitive cure is delivery and removal of all fetal-placental tissue. However, delivery may be deferred in preeclampsia without severe features to minimize neonatal complications of prematurity. Management is based on gestational age.

- **Conservative management.** Before 37 weeks' gestation as long as mother and fetus are stable, mild preeclampsia is managed in the hospital or as outpatient, watching for possible progression to severe preeclampsia. No antihypertensive agents or $MgSO_4$ are used.
- **Delivery.** At ≥37 weeks' gestation, delivery is indicated with dilute IV oxytocin induction of labor and continuous infusion of IV $MgSO_4$ to prevent eclamptic seizures.

Complications. Progression from preeclampsia without severe features to preeclampsia with severe features may occur.

Differential Diagnosis. Chronic hypertension should always be ruled out.

PREECLAMPSIA WITH SEVERE FEATURES

> A 21-year-old primigravida is seen in the outpatient prenatal clinic for a routine visit. She is at 32 weeks' gestation, confirmed by first trimester sonogram. For the past 24 h she had experienced severe, unremitting occipital headache, and mid-epigastric pain not relieved by acetaminophen, and she has also seen light flashes and spots in her vision. She has gained 10 pounds since her last visit 2 weeks ago. On examination her BP is 165/115. She has 2+ pedal edema, and her fingers appear swollen. Fundal height is 29 cm. Fetal heart tones are regular at 145 beats/min. A spot urine dipstick shows 4+ protein.

Diagnostic Tests. The diagnosis is made on the basis of the finding of at least mild elevation of BP and mild proteinuria plus any one of the following:

- **Sustained BP** elevation of ≥160/110.
- **Evidence of maternal jeopardy.** This may include symptoms (headache, epigastric pain, visual changes), thrombocytopenia (platelet count <100,000/mL), doubling of liver transaminases, pulmonary edema, serum creatinine >1.1 mg/dL, or doubling of serum creatinine.
- **Edema** may or may not be seen.

Risk Factors. These are the same as preeclampsia with the addition of diseases with small vessel disease such as systemic lupus and longstanding overt diabetes.

Etiology/Pathophysiology. Pathophysiology is the same as preeclampsia but involves **severe diffuse vasospasm** and **more intense capillary injury** to where the ischemia demonstrates itself in overt, usually multiorgan system injury.

Presenting Symptoms. Presence of new onset of persistent headache, epigastric pain, or visual disturbances is characteristic of preeclampsia with severe features.

Laboratory Abnormalities. Evidence of **hemoconcentration** will be more severe. Proteinuria is described under diagnostic tests. Evidence of DIC and hepatocellular injury is characteristic of severe preeclampsia.

Note

Preeclampsia with severe features has many presentations.

Note

Quantification of proteinuria (e.g., ≥5 g on a 24-h urine collection) is no longer used as a finding indicating a severe feature of preeclampsia. Proteinuria may even be absent, yet the diagnosis still can be made if there is new onset of hypertension with evidence of maternal jeopardy.

OB Triad

Preeclampsia with Severe Features

- Pregnancy >20 wk
- Sustained HTN (>140/90 mm Hg)
- Headache or epigastric pain or visual changes

- Pregnancy >20 wk
- Sustained HTN (>140/90 mm Hg)
- DIC or ↑ liver enzymes or pulmonary edema

Management. Aggressive prompt delivery is indicated for preeclampsia with severe features at any gestational age with evidence of maternal jeopardy or fetal jeopardy. Main goals are seizure prevention and BP control.

- **Administer IV $MgSO_4$** to prevent convulsions. Give a 5-g loading dose, then continue maintenance infusion of 2 g/h. Continue IV $MgS0_4$ for 24 hours after delivery.
- **Lower BP** to diastolic values 90–100 mm Hg with IV hydralazine and/or labetalol. More aggressive BP control may jeopardize uteroplacental fetal perfusion.
- **Attempt vaginal delivery** with IV oxytocin infusion if mother and fetus are stable.
- Cesarean section is only for obstetric indications.

Note

Because IUGR is managed similarly with and without preeclampsia, it has been removed as a finding indicating a severe feature of preeclampsia.

Conservative inpatient management may rarely be attempted in absence of maternal and fetal jeopardy with gestational age 26–34 weeks if BP can be brought <160/110 mm Hg. This should take place in an intensive care, tertiary-care setting. Continuous IV $MgSO_4$ should be administered, and maternal betamethasone should be given to enhance fetal lung maturity.

Complications. Progression from preeclampsia with severe features to eclampsia may occur.

ECLAMPSIA

A 21-year-old primigravida is brought to the emergency department after suffering from a generalized tonic-clonic seizure at 32 weeks' gestation. The seizure was preceded by a severe headache. She lost control of her bowels and bladder. She has gained 10 pounds since her last prenatal visit 2 weeks ago. On examination she is unresponsive and in a postictal state. Her BP is 185/115, and a spot urine dipstick shows 4+ protein.

Definition. Eclampsia is the presence of **unexplained generalized seizures** in a hypertensive, proteinuric pregnant woman in the last half of pregnancy.

Risk Factors. These are the same as in preeclampsia. A primary seizure disorder does not predispose to eclampsia.

Etiology/Pathophysiology. Pathophysiology is **severe diffuse cerebral vasospasm** resulting in cerebral perfusion deficits and cerebral edema.

Presenting Symptoms. In addition to those of mild and severe preeclampsia, the most significant finding is **unexplained tonic-clonic seizures.**

Laboratory Abnormalities. These are the same as found with mild and severe preeclampsia.

Diagnosis. The diagnosis is made clinically with unexplained generalized seizures occurring in a hypertensive, proteinuric pregnant woman in the last half of pregnancy.

Management. The first step is to protect the mother's airway and tongue.

- **Administer $MgSO_4$** with an IV bolus of 5 g to stop seizures, continuing maintenance infusion rate of 2 g/h. Continue IV $MgS0_4$ for 24 hours after delivery.
- **Aggressive prompt delivery** is indicated for eclampsia at any gestational age after stabilization of the mother and the fetus. Attempt vaginal delivery with IV oxytocin infusion if mother and fetus are stable.
- **Lower diastolic BP** between 90 and 100 mm Hg with IV hydralazine and/or labetalol.

Complications. Intracerebral hemorrhage can occur with even death resulting.

Table 9-1. Preeclampsia–Eclampsia Spectrum

	Preeclampsia without Severe Features	Preeclampsia with Severe Features	Eclampsia
Symptoms	None	Headache or epigastric pain or visual changes	Unexplained convulsions
Sustained ↑ blood pressure	>140/90 mm Hg <160/110 mm Hg	At least >140/90 (if other findings) or >160/110 mm Hg	At least >140/90 mm Hg
Laboratory tests	Hemoconcentration >300 mg proteinuria in 24 hrs No DIC, normal liver function tests	Hemoconcentration, or DIC, or ↑ liver function tests	Hemoconcentration At least 1-2 + proteinuria
Other findings	None	Pulmonary edema	May or may not be present
Management	<36 wk: observe in hospital, no $MgSO_4$, or blood pressure meds ≥36 wks: prompt delivery	MgSO4: prevent or treat convulsions Lower diastolic, BP to 90–100 mm Hg Prompt delivery: not necessarily Cesarean section	

CHRONIC HYPERTENSION WITH OR WITHOUT SUPERIMPOSED PREECLAMPSIA

> A 35-year-old multigravida is seen in the outpatient prenatal clinic for her first prenatal visit. She is at 12 weeks' gestation with a BP of 155/95. Chronic hypertension was diagnosed 5 years ago for which she has been treated with oral nifedipine. A spot urine dipstick protein is 2+. A recent 24-h urine collection showed 1.2 g of protein and a creatinine clearance of 85 ml/min. Serum creatinine is 1.2 mg/dl. She has no complaints of headache or visual changes.

Risk Factors. Most chronic hypertension (HTN) is **idiopathic** without specific antecedents. Risk factors are obesity, advanced maternal age, positive family history, renal disease, diabetes, and systemic lupus erythematosus.

Etiology/Pathophysiology. Pathophysiology is **vasospasm** causing **decreased end-organ perfusion**, resulting in injury and damage. The acute problems arise from excessive systolic pressures, whereas the long-term problems arise from excessive diastolic pressures.

OB Triad

Chronic HTN

- Pregnancy <20 wk or prepregnancy
- Sustained HTN (>140/90 mm Hg)
- +/– proteinuria

Diagnosis. The diagnosis of chronic HTN is made when BP ≥140/90 mm Hg with onset before the pregnancy or before 20 weeks' gestation.

Pregnancy Prognosis with Chronic HTN:

- **Good.** Favorable maternal and neonatal outcome is found when BP 140/90–179/109 mm Hg and no evidence of end-organ damage.
- **Poor.** Pregnancy complications are more common in patients with severe HTN with the following end-organ damage: cardiac, renal, and retinal.
  - **Renal disease.** Pregnancy loss rates increase significantly if serum creatinine value are >1.4 mg/dL.
  - **Retinopathy.** Longstanding HTN is associated with retinal vascular changes including hemorrhages, exudates, and narrowing.
  - **Left ventricular hypertrophy.** This is seen mostly in women with prolonged BP values >180/110 mm Hg.
- **Worst.** Tenfold higher fetal loss rate if uncontrolled HTN (before conception or early in pregnancy) and chronic HTN with superimposed preeclampsia.

OB Triad

Chronic HTN with Superimposed Preeclampsia

- Chronic HTN
- Worsening BP
- Worsening proteinuria

Chronic HTN with Superimposed Preeclampsia:

- This complication occurs in 25% of patients with chronic HTN. Risk factors include renal insufficiency, HTN for previous 4+ years, and HTN in a previous pregnancy.
- Adverse pregnancy outcomes for both mother and baby are markedly increased. Abruptio placenta incidence is markedly increased.
- The diagnosis is made on the basis of established chronic HTN along with any of the following: documented **rising BP values**; demonstrated **worsening proteinuria**; or evidence of **maternal jeopardy** (headache, epigastric pain, visual changes, thrombocytopenia [platelet count <100,000/mL], elevated liver enzymes, pulmonary edema, oliguria [<750 mL/24 h], or cyanosis). Edema may or may not be seen.

Laboratory Abnormalities. Chronic HTN patients have a spectrum of etiologies and disease severity. Those with mild HTN and no end-organ involvement have normal laboratory tests, whereas those with renal disease may have evidence of decreased renal function including proteinuria, lowered creatinine clearance, and elevated BUN, creatinine, and uric acid.

Antihypertensive Drug Therapy Issues

- **Discontinue medications.** This may be done in patients with mild-to-moderate HTN caused by the normal decrease in BP that occurs in pregnancy. Pharmacologic treatment in patients with diastolic BP <90 mm Hg or systolic BP <140 mm Hg does not improve either maternal or fetal outcome.
- **Maintain medications.** This may be necessary in patients with severe HTN. The drug of choice is methyl-dopa because of extensive experience and documented fetal safety. Labetalol and atenolol are acceptable alternatives. However, β-blocking agents are associated with intrauterine growth retardation (IUGR).
- **"Never use" medications.** Angiotensin-converting enzyme inhibitors are contraindicated in pregnancy, as they have been associated with fetal hypocalvaria, renal failure, oligohydramnios, and death. **Diuretics** should not be initiated during pregnancy owing to possible adverse fetal effects of associated plasma volume reduction.
- **BP target range.** Reduction of BP to normal levels in pregnancy may jeopardize uteroplacental blood flow. Maintain diastolic values between **90 and 100 mm Hg.**

Management

Conservative outpatient management is appropriate with uncomplicated mild-to-moderate chronic HTN.

- **Stop drug therapy.** Attempt discontinuation of antihypertensive agents. Follow guideline outlined.
- **Serial sonograms** and antenatal testing is appropriate after 30 weeks' gestation to monitor for increased risk of IUGR.
- **Serial BP and urine protein** assessment is indicated for early identification of superimposed preeclampsia.
- **Induce labor at 39 weeks** if the cervix is favorable.

Aggressive prompt delivery is indicated for chronic HTN with superimposed preeclampsia at any gestational age.

- Administer IV **$MgSO_4$** to prevent convulsions. Continue IV $MgS0_4$ for 24 hours after delivery.
- **Keep diastolic BP** between 90 and 100 mm Hg with IV hydralazine and/or labetalol.
- Attempt **vaginal delivery** with IV oxytocin infusion if mother and fetus are stable.

Complications. Progression from chronic HTN to superimposed preeclampsia, which can lead to maternal and fetal death.

HELLP SYNDROME

A 32-year-old multigravida is at 32 weeks' gestation. At a routine prenatal visit her BP was noted to be 160/105. Previous BP readings were normal. Preeclampsia workup was begun and revealed the following: elevated total bilirubin, lactate dehydrogenase, alanine aminotransferase, and aspartate aminotransferase, as well as platelet count of 85,000. She has no complaints of headache or visual changes.

OB Triad

HELLP Syndrome

- Hemolysis
- ↑ liver enzymes
- ↓ platelets

Definition. HELLP syndrome occurs in 5–10% of preeclamptic patients and is characterized by hemolysis (**H**), elevated liver enzymes (**EL**), and low platelets (**LP**).

Risk Factors. HELLP syndrome occurs twice as often in multigravidas as primigravidas.

Differential Diagnosis. It can be confused with thrombotic thrombocytopenic purpura and hemolytic uremic syndrome. HTN, although frequently seen, is not always present.

Management. Prompt delivery at any gestational age is appropriate. Use of maternal **corticosteroids** may enhance postpartum normalization of liver enzymes and platelet count.

Complications. Conditions that are associated with HELLP syndrome include DIC, abruptio placenta, fetal demise, ascites, and hepatic rupture.

Medical Complications in Pregnancy 10

Learning Objectives

- ❑ Describe the risks and special management of co-occurring medical conditions in pregnancy, including seizure disorders, DM, anemia, thyroid disease, cardiac disease, and liver disease
- ❑ Manage common infections occurring in pregnancy including urinary tract infections, pyelonephritis, cystitis, bacteriuria, and asymptomatic bacteriuria
- ❑ Give an overview of diagnosis and management of thrombophilias and antiphospholipid syndrome

CARDIAC DISEASE

A 30-year-old multigravida with a childhood history of rheumatic fever has echocardiography-diagnosed mitral stenosis. She is now at 20 weeks' gestation and has no symptoms at rest but has mild shortness of breath and dyspnea with activity. On examination she has a diastolic murmur.

Definition. General types of heart disease:

- **Coronary heart disease.** This condition is rarely found in women of childbearing age. Adverse consequences of hypoxic heart disease include miscarriage, fetal death, preterm delivery, and increased perinatal morbidity and mortality.
- **Rheumatic heart disease.** The most common **acquired lesion** in pregnancy is rheumatic heart disease. The most common rheumatic heart disease is mitral stenosis. With severe stenosis (mitral valve area <2 cm^2), the main problem is **inadequate diastolic flow** from the left atrium to the left ventricle. Obstruction to left ventricular filling may lead to left atrial enlargement, pulmonary congestion, atrial fibrillation, and subacute bacterial endocarditis (SBE) with valvular vegetations causing thromboemboli. Tachycardia and increased plasma volume, which are normal changes of pregnancy, will only exacerbate these problems. Balloon valvuloplasty may need to be performed as a last resort.
- **Congenital heart disease.** The **most common congenital** lesions are atrial (ASDs) and ventricular septal defects (VSDs). The **most common cyanotic** congenital heart disease in pregnancy is tetralogy of Fallot. ASDs and VSDs are tolerated well with pregnancy, as are any regurgitation lesions.

Maternal Mortality Risk

- **Low maternal mortality** (<1% risk of death): ASD, VSD, patent ductus arteriosus (PDA), minimal mitral stenosis, porcine heart valve, and corrected tetralogy of Fallot.
- **Intermediate maternal mortality** (5–15% risk of death): mitral stenosis with atrial fibrillation, artificial heart valve, uncorrected tetralogy of Fallot, and Marfan syndrome with normal aortic root diameter.
- **High maternal mortality** (25–50% risk of death): pulmonary hypertension, Eisenmenger's syndrome, Marfan syndrome with aortic root >40 mm diameter, and peripartum cardiomyopathy.

Unique High-Risk Conditions

Eisenmenger syndrome

This condition is characterized by pulmonary hypertension and a bidirectional intra-cardiac shunt. The normal decrease in systemic vascular resistance (SVR) in pregnancy places the patient at risk for having the pulmonary vascular resistance (PVR) exceed the SVR. When this develops, the path of least resistance for blood from the right heart is to bypass the pulmonary circulation across the shunt. This results in the left heart pumping unoxygenated blood into the systemic circulation, resulting in a 50% mortality risk. Management is by avoiding hypotension.

Marfan syndrome

This is an autosomal dominant connective tissue disorder. In pregnancy, if the aortic root diameter is >40 mm, the risk of aortic dissection is high, placing the patient at a 50% mortality risk.

OB Triad

Peripartum Cardiomyopathy

- Late pregnancy or postpartum
- Multiparity
- Biventricular cardiac failure

Peripartum cardiomyopathy

In this condition, the patient has no underlying heart disease, but develops idiopathic biventricular cardiac decompensation between the last few weeks of pregnancy and the first few months postpartum. Risk factors include advanced maternal age, multiparity, hypertension, and multiple pregnancy. Mortality rate is 75% if reversal does not occur within 6 months. Management is supportive, intensive care unit (ICU) care.

Classification of Heart Disease in Pregnancy

Following are the **New York Heart Association** (NYHA) functional classifications of heart disease in pregnancy:

- Class I—no signs or symptoms of cardiac decompensation with physical activity
- Class II—no symptoms at rest, but minor limitations with activity
- Class III—no symptoms at rest, but marked limitations with activity
- Class IV—symptoms present at rest, increasing with any physical activity

Signs of Heart Disease

- Any diastolic or continuous heart murmur
- Any systolic murmur associated with a thrill
- Any severe arrhythmias
- Unequivocal cardiac enlargement

General Principles in Pregnancy Management of Rheumatic Mitral Heart Disease

- Minimize tachycardia.
- Minimize excessive intravascular volume.

Specific Management

- **Antepartum.** Left lateral rest, 2 g sodium diet, digitalis as indicated, diuretics as indicated, avoid strenuous activity, avoid anemia, fetal echocardiogram (if patient has congenital heart disease).
- **Intrapartum.** Aim for vaginal delivery, left lateral rest, monitor intravascular volume, administer oxygen, reassurance, sedation, SBE prophylaxis, epidural, no pushing, elective forceps to shorten the second stage of labor, possible arterial line and pulmonary artery catheter (if Class III or IV status).
- **Postpartum.** Watch closely for postpartum intravascular overload caused by sudden emptying of uterine venous sinuses after placental delivery.

Table 10-1. Heart Disease in Pregnancy

Diagnosis	Problems	Management
Rheumatic mitral stenosis	↓ diastolic filling time	↓ HR; ↓ IV vol
ASD, VSD	Regurgitation	Conservative
Tetralogy of Fallot corrected	No problem	Conservative
Eisenmenger syndrome	1 Pulmonary HTN 2 Intracardiac shunt	Avoid hypotension
Marfan syndrome	Dilated aortic root External diameter ≥4 cm	Surgical reconstruction
Peripartum cardiomyopathy	Biventricular cardiac failure	Supportive care

THYROID DISEASE

> A 23-year-old primigravida is at 30 weeks' gestation. She has lost 4 pounds during the past 2 months. She states her heart "feels like it is racing," and her resting pulse is 135 beats/min. There is a noticeable tremor when she holds her arms out straight. Her eyes appear prominent and protruding. She is complaining of frequent uterine contractions.

Normal Thyroid Physiology. Increased thyroid blood flow leads to thyromegaly. Increased glomerular filtration rate (GFR) in pregnancy enhances iodine excretion, lowering plasma iodine concentrations. Estrogen causes an increase in liver-produced thyroid binding globulin (TBG), thus increasing total T3 and T4. However, **free T3 and T4 remain unchanged.** Fetal thyroid function begins as early as 12 weeks with minimal transfer of T3 or T4 across the placenta.

Hyperthyroidism

Underlying etiology may be Graves disease, toxic nodular goiter (Plummer disease), hydatidiform mole, or toxic diffuse goiter.

- **If uncontrolled**, it is associated with increased spontaneous abortions, prematurity, intrauterine growth retardation (IUGR), and perinatal morbidity and mortality.
- **If controlled**, pregnancy outcome is not altered. Clinical features include elevated resting pulse, thyromegaly, exopthalmus, inadequate weight gain or even weight loss, and markedly elevated total and free T_4.
- **Thyroid storm** is a life-threatening hypermetabolic state presenting with pyrexia, tachycardia, and severe dehydration. **Management** is propylthiouracil (PTU), β-blocking agents, steroids, and iodine.

OB Triad

Graves Disease

- ↓ TSH level
- ↑ free T_4 level
- TSHR-Ab

Graves disease

This is the most common kind of hyperthyroidism in pregnancy.

Pathophysiology. It is mediated by autoimmune production of thyrotropin-receptor antibodies (TSHR-Ab) that drives thyroid hormone production independent of thyrotropin (TSH). TSHR-Ab can cross the placenta, potentially causing fetal hyperthyroidism.

Diagnosis. The diagnosis is confirmed by elevated free T_4 and TSHR-Ab, as well as low TSH in the presence of clinical features described above.

Management

- **Antithyroid medications** are the first line of therapy in pregnancy, but can cross the placenta leading to fetal hypothyroidism. PTU and methimazole are thioamides that block thyroid hormone synthesis. Methimazole is an FDA pregnancy category D so should not be used in the first trimester, though it is acceptable in the second and third. PTU has a risk of liver failure (rare) so it should be used only in the first trimester.
- **Subtotal thyroidectomy** is primarily indicated when antithyroid medical therapy fails and is ideally performed in the second trimester.
- **Thyroid ablation** with radioactive iodine (I^{131}) is **contraindicated** because it can cross the placenta, destroying the fetal thyroid.

Hypothyroidism

This condition is most commonly a primary thyroid defect and often results in **anovulation and infertility**. If uncontrolled it is associated with spontaneous abortion; however, if pregnancy continues, the infant is healthy. If controlled with appropriate thyroid replacement, normal fertility and pregnancy outcomes are noted.

Diagnosis. Demonstration of an elevated TSH.

Management. Increase supplemental thyroid hormone by 30% in pregnancy.

OB Triad

Hypothyroidism
- ↑ TSH level
- ↓ free T_4 level
- Anovulation

Table 10-2. Thyroid Disorders in Pregnancy

	Hyperthyroid	Hypothyroid
Most common cause	Graves disease	Hashimoto's thyroiditis
Diagnostic criteria	↓ TSH, ↑ free T4 TSHR-antibody	↑ TSH, ↓ free T4
Complication if untreated	Thyroid storm, IUGR	Anovulation, spontaneous abortion
Outcome if properly treated	Normal pregnancy	Normal pregnancy
Treatment medications	1st trimester: PTU 2nd+3rd trimester: methimazole	Synthroid (↑ dose 30% above prepregnancy)

SEIZURE DISORDERS

A 25-year-old primigravida is 19 weeks' gestation. She has a 10-year history of generalized seizures poorly controlled requiring hydantoin and valproic acid. A triple marker screen result showed an elevated maternal serum alpha feto protein.

Significance. Prevalence of seizure disorders is 0.5% in women of childbearing age.

Classification:

- **Partial seizures** do not involve both hemispheres. They can be either **simple**, with no loss of consciousness, or **complex**, in which consciousness may be impaired.
- **Generalized seizures** involve both hemispheres. They can be either **absence** type, with duration <20 s (formerly called "petit mal"), or **tonic-clonic**, with duration lasting up to several minutes (formerly called "grand mal").

Effect of pregnancy on seizure disorder

- **Seizures unchanged.** Up to 25% of these women will experience deterioration of seizure control during pregnancy, with 75% seeing no change. The more severe the disorder, the more likely it will worsen.
- **Anticonvulsant metabolism increased.** Seizure medication clearance may be enhanced by higher hepatic microsomal activity, resulting in lower blood levels.

Effect of seizure disorder on pregnancy

Pregnancy complications are minimal with appropriate prenatal care and compliance with anticonvulsant medications.

Effect of anticonvulsants on fetus and infant

Congenital malformation rate is increased from 3% to >10%. In addition, cerebral palsy, seizure disorders, and mental retardation are increased in offspring of epileptic women. Maternal phenytoin use is associated with neonatal deficiency of vitamin K-dependent clotting factors: II, VII, IX, and X.

Management. Ensure extra **folic acid supplementation** before conception and during embryogenesis to minimize neural tube defects.

- **Anomaly screening.** Offer triple-marker screen and second trimester sonography to identify neural tube defects (NTDs) or other anomalies.
- **Drug monotherapy.** Use a single drug if possible, at the lowest possible dose, to ensure freedom from seizures.
- **Medication levels.** Monitor anticonvulsant levels each trimester and adjust dose as needed. Prevent seizures to minimize maternal and fetal hypoxia.

DIABETES

A 32-year-old Hispanic multigravida is at 29 weeks' gestation. Her 1-h 50-g glucose screen came back at 175 mg/dL. She is 60 inches tall and weighs 200 pounds. Her pregnancy weight gain has been 30 pounds thus far. Her previous babies weighed 3,800 and 4,200 g.

Definition. A pregnant woman is unable to maintain fasting (FBS) or postchallenge glucose values in the normal pregnant range before or after a standard 100-g glucose challenge.

Risk factors. Obesity, age >30 years, and **positive family history** are the most common risk factors for gestational diabetes. Other risk factors are fetal macrosomia, unexplained stillbirth or neonatal death, polyhydramnios, and previous traumatic delivery.

Classification by pathophysiology. Prevalence of glucose intolerance in pregnancy is 2–3%.

- Gestational diabetes mellitus (**GDM**) is the most common type with onset during pregnancy, usually diagnosed in the last half. Pathophysiology involves the diabetogenic effect of human placental lactogen (**hPL**), placental insulinase, cortisol, and progesterone. Thirty-five percent of women with GDM will develop overt diabetes within 5 to 10 years after delivery.
- **Type 1 DM** is juvenile onset, ketosis prone, insulin-dependent diabetes caused by pancreatic islet cell deficiency.
- **Type 2 DM** is adult onset, ketosis resistant, non–insulin-dependent diabetes caused by insulin resistance.

Table 10-3. Classification of Diabetes Mellitus by Pathophysiology

Gestational	Pregnancy onset	Insulin resistance
Type 1	Juvenile onset	Ketosis prone
Type 2	Adult onset	Insulin resistance

Table 10-4. White Classification of Diabetes in Pregnancy

Class A1	GDM with normal FBS not requiring insulin
Class A2	GDM with elevated FBS requiring insulin
Class B	Overt DM onset after age 20 years and duration <10 years
Class C	Overt DM onset age 10–19 years or duration 10–19 years
Class D	Overt DM onset before age 10 years or duration ≥20 years
Class E	Overt DM with calcified pelvic vessels
Class F	Overt DM with nephropathy
Class R	Overt DM with proliferative retinopathy

Screening. Screening is performed on **all pregnant women** 24–28 weeks' gestation when the anti-insulin effect of hPL is maximal. On patients with **risk factors** it is performed on the first prenatal visit then repeated at 24–28 weeks if initially negative.

- The screening test is a 1-h 50-g oral glucose challenge test (OGTT) with normal values being <140 mg/dL. This does not need to be in a fasting state.
- If screening value ≥140 mg/dL, then proceed to a definitive 3-h 100-g OGTT. If screening value ≥200 mg/dL, and an FBS is ≥95 mg/dl, GDM is diagnosed and no further OGTT testing is needed.

Diagnosis. The 3-h OGTT is performed on **all patients with an abnormal screening test.** Definitive diagnosis is based on an abnormal 3-h 100-g OGTT performed after an overnight fast. Four glucose values are obtained.

- Normal pregnant values are FBS <95 mg/dL, 1 h <180 mg/dL, 2 h <155 mg/dL, 3 h <140 mg/dL. **Impaired glucose tolerance** is diagnosed if only one value is abnormal. **GDM** is diagnosed if ≥2 values are abnormal.
- If the FBS is ≥125, overt diabetes is diagnosed and the 100-g glucose load should not be given.

Antepartum General Management

The most significant factor in management of diabetic pregnancies is achieving maternal euglycemia.

- **American Diabetes Association diet.** Educate patient regarding spreading calories evenly throughout the day, encourage complex carbohydrates. Eighty percent of patients with GDM can maintain glucose control with diet therapy.

- **Home blood glucose monitoring.** Patient checks her own blood glucose values at least four times a day with target values of FBS <90 mg/dL and 1 h after meal of <140 mg/dL.
- **Insulin therapy.** Start subcutaneous insulin with type 1 and type 2 DM and with GDM if home glucose values are consistently above the target range. Initial dose is based on pregnancy trimester.

  Total daily insulin units = actual body weight in kilograms × 0.8 (first trimester), 1.0 (second trimester), or 1.2 (third trimester)

  Insulin is divided with two thirds of total daily dose in morning (split into 2/3 NPH and 1/3 regular) and one third of total daily dose in evening (split into 1/2 NPH and 1/2 regular). Insulin is a large molecule and **does not cross the placenta**. Insulin requirements will normally increase through the course of the pregnancy. 15% of patients with GDM will require insulin.
- **Oral hypoglycemic agents.** These were contraindicated in the past because of concern that they would cross the placenta and cause fetal or neonatal hypoglycemia. **Glyburide** appears to cross the placenta minimally, if at all, and is being used for patients with GDM who cannot be controlled by diet alone.

Table 10-5. Gestational Diabetes

Questions	Criteria/Problems	Diag/Mgmt
1-hr 50g OGTT Screening test	<140 mg/dL	GDM ruled out
3-hr 100g OGTT Definitive diagnosis	≥2 values ↑	GDM diagnosed
Home glucose monitoring	Mean glucose values FBS >90; 1 hr pp >140	Start insulin or glyburide
Fetal demise risk factors	1: needs insulin or glyburide 2: HTN 3: previous demise	Starting 32 wk NST & AFI 2/wk
L&D problems	Arrest stage 1 or 2 Shoulder dystocia	CS if estimated fetal weight >4500 g
Post partum management	Prevent postpartum hemorrhage	FBS ≥126 mg/dL 2 hr 75 gm OGTT

Antepartum Overt Diabetes Management

- **Hemoglobin A_{1C}.** Obtain a level on the first visit to ascertain degree of glycemic control during the previous 60–120 days. Repeat levels each trimester.
- **Renal status.** Obtain an early pregnancy baseline 24-h urine collection for total protein and creatinine clearance.
- **Retinal status.** Obtain an early pregnancy ophthalmologic funduscopic evaluation for proliferative retinopathy.
- **Home blood glucose monitoring.** Patient checks her own blood glucose values at least 4 times a day with target values of FBS 60–90 mg/dL and 1 h after a meal of <140 mg/dL.

Preconception Anomaly Prevention

- **Anomaly risk.** Women with overt diabetes are at increased risk of fetal anomalies. This risk can be minimized by lifestyle modification.
- **Euglycemia.** Maintaining glucose values at normal levels reduces anomaly risk close to that of nondiabetes; start 3 months prior to discontinuing contraception.
- **Folate supplementation.** Folic acid, 4 mg a day, should be started 3 months prior to conception to prevent both fetal neural tube defects, as well as congenital heart defects.

Antepartum Fetal Assessment

- **Anomaly screening.** Anomalies are mediated through hyperglycemia and are highest with poor glycemic control during embryogenesis. **Anomalies are not increased in GDM** because hyperglycemia is not present in the first half of pregnancy. Most common fetal anomalies with overt DM are **NTD and congenital heart disease**. An uncommon anomaly, but one highly specific for overt DM, is **caudal regression syndrome**. Obtain a **quadruple-marker screen** at 16–18 weeks to assess for NTD as well as a targeted ultrasound at 18–20 weeks to look for structural anomalies. If the glycosylated hemoglobin is elevated, order a fetal echocardiogram at 22–24 weeks to assess for congenital heart disease.
- **Fetal growth.** Monthly sonograms will assess fetal macrosomia (most commonly seen) or IUGR (seen with longstanding DM and vascular disease).
- **Fetal surveillance.** Start weekly NSTs and amniotic fluid index (AFIs) at **32 weeks** if taking insulin, macrosomia, previous stillbirth, or hypertension. Start NSTs and AFIs at **26 weeks** if small vessel disease is present or there is poor glycemic control. Biophysical profiles can be performed at the time of monthly sonograms.

Intrapartum Management

- **Timing of delivery.** Fetal maturity is often delayed in fetuses of diabetic mothers, yet prolonging the pregnancy may increase the risk of stillbirth; delivery planning is a result of balancing these factors. The target delivery gestational age is 40 weeks, but may be necessary earlier in the presence of fetal jeopardy and poor maternal glycemic control. An amniotic fluid lecithin to sphingomyelin **(L/S) ratio of 2.5** in the presence of **phosphatidyl glycerol** assures fetal lung maturity.
- **Mode of delivery.** The cesarean section rate in diabetic pregnancies approaches 50% because of fetal macrosomia, arrest of labor, and concern regarding shoulder dystocia.
- **Glycemic control.** Maintain maternal blood glucose levels between 80 and 100 mg/dL using 5% dextrose in water and an insulin drip.

Postpartum Management

- **Postpartum hemorrhage.** Watch for uterine atony related to an overdistended uterus.
- **Hypoglycemia.** Turn off any insulin infusion because insulin resistance decreases with rapidly falling levels of hPL after delivery of the placenta. Maintain blood glucose levels with a sliding scale.

Neonatal Problems

- **Hypoglycemia** caused by persistent hyperinsulinemia from excessive prenatal transplacental glucose.
- **Hypocalcemia** caused by failure to increase parathyroid hormone synthesis after birth.
- **Polycythemia** caused by elevated erythropoietin from relative intrauterine hypoxia.
- **Hyperbilirubinemia** caused by liver immaturity and breakdown of excessive neonatal red blood cells (RBCs).
- **Respiratory distress syndrome** caused by delayed pulmonary surfactant production.

ANEMIA

An 18-year-old woman G3 P2 had prenatal laboratory tests drawn when she was seen for her first prenatal visit at 18 weeks' gestation. The complete blood count showed the following: hemoglobin 9.5 g/dL, hematocrit 28%, MCV 75, and RDW 17.0. Her first child was delivered 2 years ago, with her second child born 1 year ago.

Definition. A hemoglobin concentration of <10 g/dL during pregnancy or the puerperium. This is less than the 12 g/dL, which is the lower limits of normal in the nonpregnant woman.

OB Triad

Iron Deficiency Anemia

- Hemoglobin <10 g
- MCV <80 μm^3
- RDW >15%

Iron Deficiency Anemia

This is a nutritional anemia resulting in decreased heme production. It is the **most common** anemia in women because of **menstrual and pregnancy** needs.

Diagnosis. RBCs are microcytic and hypochromic. Hemoglobin <10 g/dL, MCV <80, RDW >15.

Pathophysiology. Falling hemoglobin values do not occur until complete depletion of iron stores in the liver, spleen, and bone marrow, which is followed by a decrease in serum iron with increase in total iron binding capacity (TIBC).

Pregnancy Requirements. A pregnant woman needs 800 mg of elemental iron, of which 500 mg goes to expand the RBC mass and 300 mg goes to the fetal-placental unit.

Risk Factors. Chronic bleeding, poor nutrition, and frequent pregnancies.

Symptoms. Findings may vary from none to general malaise, palpitations, and ankle edema.

Fetal Effects. Increased IUGR and Preterm birth.

Treatment. $FeSO_4$ 325 mg po tid.

Prevention. Elemental iron 30 mg per day.

Folate Deficiency Anemia

This is a nutritional anemia resulting in decreased hemoglobin production.

Diagnosis. RBCs are macrocytic. Hemoglobin ≤10 g/dL, MCV >100, RDW >15. RBC folate levels are low. Peripheral smear may show hypersegmented neutrophils.

Pathophysiology. Folate stores in the body are usually enough for 90 days. Falling hemoglobin values do not occur until complete depletion of folate stores.

Risk Factors. Chronic hemolytic anemias (e.g., sickle cell disease), anticonvulsant use (phenytoin, phenobarbital), and frequent pregnancies.

Symptoms. Findings may vary from none to general malaise, palpitations, and ankle edema.

Fetal Effects. Increased IUGR ,Preterm birth and NTD.

Treatment. Folate 1 mg po daily.

Prevention. Folate 0.4 mg po daily for all women; 4 mg po daily for those at high risk for NTDs.

OB Triad

Folate Deficiency Anemia

- Hemoglobin <10 g
- MCV >100 μm³
- RDW >15%

Sickle Cell Anemia

This is an inherited autosomal recessive disease resulting in normal production of abnormal globin chains.

Screening Test. These are peripheral blood tests used to detect the presence or absence of hemoglobin S. They do not differentiate between disease and trait.

Diagnostic Test. A hemoglobin electrophoresis will differentiate between SA trait (<40% hemoglobin S) or SS disease (>40% hemoglobin S).

Risk Factors. African and Mediterranean descent is the only significant risk factor for sickle cell anemia.

Effects on Pregnancy.

- **With SA,** the patient may have increased urinary tract infections (UTIs) but pregnancy outcome is not changed.
- **With SS**, the pregnancy may be complicated by increased spontaneous abortions, IUGR, fetal deaths, and preterm delivery.

Treatment. Avoid hypoxia, take folate supplements, and monitor fetal growth and well-being.

LIVER DISEASE

Intrahepatic Cholestasis of Pregnancy

A 31-year-old primigravida woman with a history of infertility underwent ovulation induction. She is now at 20 weeks' gestation with dizygotic twins of different genders. She is of Swedish descent and complains of intense skin-itching. She has not experienced these symptoms previously. Her sister experienced similar complaints when she was pregnant, and delivered her baby prematurely. No identifiable rash is noted on physical examination. She states that her urine appears dark-colored.

Pathophysiology. Intrahepatic cholestasis is stimulated by estrogen in genetically predisposed women in the second half of pregnancy. Risk is increased with twins.

Bile acids are incompletely cleared by the liver and accumulate in the plasma. The overall prevalence is 0.5% in North America and Europe. There is a high recurrence rate with subsequent pregnancies.

Findings. The most significant symptom is intractable pruritus on the palms and soles of the feet, worse at night, without specific skin findings.

- Laboratory tests show a mild elevation of bilirubin but diagnostic findings are serum bile acids increased 10- to 100-fold.

Outcome. No adverse effect on maternal outcome, but preterm births and stillbirths are increased

Management

- Oral antihistamines can be helpful in mild cases.
- Cholestyramine has been used to decrease enterohepatic circulation.
- Ursodeoxycholic acid is the treatment of choice. Antenatal fetal testing should be initiated at 34 weeks. Symptoms disappear after delivery.
- Induce labor at 38 weeks gestation.

Acute Fatty Liver

A 29 year-old primagravida is at 33 weeks' gestation. She is brought to the maternity unit by her husband who states she is becoming mentally confused. He reports she started experiencing nausea and vomiting 3 days ago which are becoming worse, associated with lack of appetite. Fundal height is 30 cm. Fetal heart rate is 145/min with non-reactive non-stress test. Her BP is 150/95 mm Hg. Random blood glucose is 52 mg/dL. Platelet count is 75,000. PTT is prolonged at 64.7 seconds. Creatinine is 2.1 mg/dL. Uric acid is 11.9 mg/dL, lactic dihydrogenase 1063 U/l, ALT 220 U/l, AST 350 U/l, total bilirubin 8.4 mg/dL. Serum ammonia is elevated. Urine protein dipstick is 3+.

Description. This is a rare life-threatening complication of pregnancy that usually occurs in the third trimester. Prevalence is 1 in 15,000. Maternal mortality rate is 20%. It is thought to be caused by a disordered metabolism of fatty acids by mitochondria in the fetus, caused by deficiency in the long-chain 3-hydroxyacyl-coenzyme A dehydrogenase (LCHAD) enzyme.

Findings. Symptom onset is gradual, with nonspecific flulike symptoms including nausea, vomiting, anorexia, and epigastric pain.

- Jaundice and fever may occur in as many as 70% of patients.
- Hypertension, proteinuria, and edema can mimic preeclampsia.
- This may progress to involvement of additional systems, including acute renal failure, pancreatitis, hepatic encephalopathy, and coma. Laboratory findings may include: moderate elevation of liver enzymes (e.g., ALT, AST, GGT), hyperbilirubinemia, DIC.
- **Hypoglycemia** and **increased serum ammonia** are unique laboratory abnormalities.

Management. Intensive care unit stabilization with acute IV hydration and monitoring is essential.

- Prompt delivery is indicated.
- Resolution follows delivery if mother survives.

URINARY TRACT INFECTION, PYELONEPHRITIS, AND BACTERIURIA

A 23-year-old primigravida at 31 weeks' gestation comes to the birthing unit with complaints of flank pain, nausea, vomiting, and shaking chills for the past 12 h. She has been diagnosed with sickle cell trait. On examination her temperature is 103°F, pulse 125 beats/min, and respirations 30 breaths/min. Her skin is grossly diaphoretic and she has exquisite right costovertebral angle tenderness. Electronic fetal monitoring shows baseline heart rate 170/min with reactivity. Uterine contractions are noted every 10 min.

Definition. UTI may involve either the **lower tract** (including the bladder or urethra) or the **upper tract** (including the kidney). The most common organisms are **gram-negative enteric bacteria** with *Escherichia coli* the most frequent.

Risk Factors. Pregnancy is a risk factor. Others include mechanical urinary obstructions and systemic diseases (such as sickle cell trait/disease, diabetes mellitus, and gout).

Asymptomatic Bacteriuria

This is the **most common** UTI in pregnancy.

Clinical Findings. No symptoms or signs are present.

Significance. If not treated, 30% of cases will develop acute pyelonephritis.

Diagnosis. Made with a positive urine culture showing >100K colony-forming units (CFU) of a single organism.

Treatment. Single-agent, outpatient oral antibiotics.

OB Triad

Asymptomatic Bacteriuria

- No urgency, frequency, or burning
- No fever
- Urine culture (+)

Acute Cystitis

This is a UTI localized to the bladder without systemic findings.

Clinical Findings. Urgency, frequency, and burning are common.

Significance. If not treated, 30% of cases will develop acute pyelonephritis.

Diagnosis. Made with a positive urine culture showing >100 K CFU of a single organism.

Treatment. Single-agent, outpatient oral antibiotics.

OB Triad

Acute Cystitis

- Urgency, frequency, and burning
- No fever
- Urine culture (+)

Acute Pyelonephritis

This is a UTI involving the upper urinary tract with systemic findings. This is one of the **most common** serious medical complications of pregnancy.

Symptoms. Include shaking chills, anorexia, nausea, vomiting, and flank pain.

Signs. Include high fever, tachycardia, and costovertebral angle tenderness (R>L).

Significance. Preterm labor and delivery can occur. Severe cases are complicated by sepsis, anemia, and pulmonary dysfunction, sometimes requiring ICU care, including intubation.

Diagnosis. Confirmed with a positive urine culture showing >100 K CFU of a single organism.

Treatment. Hospital admission, generous IV hydration, parenteral antibiotics e.g., ceftriaxone, and tocolysis as needed.

OB Triad

Acute Pyelonephritis

- Urgency, frequency, and burning
- Fever and costovertebral angle tenderness (CVAT)
- Urine culture (+)

THROMBOPHILIAS

> A 26-year-old G4 P1 Ab2 woman comes in for her first prenatal visit at 8 weeks' gestation by dates. Her first pregnancy was a spontaneous first-trimester loss, for which she underwent a D&C. In her second pregnancy she developed right lower extremity deep venous thrombosis at 29 weeks, which was followed by an unexplained fetal demise at 30 weeks. Labor was induced with PGE2. The fetus was normal in appearance, without congenital anomalies. Autopsy on the fetus was unremarkable. Her last pregnancy was also a spontaneous first-trimester loss. Her sister has a history of recurrent deep venous thrombosis.

Description. The thrombophilias are a group of disorders that promote blood clotting, because of either an excess of clotting factors or a deficiency of anticlotting proteins that limit clot formation. Prevalence is as high as 20% of the population, but most individuals are asymptomatic. Some will develop deep vein thrombosis or venous thromboembolism (VTE) that can become life-threatening. Risk factors include immobilization, surgery, or pregnancy.

Pregnant women with a thrombophilia are also at higher risk than other pregnant women of developing a VTE. Pulmonary embolus is the leading cause of maternal death in the United States. More than half of pregnant women who develop a pulmonary embolus or other VTE have an underlying thrombophilia.

Diagnosis. Indications for testing are history of VTE or first-degree relative with high-risk thrombophilia or VTE age <50 years.

- **Inherited thrombophilias to test for**: Factor V Leiden (FVL) mutation, prothrombin gene mutation (PGM) G2021 OA, protein C deficiency (PCD), protein S deficiency (PSD), antithrombin deficiency (ATD)
  - **High risk** thrombophilias include homozygous FVL or PGM; compound heterozygote FVL & PTM; and all ATD
  - **Low risk** thrombophilias include heterozygous FVL or PGM; and all PCD & PSD
- **Acquired thrombophilias to test for:** Antiphospholipid Syndrome (APS).

  One or more of the following 3 antiphospholipid antibodies must be positive on ≥2 occasions at least 12 weeks apart.
  - Lupus anticoagulant
  - Anticardiolipin antibody (lgG & IgM)
  - Anti-β_2-glycoprotein 1 (lgG & IgM)

Treatment. Anticoagulation options:

- **Unfractionated heparin** (UFH) can be used antepartum & postpartum
  - Advantages: inexpensive, can be reversed with protamine sulfate,
  - Disadvantages: cannot use orally, short half-life, needs monitoring with aPTT levels, heparin-induced osteopenia, heparin-induced thrombocytopenia (HIT)
- **Low molecular weight heparin** (LMWH) can be used antepartum & postpartum
  - Advantages: longer half-life, less need for monitoring with antifactor Xa levels
  - Disadvantages: cannot use orally, higher cost, can not be reversed
- **Warfarin/coumadin** can be used only postpartum
  - Advantages: oral administration, long half-life, inexpensive, OK for breast feeding
  - Disadvantages: crosses placenta, needs monitoring with INR,

For anticoagulation medications, use the following guidelines:

Antepartum: Use LMWH from first trimester to 36 weeks; then at 36 weeks transition to UFH until delivery

- **None or prophylactic dose**
  - Low-risk thrombophilia without VTE episode
- **Prophylactic or intermediate-dose**
  - Low-risk thrombophilia with single VTE episode
  - High-risk thrombophilia without VTE episode
- **Therapeutic dose**
  - High-risk thrombophilia with single VTE episode
  - Any thrombophilia with VTE in current pregnancy

Intrapartum

- Discontinue UFH during immediate peripartum interval to decrease risk of hemorrhage and permit regional anesthesia
- Protamine sulfate can be used to reverse UFH effect

Postpartum

- VTE risk increased 20-fold in the first week postpartum.
- All patients at risk should be receive postpartum anticoagulation even if they did not receive it antepartum.
- Resume anticoagulation 6 hours after vaginal delivery and 12 hours after cesarean section.
- Coumadin is safe for breastfeeding moms

ANTIPHOSPHOLIPID SYNDROME (APS)

Definition: This is an autoimmune disorder defined by both the presence of characteristic clinical features and circulating antiphospholipid antibodies. Diagnosis requires that at least one clinical and one laboratory criterion are met.

Clinical Criteria for Diagnosis / Indications for Laboratory testing

- **Vascular thrombosis:** 1 or more clinical thrombotic episodes (arterial, venous, or small vessel)
- **Pregnancy morbidity (unexplained):** fetal demise: 1 or more at ≥10 weeks; consecutive miscarriages: 3 or more at <10 weeks

Laboratory criteria: 1 or more of the following 3 anti-phospholipid antibodies must be positive on ≥2 occasions at least 12 weeks apart.

- Lupus anticoagulant
- Anticardiolipin antibody (lgG & IgM)
- Anti-132-glycoprotein I (lgG & IgM)

Management:

Antepartum anticoagulation management:

- APS without a thrombotic event: no heparin or only prophylactic heparin
- APS with a thrombotic event: prophylactic heparin

General management for all women with APS:

- Antepartum: sono assessment of fetal growth monthly; modified Biophysical Profile weekly starting at 32 weeks
- Intrapartum: stop anticoagulation
- Postpartum: resume or start anticoagulation in 6 hours (after vaginal delivery) or 12 hours (after cesarean section); continue anticoagulation for 6 weeks using either heparin or coumadin (safe for breastfeeding moms); avoid estrogen-containing contraceptives

THROMBOEMBOLISM

The mediating factor is frequently endothelial injury from traumatic delivery or cesarean section. In the postpartum period, the risk is increased fivefold. Vascular stasis is the strongest predisposing factor with decreased pelvic and lower extremity blood flow. Enhanced blood coagulability in pregnancy is due to increased factors II, VII, VIII, IX, and X. Risk is even more elevated if the patient has coagulation protein deficiencies: antithrombin III, protein C, protein S, and plasminogen.

Superficial Thrombophlebitis

Superficial thrombophlebitis does not predispose to thromboembolism but may mimic more severe disease.

- **Findings:** Symptoms include localized pain and sensitivity. Signs include erythema, tenderness, and swelling. Diagnosis is one of exclusion after ruling out DVT.
- **Management**: Treatment is conservative: bed rest, local heat, NSAIDs.

Deep Venous Thrombosis (DVT)

DVT **does** predispose to thromboembolic disease. The site of thrombosis is typically in the lower half of the body. Half of cases occur in the pelvic veins and half occur in the lower extremities.

- **Findings:** Symptoms may include pain and increased skin sensitivity, but there may be no complaints. Signs may include calf pain on foot dorsiflexion (Homan sign), although these findings are not highly sensitive or specific. Diagnosis is by duplex Doppler.
- **Management:** Treatment is full anticoagulation with IV heparin to increase PTT by 1.5 to 2.5 times the control value. Subcutaneous heparin is used once therapeutic levels are achieved. No warfarin is used antepartum because of teratogenicity concerns with the fetus. Thrombophilia workup should be performed.

Pulmonary Embolus (PE)

PE is a potentially fatal result of DVT in which emboli travel through the venous system to the lungs. The source of the emboli is most commonly in the lower extremities or pelvis.

- **Findings:** Symptoms include chest pain and dyspnea (80%) but no single symptom(s) predominate because thrombi location varies. Physical and imaging findings include:
  - Tachypnea (90%)
  - **Chest x-ray** often normal
  - **ABG** showing low pO_2 (but often in the normal range)
  - **EKG** that may show tachycardia
  - Right axis deviation (but usually is normal)
- **Diagnosis** depends on the pulmonary imaging modalities used. Spiral CT scan of the chest is the best initial test for suspected PE. **Pulmonary angiography** is the most definitive diagnostic method; most common indication is a negative spiral CT scan in a high-risk and symptomatic patient.
- **Management**: Treatment is full anticoagulation (IV, SQ) heparin to increase PTT by 1.5 to 2.5 times the control value. No warfarin is used antepartum due to teratogenic concerns. Thrombophilia workup should be performed.

Disproportionate Fetal Growth 11

Learning Objectives

- ❑ Demonstrate understanding of intrauterine growth restriction
- ❑ Answer questions about macrosomia

INTRAUTERINE GROWTH RESTRICTION (IUGR)

Common Definition. Fetus with estimated fetal weight (EFW) <5–10th percentile for gestational age. This assumes the fetus is not growing to its genetic potential.

Birth Weight. Another definition is <2,500 grams (5 lb, 8 oz). Clearly, neonatal morbidity and mortality are affected by lowering birth weight. However, **70% of these fetuses are constitutionally small.**

Dating. Accurate early pregnancy dating is essential for making the diagnosis. An early sonogram (<20 weeks) is most accurate if conception date is unknown. **Don't change gestational age based on a late sonogram.**

Fetal Causes. Examples include aneuploidy (e.g., T21, T18, T13); infection (e.g., TORCH), structural anomalies (e.g., congenital heart disease, neural tube defects, ventral wall defects). These causes typically lead to **symmetric** IUGR.

Placental Causes. Examples include infarction, abruption, twin-twin transfusion syndrome (TTTS), velamentous cord insertion. These causes typically lead to **asymmetric** IUGR.

Maternal Causes. Examples include hypertension (e.g., chronic, preeclampsia), small vessel disease (e.g., SLE, long-standing type 1 diabetes), malnutrition, tobacco, alcohol, street drugs. These causes typically lead to **asymmetric** IUGR.

Symmetric IUGR

- All ultrasound parameters (HC, BPD, AC, FL) are smaller than expected.
- Etiology is **decreased growth potential**, i.e., aneuploidy, early intrauterine infection, gross anatomic anomaly.
- Workup should include detailed sonogram, karyotype, and screen for fetal infections.
- **Antepartum tests are usually normal.**

OB Triad

Symmetric IUGR

- Head and abdomen both small
- Etiology: fetal (aneuploidy, infection, anomaly)
- Decreased growth potential

OB Triad

Asymmetric IUGR

- Head normal; abdomen small
- Etiology: maternal-fetal (inadequate nutritional substrates)
- Decreased placental perfusion

Asymmetric IUGR

- Ultrasound parameters show **head sparing**, but **abdomen is small.**
- Etiology is **decreased placental perfusion** due to chronic maternal diseases (hypertension, diabetes, SLE, cardiovascular disease) or abnormal placentation (abruption and infarction).
- Amniotic fluid index is often decreased, especially if uteroplacental insufficiency is severe.
- **Monitoring** is with serial sonograms, non-stress test, amniotic fluid index, biophysical profile, and umbilical artery Dopplers.

MACROSOMIA

Definition. Fetus with estimated fetal weight (EFW) >90–95th percentile for gestational age. Birth weight ≥4,000–4,500 grams (8 lb, 13 oz to 9 lb, 15 oz).

Sonogram EFW. Accuracy in estimating birth weight is poor. Errors in prediction of EFW at term are ±400 grams.

Risk Factors. Gestational diabetes mellitus, overt diabetes, prolonged gestation, increase in BMI (obesity), increase in pregnancy weight gain, multiparity, male fetus.

Maternal Hazards. Operative vaginal delivery, perineal lacerations, postpartum hemorrhage (uterine atony), emergency cesarean section, pelvic floor injury.

Fetal Hazards. Shoulder dystocia, birth injury, asphyxia.

Neonatal Hazards. Neonatal intensive care admission, hypoglycemia, Erb palsy.

Prevention. No accurate ways of predicting or prevention are currently available.

Management. Consider elective cesarean (if EFW >4,500 g in diabetic mother or >5,000 g in nondiabetic mother) or early induction, but this may result in increased cesarean delivery rate due to failure of induction.

Antepartum Fetal Testing 12

Learning Objectives

- ❏ Describe the appropriate use antepartum fetal testing including nonstress test, amniotic fluid index, biophysical profile, contraction stress test, and umbilical artery Doppler

OVERVIEW

A 37-year-old multipara with systemic lupus erythematosus is at 31 weeks' gestation. She has chronic hypertension that is being controlled with methyldopa. She comes to the office stating her fetus is not moving as much as it used to.

Antenatal fetal tests are highly accurate in confirming fetal well-being but are poor predictors of fetal jeopardy. The most common reasons for fetal testing are decreased fetal movements, diabetes, post dates, chronic hypertension, and IUGR.

NONSTRESS TEST (NST)

This test assesses the frequency of fetal movements using an external fetal heart rate (FHR) monitoring device to detect the presence or absence of accelerations. These are abrupt increases in FHR above the baseline lasting <2 min and are unrelated to contractions. The criteria vary by gestational age:

- <32 weeks, the increase should be ≥10 beats/min lasting ≥10 s
- >32 weeks, the increase should be ≥15 beats/min lasting ≥15 s

They are mediated by the **sympathetic** nervous system and always occur in response to **fetal movements. Interpretation: accelerations are always reassuring.**

- **Reactive NST** requires the presence of 2 accelerations in a 20-min window of time meeting the above criteria. This is reassuring and highly predictive for fetal well-being. Fetal death rate is only 3 per 1,000 in the next week. **Management** is weekly NST.
- **Nonreactive NST** is diagnosed when any criteria for reactivity are not met: either the number of accelerations in 20 min or the amplitude or duration of the acceleration. Eighty percent of nonreactive NSTs are false positives (meaning the fetus is not hypoxemic). Nonhypoxemic causes include fetal sleep, prematurity, drug effects, and CNS anomalies. **Management** is fetal vibroacoustic stimulation to see whether this results in reactivity. If the NST is persistently nonreactive, perform a biophysical profile.

Table 12-1. Nonstress Test (NST)

Reactive NST	**Criteria:** ≥2 accelerations in 20 min: ↑ FHR ≥15 beats/min and lasting ≥15 seconds
	Assessment: reassuring of fetal well-being
	Follow-up: repeat weekly/biweekly
Nonreactive NST	**Criteria:** no FHR accelerations or did not meet criteria
	Assessment: sleeping, immature, or sedated fetus; acidotic, compromised fetus?
	Follow-up: VAS
	If still NR: do CST or BPP

Definition of abbreviations: BPP, biophysical profile; CST, contraction stress test; FHR, fetal heart rate; VAS, vibroacoustic stimulation.

AMNIOTIC FLUID INDEX

The 4-quadrant amniotic fluid index test assesses in centimeters the deepest single vertical amniotic fluid pocket in each of the 4 quadrants of the uterus. The sum of the pockets is known as the amniotic fluid index, or AFI. Interpretation is as follows:

<5 cm—oligohydramnios

5–8 cm—borderline

9–25 cm—normal

>25 cm—polyhydramnios

BIOPHYSICAL PROFILE (BPP)

A complete BPP measures **5 components of fetal well-being:** NST, amniotic fluid volume, fetal gross body movements, fetal extremity tone, and fetal breathing movements. The last 4 components are assessed using obstetric ultrasound. Scores given for each component are 0 or 2, with maximum possible score of 10 and minimum score of 0.

- **Score of 8 or 10**—highly **reassuring** of fetal well-being. Management is to repeat the test weekly or as indicated. Fetal death rate is only 1 per 1,000 in the next week.
- **Score of 4 or 6—worrisome**. Management is delivery if the fetus is ≥36 weeks or repeat the biophysical profile in 12–24 h if <36 weeks. An alternative is to perform a CST.
- **Score of 0 or 2**—highly predictive of fetal **hypoxia** with low probability of false positive. Management is prompt delivery regardless of gestational age.

A **modified BPP** includes only the NST and amniotic fluid volume. Its predictive value is almost as high as a complete BPP.

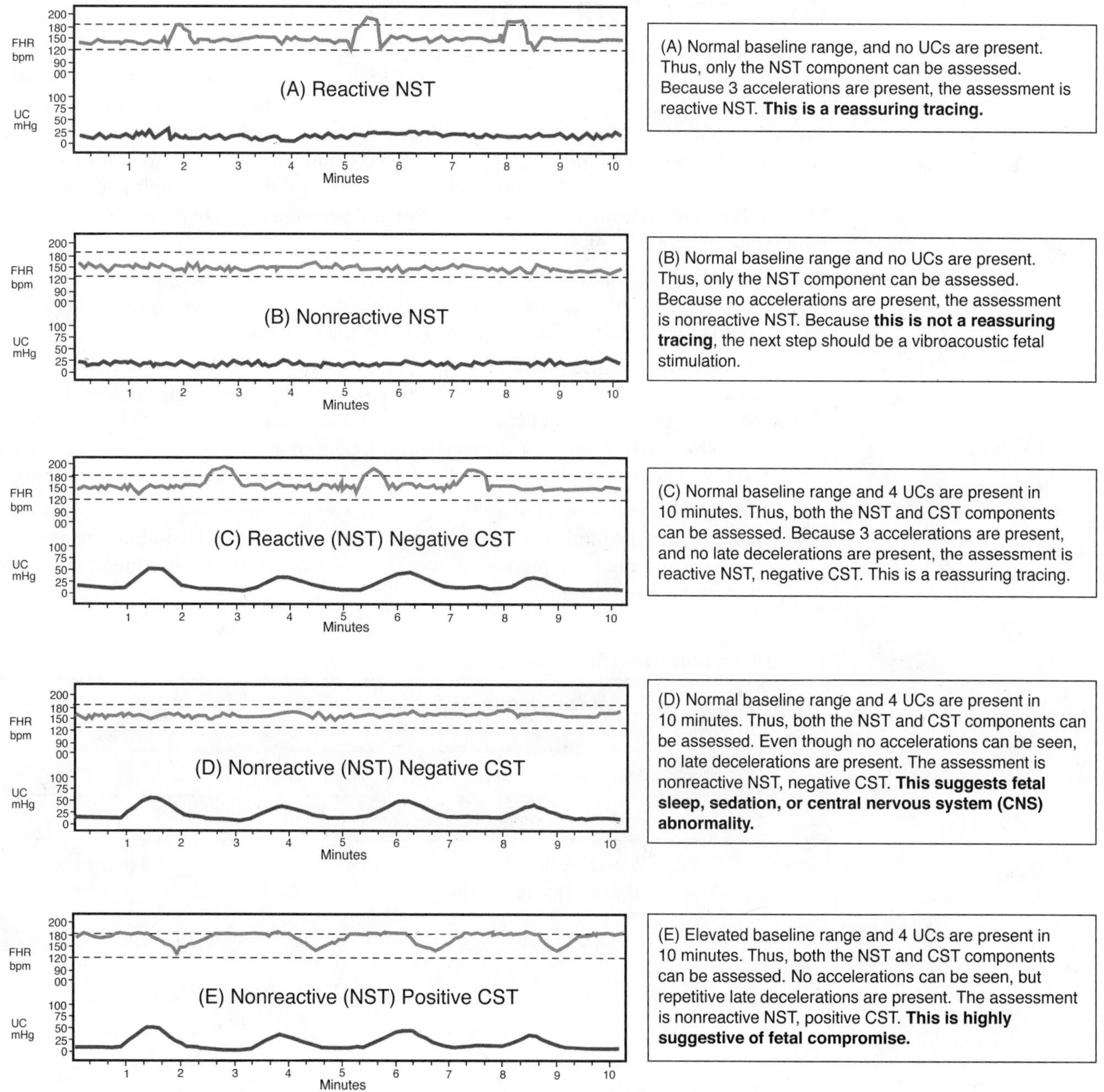

Figure I-12-1. Antepartum Electronic Fetal Monitor (EFM) Tracings

All EFM tracings should be evaluated for the nonstress test (NST) and the contraction stress test (CST). If a technically adequate fetal heart rate (FHR) tracing is present, the NST component can be assessed as reactive or nonreactive. If 3 or more uterine contractions (UCs) are present in 10 minutes, the CST components can be assessed as negative or positive.

CONTRACTION STRESS TEST (CST)

This test assesses the ability of the fetus to tolerate transitory decreases in intervillous blood flow that occur with uterine contractions. It uses both external FHR and contraction monitoring devices and is based on the presence or absence of **late decelerations**. These are **gradual** decreases in FHR below the baseline with onset to nadir of ≥30 s. The deceleration onset and end is **delayed** in relation to contractions. If 3 contractions in 10 min are not spontaneously present, they may be induced with either IV oxytocin infusion or nipple stimulation. This test is **rarely performed** because of the cost and personnel time required. The most common indication is a **BPP of 4 or 6.**

- **Negative CST** requires absence of any late decelerations with contractions. This is reassuring and highly reassuring for fetal well-being. Management is to repeat the CST weekly. Fetal death rate is only 1 per 1,000 in the next week.
- **Positive CST** is worrisome. This requires the presence of late decelerations associated with at least 50% of contractions. Fifty percent of positive CSTs are false positive (meaning the fetus is not hypoxemic). They are associated with good FHR variability. The 50% of true positives are associated with poor or absent variability. Management is prompt delivery.
- **Contraindications**—CST should not be performed whenever contractions would be hazardous to the mother or fetus. Examples include previous classical uterine incision, previous myomectomy, placenta previa, incompetent cervix, preterm membrane rupture, and preterm labor.

Table 12-2. Contraction Stress Test (CST)

Negative CST	No **late decelerations** are seen in the presence of 3 uterine contractions in 10 min
	Assessment: reassuring of fetal well-being
	Follow-up: repeat CST weekly as needed
Positive CST	Repetitive **late decelerations** are seen in the presence of 3 uterine contractions in 10 min
	Assessment: worrisome, especially if nonreactive non-stress test
	Follow-up: prompt delivery

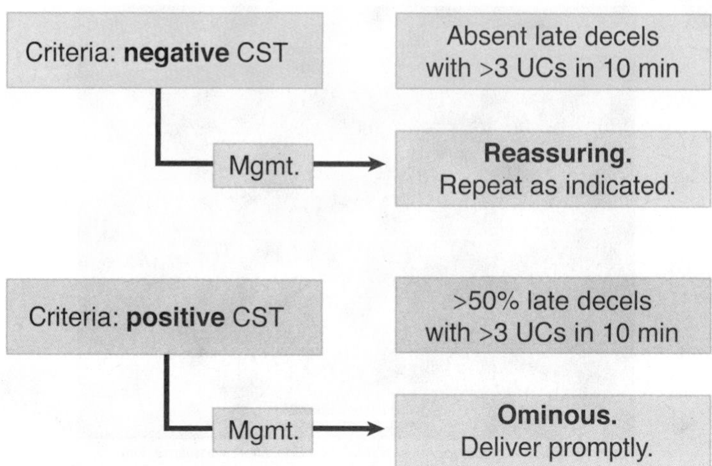

Figure I-12-2. Contraction Stress Test

UMBILICAL ARTERY DOPPLER

This test measures the ratio of systolic and diastolic blood flow in the umbilical artery. The umbilical circulation normally has low resistance, so significant diastolic blood flow is expected. The systolic/diastolic (S/D) ratio normally decreases throughout pregnancy.

This test is predictive of poor perinatal outcome only in IUGR fetuses. Nonreassuring findings, which may indicate need for delivery, are absent diastolic flow and reversed diastolic flow.

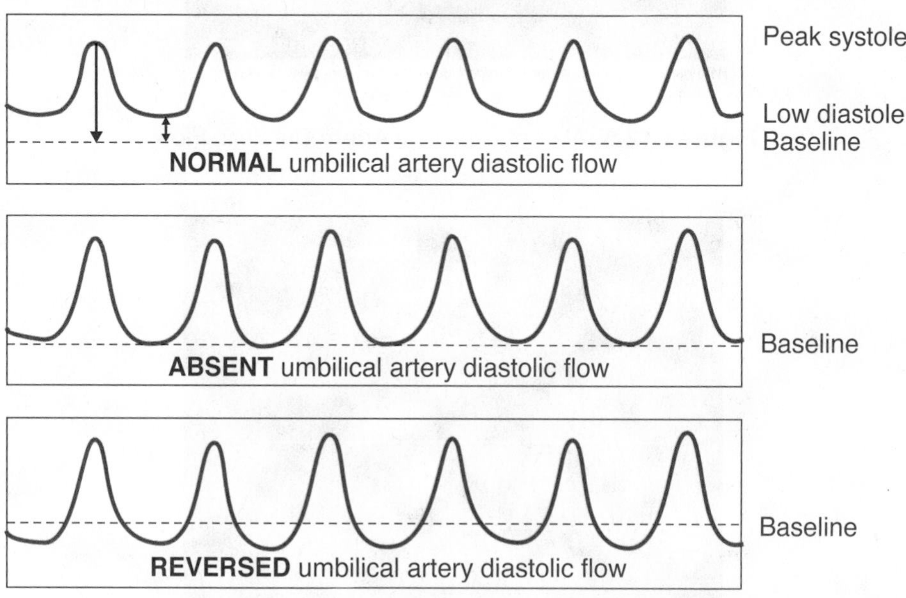

Figure I-12-3. Umbilical Artery Doppler Waveform Patterns

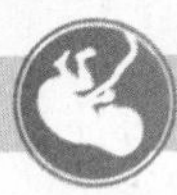

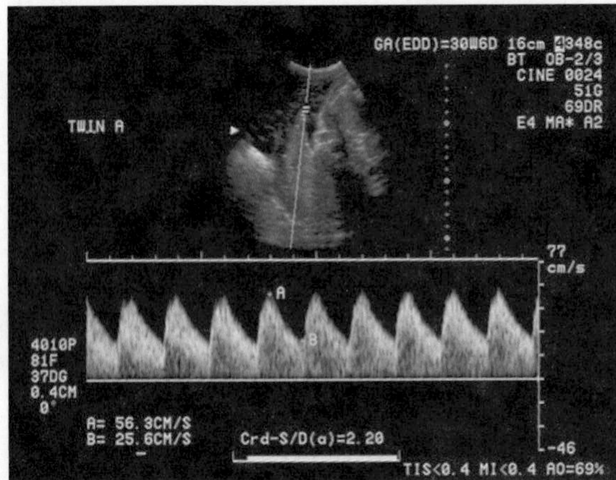

With permission, Institute for Advanced Medical Education, www.iame.com

Figure I-12-4. Normal Umbilical Artery Diastolic Flow

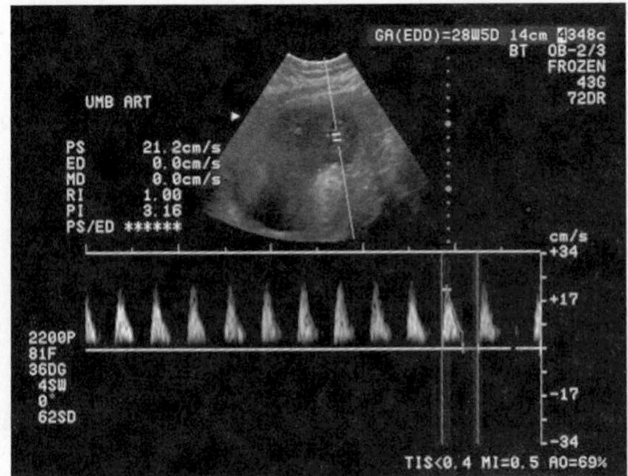

With permission, Institute for Advanced Medical Education, www.iame.com

Figure I-12-5. Absent Umbilical Artery Diastolic Flow

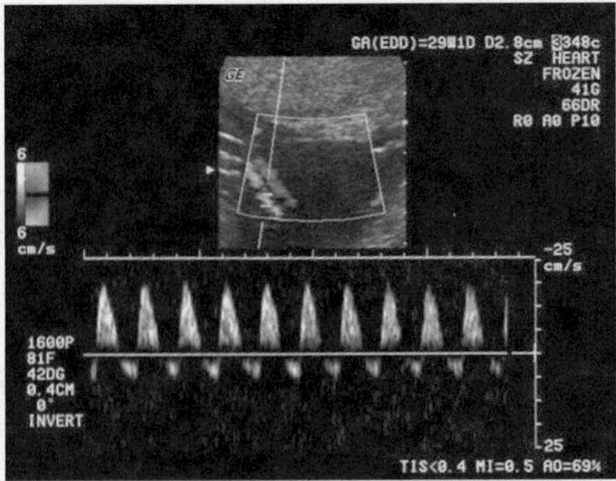

With permission, Institute for Advanced Medical Education, www.iame.com

Figure I-12-6. Reversed Umbilical Artery Diastolic Flow

Fetal Orientation in Utero 13

Learning Objectives

- ❑ List the possible fetal orientations in utero and their relation to potential complications of delivery

ANATOMY OF THE BONY PELVIS

The **pelvis** is constructed of **4 bones:** ileum superior-laterally, ischium inferior-laterally, pubis anteriorly, and the sacrum and coccyx posteriorly. It is held together by the following **4 joints: bilateral sacroiliac joints**, the **symphysis pubis**, and the **sacrococcygeal joint**. The sacrum has 5 vertebrae joined together. The anterior superior edge of the first sacral vertebra is called the **sacral promontory**.

Landmarks. The pelvis is divided by the **linea terminalis** into the false pelvis above and the true pelvis below. The **false pelvis** is bordered by lumbar vertebrae posteriorly, by the iliac fossa laterally, and by the abdominal wall anteriorly. The **true pelvis** is a bony canal formed by posterior sacrum and coccyx, lateral ischial, and anterior pubis.

Types of Pelvic Shapes

Gynecoid shape is the classic female pelvis and is found in 50% of women. The inlet is a round oval with largest diameter transverse. It has straight side walls, well-curved sacrum, and spacious subpubic arch with a 90° angle. **Assessment:** This pelvis is **spacious** for the fetal head to pass through.

Android shape is the typical male pelvis and is found in 30% of women. The inlet is triangular with convergent side walls, shallow sacral curve, and narrow subpubic arch. **Assessment:** This pelvis is **restricted** at all levels. Arrest of descent in labor is common.

Anthropoid shape resembles that of anthropoid apes and is found in 20% of women. The inlet is larger anterior-posteriorly with side walls that converge. Subpubic arch is narrow. **Assessment:** The fetal head **engages anterior-posteriorly**, often in occiput posterior position, making **delivery difficult**.

Platypelloid shape is like a flattened gynecoid pelvis. The inlet is an elongated transverse oval. It has straight side walls with deep sacral curve and wide subpubic arch. **Assessment:** The fetal head **engages transversely and delivers occiput transverse position.**

ORIENTATION IN UTERO

Lie

Orientation of the long axis of the fetus to the long axis of the uterus. The **most common lie is longitudinal**. 99% of fetuses at term.

- **Longitudinal:** fetus and mother are in same vertical axis
- **Transverse:** fetus at right angle to mother
- **Oblique:** fetus at 45° angle to mother

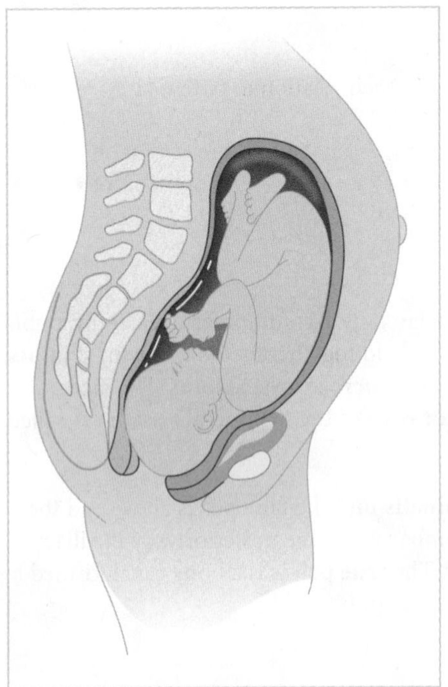

Figure I-13-1. Longitudinal Fetal Lie

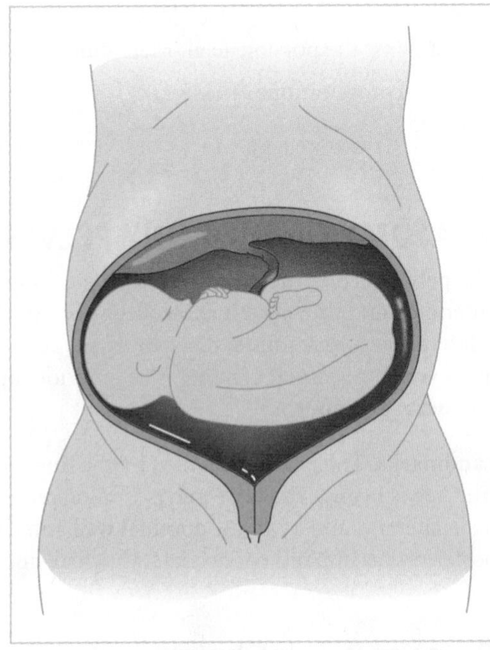

Figure I-13-2. Transverse Fetal Lie

Presentation

Portion of the fetus overlying the pelvic inlet. The **most common presentation is cephalic.** This is 96% of fetuses at term.

- **Cephalic:** head presents first
- **Breech:** feet or buttocks present first. The major risk of vaginal breech delivery is entrapment of the after-coming head.
  - **Frank** breech means thighs are flexed and legs extended. This is the only kind of breech that potentially could be safely delivered vaginally.
  - **Complete** breech means thighs and legs flexed.
  - **Footling** breech means thighs and legs extended.
- **Compound:** more than one anatomic part is presenting (e.g., head and upper extremity)
- **Shoulder:** presents first

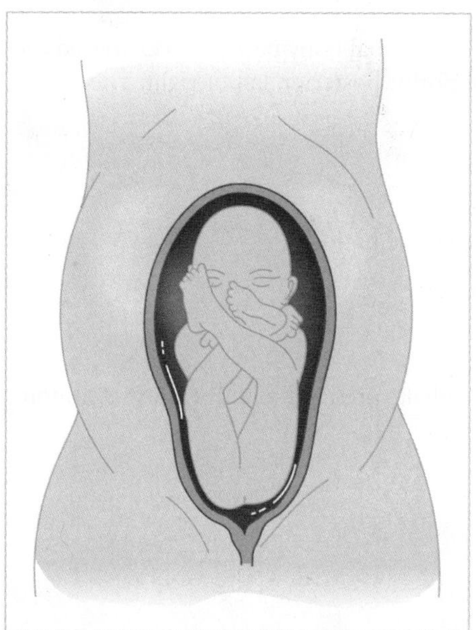

Figure I-13-3. Frank Breech

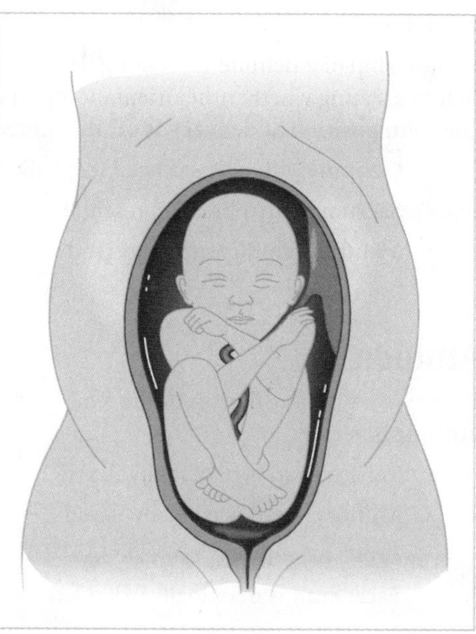

Figure I-13-4. Complete Breech

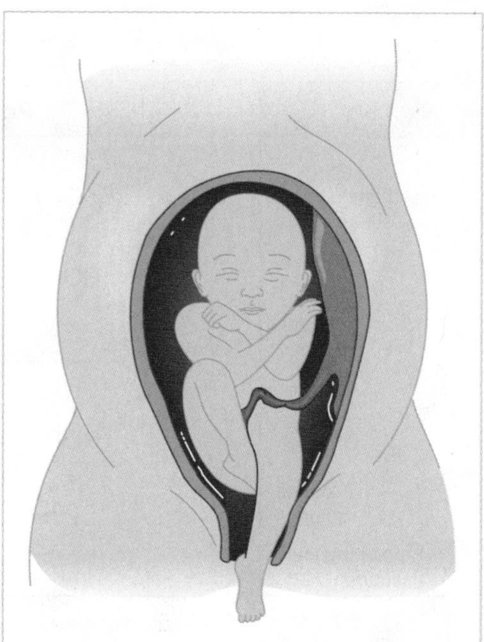

Figure I-13-5. Footling Breech

OB Triad

Breech Presentations

- Frank: thighs flexed, legs extended
- Complete: thighs and legs flexed
- Footling: thighs and knees extended

Position

Relationship of a definite presenting fetal part to the maternal bony pelvis. It is expressed in terms stating whether the orientation part is anterior or posterior, left or right. The **most common position at delivery is occiput anterior**.

- **Occiput:** with a flexed head (cephalic presentation)
- **Sacrum:** with a breech presentation
- **Mentum (chin):** with an extended head (face presentation)

Attitude

Degree of extension-flexion of the fetal head with cephalic presentation. The **most common attitude is vertex.**

- **Vertex:** head is maximally flexed
- **Military:** head is partially flexed
- **Brow:** head is partially extended
- **Face:** head is maximally extended

Station

Degree of descent of the presenting part through the birth canal; expressed in centimeters above or below the maternal ischial spine.

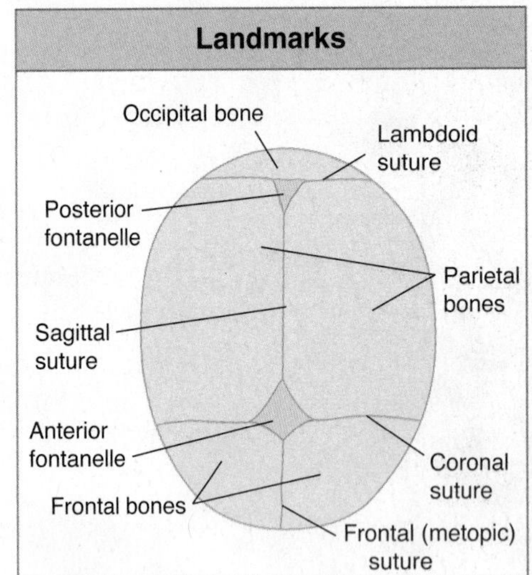

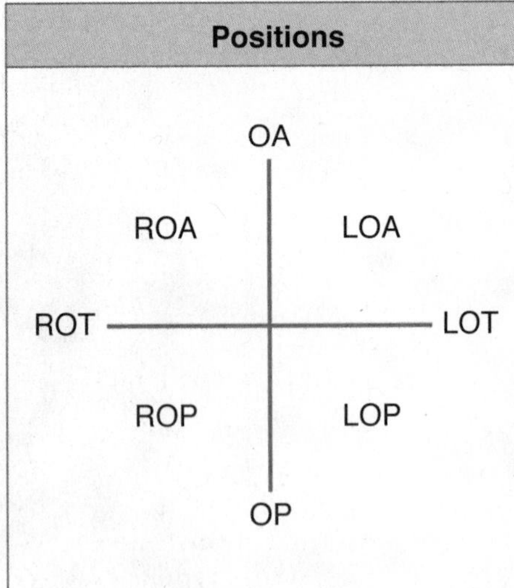

Figure I-13-6. Landmarks and Positions

Synclitism

The condition of parallelism between the plane of the pelvis and that of the fetal head.

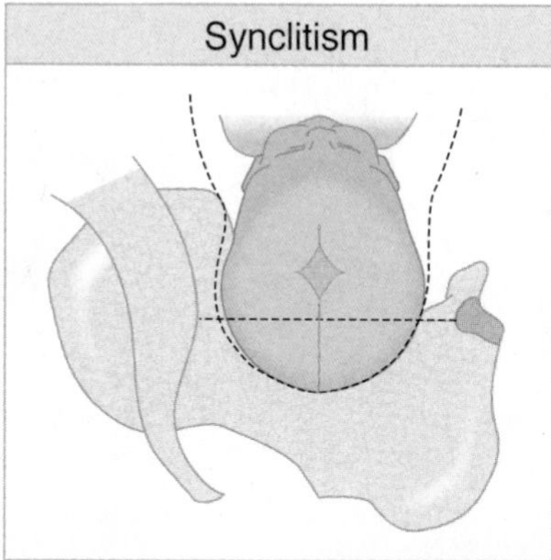

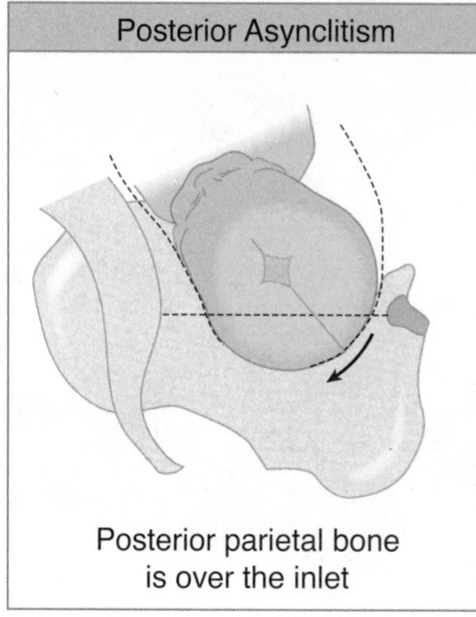

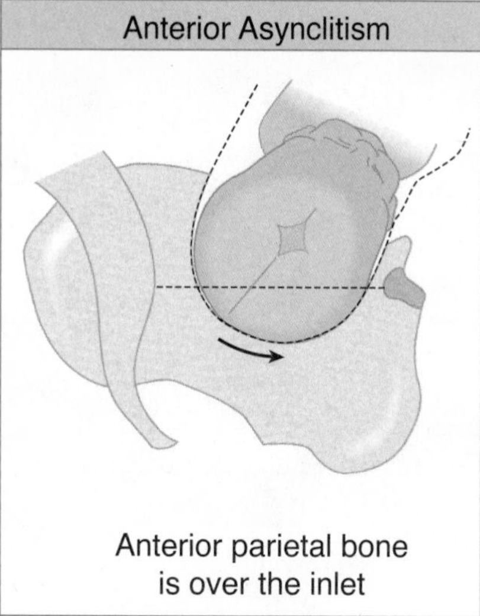

Figure I-13-7. Synclitism

Normal and Abnormal Labor 14

Learning Objectives

- ❑ List the normal stages of labor and abnormalities that can occur in the process
- ❑ Describe the risks and management of obstetric complications during labor

OVERVIEW OF LABOR

Labor is a process whereby over time regular uterine contractions bring about progressive effacement and dilation of the cervix, resulting in delivery of the fetus and expulsion of the placenta. Contractions will occur at least every 5 min lasting 30 s.

Physiology. Increasing frequency of contractions is associated with the formation of **gap junctions** between uterine myometrial cells. These events are correlated with increasing levels of **oxytocin** and **prostaglandins** along with multiplication of specific **receptors**.

Uterine Changes. The contractile **upper uterine segment**, containing mostly smooth muscle fibers, becomes thicker as labor progresses, exerting forces that expel the fetus down the birth canal. The **lower uterine segment**, containing mostly collagen fibers, passively thins out with contractions of the upper segment.

Cervical Effacement. Cervical softening and thinning occur as increasing levels of oxytocin and prostaglandins lead to breakage of **disulfide linkages** of collagen fibers, resulting in increasing water content. Effacement is often expressed in percentages with the uneffaced (0%) cervix assumed to be 2 cm long and 2 cm wide. Progressive shortening and thinning lead to full effacement (100%) in which the cervix has no length and is paper-thin.

Cervical Dilation. This occurs as the passive lower uterine segment is thinned and pulled up by the contractile upper segment. In early labor (latent phase), the rate of dilation is slow, but at 6 cm of dilation, the rate accelerates to a maximum rate in the active phase of labor. Complete dilation is expressed as 10 cm.

Cardinal Movements of Labor. The first 3 steps occur simultaneously.

- **Engagement:** movement of the presenting part below the plane of the pelvic inlet.
- **Descent:** movement of the presenting part down through the curve of the birth canal.
- **Flexion:** placement of the fetal chin on the thorax.

(simultaneous)

The next 4 steps occur in order.

- **Internal rotation:** rotation of the position of the fetal head in the mid pelvis from transverse to anterior-posterior.
- **Extension:** movement of the fetal chin away from the thorax.

- **External rotation:** rotation of the fetal head outside the mother as the head passes through the pelvic outlet.
- **Expulsion:** delivery of the fetal shoulders and body.

STAGES OF LABOR

Labor refers to the complex process through which uterine contractions bring about progressive dilation/opening and effacement/thinning of the cervix leading to descent of the fetus through the birth canal ending with expulsion of the neonate from the mother's body.

The classic studies in defining normal labor (Friedman, 1954) were conducted on 500 women at a single U.S. hospital in the 1950s. These studies established norms for various parts of labor that have been used by obstetricians for decades. Friedman's labor curves have dominated the obstetrical literature for 60 years. "Normal" labor was characterized as:

- Transition from latent to active labor occurring at 3-4 cm dilation
- Progress in active phase of labor was ≥1.2 cm/hr for nulliparas; ≥1.5 cm/hr for multiparas
- Length of second stage of labor was ≤3 hr for nulliparas; ≤1 hr for multiparas

Note

These Notes use current evidence-based management based on the Zhang labor data.

Over the past half-century, however, there have been marked increases in the average pregnant women's body-mass-index (BMI), along with modifications in obstetrical and anesthesia practices resulting in alterations in the typical progress of labor. These changes suggest the criteria for normal labor progress needs to be revised.

More recent studies (**Zhang et al, 2010**) are based on over 60,000 women in labor at 19 U.S. medical centers producing contemporary labor curves and norms that differ significantly from the older Friedman data.

Stage 1 begins with onset of regular uterine contractions and ends with complete cervical dilation at 10 cm. The precise identification when regular contractions began is often difficult. The first stage of labor is divided into a **latent** and an **active** phase.

Latent phase begins with onset of regular contractions and ends with the acceleration of cervical dilation. Its **purpose** is to soften and efface the cervix preparing it for rapid dilation. Minimal descent of the fetus through the birth canal occurs in this phase. The main abnormality is prolonged latent phase. **Latent phase rate of dilation is slower than previous studies showed and is similar in both multiparas and nulliparas.**

- Both nulliparas and multiparas may take more than 6 hours to dilate from 4 to 5 cm; and more than 3 hours to dilate from 5 to 6 cm.
- The upper limit of latent phase **duration** may be up to 20 h in a primipara and up to 14 h in a multipara.

Active phase begins with cervical dilation acceleration, usually by 6 cm of dilation, ending with complete cervical dilation. Its **purpose** is rapid cervical dilation. The **cardinal movements of labor occur** in the active phase with beginning descent of the fetus in the latter part. The main abnormality is Arrest of Active Phase. **The active phase dilation rate is more rapid in multiparas than nulliparas.**

- In a nullipara the average **rate of dilation** is 2 cm/h (abnormal would be <0.7 cm/hr)
- In a multiipara the average **rate of dilation** is 3 cm/h (abnormal would be <1.0 cm/hr)

Stage 2 begins with complete cervical dilation and ends with delivery of the fetus. Its **purpose** is descent of the fetus through the birth canal. Whereas in Stage 1 uterine contractions are the only force that acts on cervical dilation, in Stage 2 maternal pushing efforts are vitally important to augment the uterine contractions to bring about descent of the fetal presenting part. The **duration of stage 2** may be up to 3 h in a primipara and 2 h in a multipara. The main abnormality is prolonged second stage or arrest of descent.

Stage 3 begins with delivery of the fetus and ends with expulsion of the placenta. The mechanism of placental separation from the uterine wall is dependent on myometrial contractions shearing off the anchoring villi. This is usually augmented with IV oxytocin infusion. **Signs of the third stage** include gush of blood vaginally, change of the uterus from long to globular, "lengthening" of the umbilical cord. **Duration** may be up to 30 min in all women. The main abnormality is prolonged third stage.

Stage 4 is not an official stage of labor, but is a critical 2-h period of close observation of the parturient immediately after delivery. Vital signs and vaginal bleeding are monitored to recognize and promptly treat preeclampsia and postpartum hemorrhage.

Table 14-1. Stages of Labor

Labor Stage	Definition	Function	Duration
Stage 1—Latent phase Effacement	Begins: onset of regular uterine contractions Ends: acceleration of cervical dilation	**Prepares cervix for dilation**	<20 hours in primipara <14 hours in multipara
Stage 1—Active phase Dilation	Begins: acceleration of cervical dilation Ends: 10 cm (complete)	**Rapid cervical dilation**	≥0.7 cm/hours primipara ≥1.0 cm/hours multipara
Stage 2 Descent	Begins: 10 cm (complete) Ends: delivery of baby	**Descent of the fetus**	<3 hours in primipara <2 hours in multipara Add 1 hour if epidural
Stage 3 Expulsion	Begins: delivery of baby Ends: delivery of placenta	**Delivery of placenta**	<30 minutes

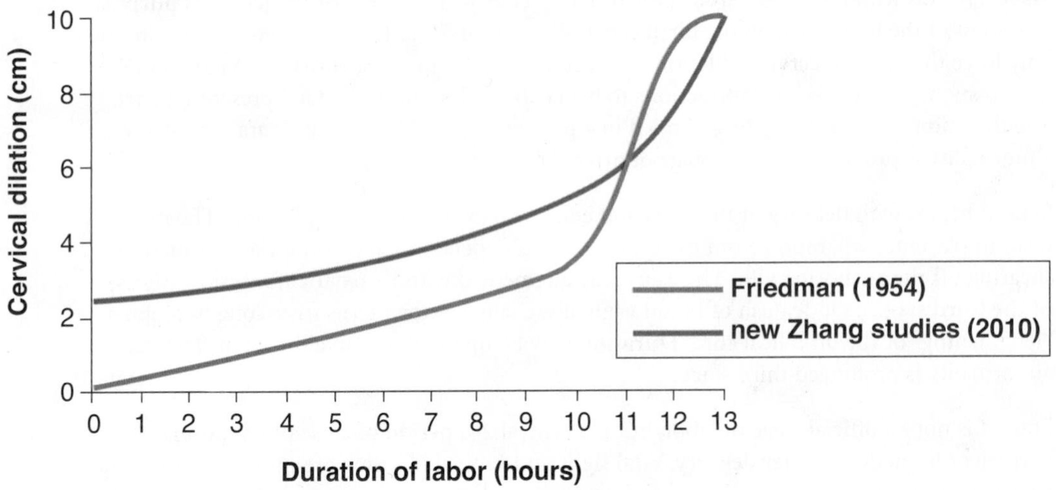

Figure I-14-1. Old versus New Labor Curves

CONDUCT OF NORMAL SPONTANEOUS LABOR

A 20-year-old primigravida comes to the maternity unit at 39 weeks' gestation complaining of regular uterine contractions every 3 min for the past 6 h. The contractions are becoming more frequent. She denies any vaginal fluid leakage. Vital signs are blood pressure is 125/75 mm Hg, pulse 80 beats/min, respirations 17 breaths/min. On pelvic examination the fetus is cephalic presentation at –1 station. Her cervix is 5 cm dilated, 90% effaced, and soft and anterior in position. On the electronic fetal monitor (EFM) the fetal heart rate baseline is 135 beats/min with moderate variability, frequent accelerations, and no decelerations. How will you manage this patient?

Preadmission

The parturient is not admitted to the maternity unit until cervical dilation is at least 3 cm, unless premature membrane rupture has occurred. Fetal presentation is confirmed to be cephalic.

Admission

On admission intravenous access is established, and oral clear liquid may be ingested. The patient is allowed whatever position is comfortable; however, the lateral recumbent position is encouraged as it optimizes uteroplacental blood flow.

First Stage

The fetal heart rate is assessed, usually with continuous electronic monitoring. Cervical dilation and fetal head descent are followed through appropriately spaced vaginal examinations. Amniotomy is performed in the active phase when the fetal head is well applied to the cervix. Obstetric analgesia is administered at patient request.

Second and Third Stages

Maternal pushing efforts augment uterine contractions in the second stage of labor. An episiotomy is not routine, but is performed as indicated. After delivery of the fetus, the placenta is allowed to spontaneously separate, after which IV oxytocin is administered to prevent uterine atony and bleeding.

Recovery Period

For the first 2 hours postpartum, the parturient is observed closely for excessive bleeding and development of preeclampsia.

ABNORMAL LABOR

Prolonged Latent Phase

> A 29-year-old multigravida at 40 weeks' gestation is being observed in the maternity unit. She states she has been having regular uterine contractions for 24 h but cervical dilation remains at 1–2 cm. Her vital signs are stable. EFM tracing is reassuring regarding fetal status.

Diagnosis. Prolonged latent phase requires that, in the face of regular uterine contractions, the cervical dilation is <6 cm for a duration of >20 h in a primipara or >14 h in a multipara.

Cause. Latent-phase abnormalities are most commonly caused by injudicious analgesia. Other causes are contractions, which are hypotonic (inadequate frequency, duration, or intensity) or hypertonic (high intensity but inadequate duration or frequency).

Management. This involves (a) therapeutic rest with narcotics or sedatives, (b) oxytocin administration or (c) amniotomy. Cesarean delivery is never appropriate management for prolonged latent phase.

OB Triad

Prolonged Latent Phase

- Pregnant with regular uterine contractions
- Cervix dilated 2 cm
- No cervical change in 14 h

Arrested Active Phase

> A 22-year-old primigravida at 39 weeks' gestation has progressed in labor to 8 cm of cervical dilation but has not changed for 3 h. Her vital signs are stable. EFM tracing is reassuring regarding fetal status.

Diagnosis. Arrested active phase is diagnosed if membranes are ruptured and cervical dilation has not changed for (a) ≥4 h with adequate uterine contractions or (b) ≥6 h of IV oxytocin administration with inadequate uterine contractions.

OB Triad

Active Phase Arrest

- Pregnant with regular uterine contractions
- Cervix dilated 8 cm
- No cervical change in 4 h

Causes. Active-phase abnormalities may be caused by either abnormalities of the **passenger** (excessive fetal size or abnormal fetal orientation in the uterus), abnormalities of the **pelvis** (bony pelvis size), or abnormalities of **powers** (dysfunctional or inadequate uterine contractions).

Management. This is directed at assessment of uterine contraction quality. Contractions should occur every 2–3 min, last 45–60 s with 50 mm Hg intensity. If contractions are hypotonic, IV oxytocin is administered. If contractions are hypertonic, give morphine sedation. If contractions are adequate, proceed to emergency cesarean section.

OB Triad

Second-Stage Arrest

- Pregnant with regular uterine contractions
- 10 cm dilation at +1 station
- No descent change in 3 h

Prolonged Second Stage

A 20-year-old primigravida at 41 weeks' gestation has progressed in labor to 10 cm of cervical dilation and has been pushing for the past 3 hrs. The fetus is cephalic presentation, right occiput transverse position. The fetal head has not descended below +2 station. Her vital signs are stable. EFM tracing is reassuring regarding fetal status.

Diagnosis.

- **Nulliparous** women: After complete dilation, no progress in either **descent or rotation** of the fetus after $\geq$3 h without epidural anesthesia and $\geq$4 h with epidural anesthesia.
- **Multiparous** women: After complete dilation, no progress in either **descent or rotation** of the fetus after $\geq$2 h without epidural anesthesia and $\geq$3 h with epidural anesthesia.

Management. This involves assessment of uterine contractions and maternal pushing efforts. IV oxytocin can strengthen the contractions. Enhanced coaching to optimize maternal pushing should be utilized as needed. If they are both adequate, assess whether the fetal head is engaged. If the head is not engaged, proceed to emergency cesarean. If the head is engaged, consider a trial of either obstetric forceps or a vacuum extractor delivery.

Prolonged Third Stage

A 20-year-old primigravida at 39 weeks' gestation underwent a spontaneous vaginal delivery 40 min ago of a healthy 3,500-g daughter. However, the placenta has still not delivered. Her vital signs are stable.

Diagnosis. Failure to deliver the placenta within 30 minutes.

Cause. May be inadequate uterine contractions. If the placenta does not separate, in spite of IV oxytocin stimulation of myometrium contractions, think of abnormal placental implantation (e.g., placenta **accreta**, placenta **increta,** and placenta **percreta**).

Management. May require manual placental removal or rarely even hysterectomy.

OBSTETRIC COMPLICATIONS DURING LABOR

Prolapsed Umbilical Cord

A 34-year-old multigravida with a known uterine septum comes to the maternity unit at 34 weeks' gestation complaining of regular uterine contractions. She underwent a previous cesarean at 37 weeks' gestation for breech presentation. Pelvic examination determines that the fetus is a footling breech. Her cervix is 6 cm dilated with bulging membranes. During the examination, the patient's bag of waters suddenly ruptures, and a loop of umbilical cord protrudes through the cervix between the fetal extremities.

Umbilical cord prolapse is an obstetric emergency because if the cord gets compressed, fetal oxygenation will be jeopardized, with potential fetal death.

Prolapse can be **occult** (the cord has not come through the cervix but is being compressed between the fetal head and the uterine wall), partial (the cord is between the head and the dilated cervical os but has not protruded into the vagina), or **complete** (the cord has protruded into the vagina).

Risk Factors. Rupture of membranes with the presenting fetal part not applied firmly to the cervix, malpresentation.

Management. Do not hold the cord or try to push it back into the uterus. Place the patient in knee-chest position, elevate the presenting part, avoid palpating the cord, and perform immediate cesarean delivery.

OB Triad

Prolapsed Umbilical Cord

- Pregnant with regular uterine contractions
- Amniotomy at –2 station
- Severe variable decelerations

Shoulder Dystocia

A 20-year-old primigravida at 39 weeks' gestation was pushing in the second stage of labor for 90 min and has just delivered the fetal head. However, in spite of vigorous pushing efforts by the mother, and moderate traction on the fetal head, you are unable to deliver the anterior shoulder. Since delivery of the fetal head, 30 s has passed. The fetal heart rate is now 70 beats/min.

Diagnosis. This diagnosis is made when delivery of the fetal shoulders is delayed after delivery of the head. It is usually associated with fetal shoulders in the anterior-posterior plane, with the anterior shoulder impacted behind the pubic symphysis. It occurs in 1% of deliveries and may result in permanent neonatal neurologic damage in 2% of cases.

Risk Factors. Include **maternal diabetes**, obesity, and postdates pregnancy, which are associated with fetal macrosomia. Even though incidence increases with birth weight, half of shoulder dystocias occur in fetuses <4,000 grams.

Management. Includes suprapubic pressure, maternal thigh flexion (McRobert's maneuver), internal rotation of the fetal shoulders to the oblique plane (Wood's "corkscrew" maneuver), manual delivery of the posterior arm, and Zavanelli maneuver (cephalic replacement).

OB Triad

Shoulder Dystocia

- Second stage of labor
- Head has delivered
- No further delivery of body

Obstetric Lacerations

Perineal lacerations are classified by the extent of tissue disruption between the vaginal introitus and the anus.

- **First degree:** involve only the vaginal mucosa. Suture repair is often not needed.
- **Second degree:** involve the vagina and the muscles of the perineal body but do not involve the anal sphincter. Suturing is necessary.
- **Third degree:** involve the vagina, the perineal body, and the anal sphincter but not the rectal mucosa. Suturing is necessary to avoid anal incontinence.
- **Fourth degree:** involve all the way from the vagina through to the rectal mucosa. Complications of faulty repair or healing include rectovaginal fistula.

Episiotomy

This is a surgical incision made in the perineum to enlarge the vaginal opening and assist in childbirth. It is one of the most common female surgical procedures. American trained physicians tend to prefer a midline episiotomy whereas British trained physicians tend to perform mediolateral episiotomies. It is not practiced routinely in the United States today because the arguments made in its favor **have not been shown** to have scientific support.

- **False arguments:** less perineal pain; more rapid return of sexual activity; less urinary incontinence; less pelvic prolapse.
- **Disadvantages:** more perineal pain than with lacerations; longer return to sexual activity; more extensions into the anal sphincter and rectum.
- **Possible indications:** shoulder dystocia, non-reassuring fetal monitor tracing, forceps or vacuum extractor vaginal delivery, vaginal breech delivery, narrow birth canal.

Obstetric Anesthesia 15

Learning Objectives

- ❑ Differentiate the physiology of anesthesia as applied to a pregnant versus a non-pregnant woman
- ❑ Describe possible anesthetic complications and management strategies

PHYSIOLOGY

Pain relief from uterine contractions and cervical dilation in **stage 1 of labor** involves thoracic nerve roots, T10 to T12. Pain relief from perineal distention in **stage 2 of labor** involves sacral nerve roots, S2 to S4.

- Pregnancy predisposes to hypoxia because of decreased functional residual capacity.
- Placental transfer of medications exposes the fetus to lipid-soluble anionic substances.
- Antacids should be given prophylactically because of delayed gastric emptying time in pregnancy.
- Uterus should be laterally displaced to avoid inferior vena cava compression in the supine position.

ANESTHETIC OPTIONS DURING LABOR

Intravenous Agents

This includes narcotics and sedatives, which are frequently given in the active phase of labor. **Advantages** include ease of administration and inexpensive cost. **Disadvantages** include neonatal depression if given close to delivery. The neonate may need administration of **naloxone** to reverse the effect.

Paracervical Block

This is a mode of conduction anesthesia that involves bilateral transvaginal local anesthetic injection to block **Frankenhauser's ganglion** lateral to the cervix. It is administered in the active phase of labor. **Disadvantages** include temporary high levels of local anesthetic in the uterus which may lead to **transitory fetal bradycardia**, which is managed conservatively.

OB Triad

Paracervical Block Effect

- Term pregnancy in active labor
- Local anesthetic injection into cervix
- Immediate fetal bradycardia

Pudendal Block

This is a mode of conduction anesthesia that involves bilateral transvaginal local anesthetic injection to block the pudendal nerve as it passes by the ischial spines. It is administered in stage 2 of labor to provide perineal anesthesia.

OB Triad

Epidural Block Side Effect

- Pregnancy in active labor
- Conduction anesthesia given
- ½ body numb; ½ body pain

Epidural Block

This is a mode of conduction anesthesia that involves injection of local anesthetic into the epidural space to block the lumbosacral nerve roots during both stages 1 and 2 of labor. **Advantages** include use for either vaginal delivery or cesarean section. **Disadvantages** include patchy block from nonuniform spread of the local anesthetic around the nerve roots. **Complications** include hypotension from peripheral vascular dilation owing to sympathetic blockade and spinal headache from inadvertent dural puncture, as well as CNS bleeding or infection (rare). Hypotension is treated with IV fluids and IV ephedrine. Spinal headache is treated with IV hydration, caffeine, or blood patch.

OB Triad

High Spinal (Intrathecal)

- Pregnancy in active labor
- Conduction anesthesia given
- Patient stops breathing

Spinal Block

This is a mode of conduction anesthesia that involves injection of local anesthetic into the subarachnoid space to block the lumbosacral nerve roots. It is used as a saddle block for stage 2 of labor and for cesarean delivery. **Advantages** are complete predictable anesthesia. **Complications** include hypotension from peripheral vascular dilation because of sympathetic blockade (common) and spinal headache (rare), as well as CNS bleeding or infection (rare).

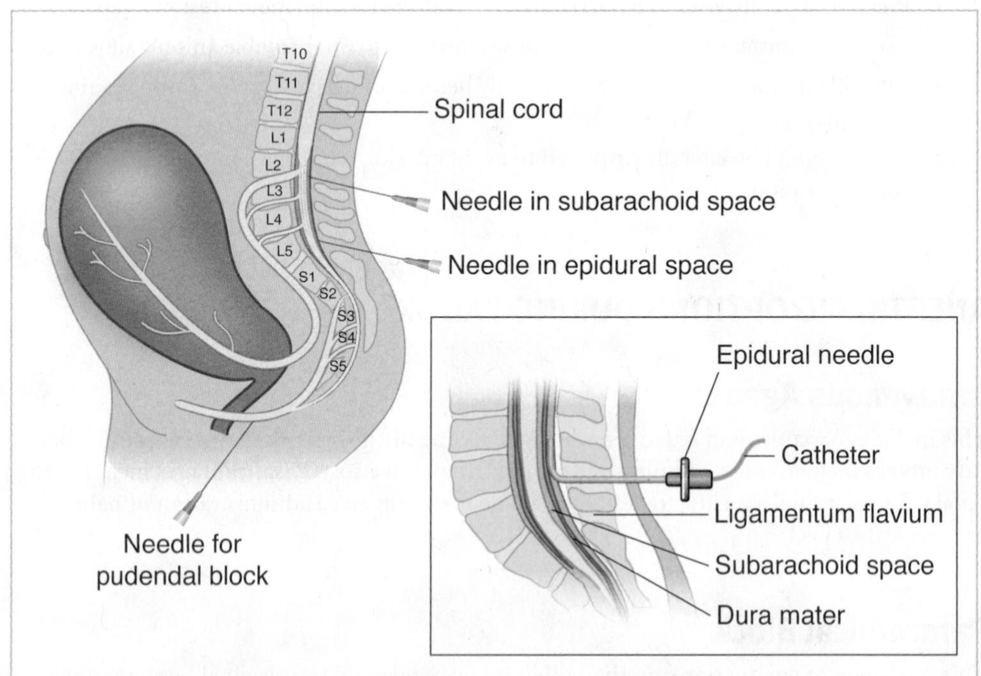

Figure I-15-1. Anesthetic Options During Labor

General Anesthesia

This is seldom used for vaginal delivery and rarely for cesarean section. **Indications** include need for rapid emergency delivery, maternal medical conditions in which conduction anesthesia is unsafe (e.g., blood dyscrasia, thrombocytopenia). **Complications** include aspiration pneumonia, atelectasis, and uterine atony (associated with inhalation agents, e.g., halothane, enflurane).

Intrapartum Fetal Monitoring 16

Learning Objectives

- ❑ Describe the appropriate use of intrapartum fetal monitoring including FHR monitoring, fetal pH assessment, and category III fetal monitoring tracings
- ❑ Describe intrauterine resuscitation

FETAL HEART RATE (FHR) MONITORING

Normal FHR findings are highly reassuring of fetal well-being. Abnormal FHR findings are poor predictors of fetal compromise. Wide usage of electronic FHR monitoring has not lowered the rate of cerebral palsy (CP) because the antecedents of CP appear not to be intrapartum events but rather antenatal events. The false-positive rate for electronic FHR monitoring for predicting CP is >99%.

Modalities of Labor Monitoring

Both of the following modalities are equivalent in predicting fetal outcome.

- **Intermittent auscultation** of FHR is performed with a fetoscope using auditory FHR counting averaged for 10–15 s.
- **Electronic monitoring** measures the milliseconds between consecutive cardiac cycles giving an instantaneous FHR continuously.

External Devices

These are placed on the uterine fundus and are the **most common device** used. **Advantages** are utilization before significant cervical dilation and membrane rupture. **Disadvantages** are poor quality tracing with maternal obesity and maternal discomfort from the device belts.

- **Fetal.** A continuous ultrasound transducer picks up fetal cardiac motion but also can register maternal great vessel pulsations.
- **Contractions.** A tocographic transducer device senses the change in uterine wall muscle tone. It can measure the beginning and ending of contractions but cannot assess contraction intensity.

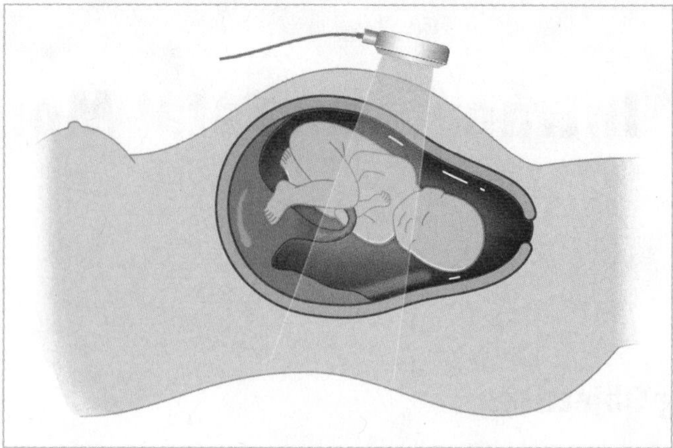

Figure I-16-1. Electronic Fetal Heart Rate Monitor

Internal Devices

These are placed through the dilated cervix. **Advantages** include optimum signal quality, which is unaffected by maternal obesity. **Disadvantages** include limitation to labor when cervical dilation and membrane rupture have occurred.

- **Fetal.** A direct scalp electrode precisely senses each QRS complex of the fetal cardiac cycle. Complications can include fetal scalp trauma and infection.
- **Contractions.** An intrauterine pressure catheter (IUPC), placed into the uterine cavity, precisely registers intrauterine hydrostatic changes with each contraction.

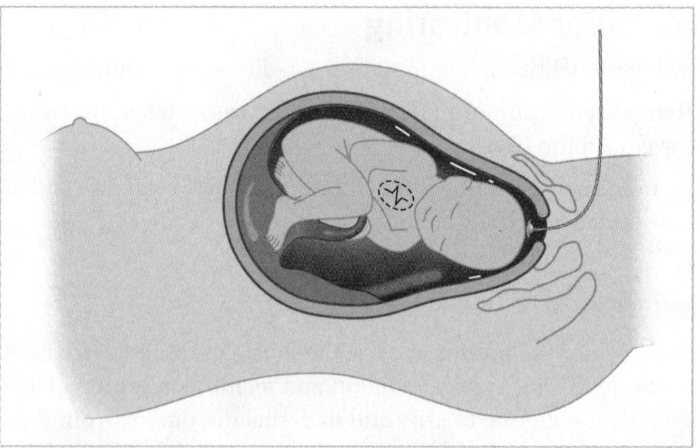

Figure I-16-2. Internal Fetal Heart Rate Monitoring

INTRAPARTUM FETAL HEART RATE MONITORING

Electronic Fetal Monitoring (EFM) Definitions

Baseline Fetal Heart Rate (FHR): The mean FHR rounded to increments of 5 beats/min during a 10-minute segment. Normal FHR baseline: 110–160 beats/minute

Tachycardia: FHR baseline is >160 beats/min

- Non-hypoxic explanations include:
  - **Maternal:** medications (β-adrenergic agonists [terbutaline], atropine, scopolamine), fever, thyrotoxicosis
  - **Fetal:** repetitive accelerations (from fetal movements), fetal tachyarrythmias, prematurity

Bradycardia: FHR baseline is <110 beats/min

- Non-hypoxic explanations include:
  - **Maternal medications:** β-adrenergic blockers, local anesthetics
  - **Fetal arrhythmia:** congenital heart block (associated with maternal lupus)

Baseline variability: Fluctuations in the baseline FHR that are irregular in amplitude and frequency. It is a reflection of the autonomic interplay between the sympathetic and parasympathetic nervous system.

- **Absent** amplitude range undetectable
- **Minimal** amplitude range detectable but ≤5 beats/min
- **Moderate** (normal): amplitude range 6-25 beats/min
- **Marked:** amplitude range >25 beats/min

Acceleration: A visually apparent **abrupt** increase (onset to peak in <30 seconds) in the FHR. These are mediated by the sympathetic nervous system in response to fetal movements or **scalp stimulation**.

- **At ≥32 weeks gestation,** an acceleration has a peak of >15 beats/min above baseline, with a duration of >15 seconds but < 2 min from onset to return.
- **At <32 weeks gestation**, an acceleration has a peak of ≥10 beats/min above baseline, with a duration of ≥10 sec but <2 min from onset to return.

Early deceleration: A visually apparent usually symmetrical **gradual** decrease and return of the FHR associated with a uterine contraction. These are mediated by parasympathetic stimulation and occur in response to **head compression**.

- A gradual FHR decrease is defined as from the onset to the FHR nadir of ≥30 seconds.
- The decrease in FHR is calculated from the onset to the nadir of the deceleration.
- The nadir of the deceleration occurs at the same time as the peak of the contraction.

Late deceleration: A visually apparent usually symmetrical **gradual** decrease and return of the FHR associated with a uterine contraction. These are mediated by either vagal stimulation or myocardial depression and occur in response to **placental insufficiency**.

- A gradual FHR decrease is defined as from the onset to the FHR nadir of ≥30 seconds.
- The decrease in FHR is calculated from the onset to the nadir of the deceleration.
- The deceleration is delayed in timing, with the nadir of the deceleration occurring after the peak of the contraction.

OB Triad

Early Decelerations

- Gradual drop of FHR
- Gradual return of FHR
- Mirror image of contraction

OB Triad

Late Decelerations

- Gradual drop of FHR
- Gradual return of FHR
- Delayed in relation to contractions

OB Triad

Variable Decelerations

- Abrupt drop of FHR
- Sudden return of FHR
- Variable in relation to contractions

Variable deceleration: A visually apparent **abrupt** decrease in FHR. These are mediated by **umbilical cord compression.**

- An abrupt FHR decrease is defined as from the onset of the deceleration to the beginning of the FHR nadir of <30 seconds.
- The decrease in FHR is calculated from the onset to the nadir of the deceleration.
- The decrease in FHR is ≥15 beats per minute, lasting ≥15 seconds, and<2 minutes in duration.

Sinusoidal pattern:

- A visually apparent, smooth, sine wave-like undulating pattern in FHR baseline with a cycle frequency of 3–5/min which persists for ≥20 min.

FHR Categories

A 3-tiered system for the categorization of FHR patterns is recommended. It is important to recognize that FHR tracing patterns provide information only on the current acid–base status of the fetus.

- Categorization of the FHR tracing evaluates the fetus at that point in time; tracing patterns can and will change.
- FHR tracing may move back and forth between the categories depending on the clinical situation and management strategies used.

Category I: FHR tracings are normal

Criteria include all of the following:

- **Baseline rate:** 110-160 beats/min
- **Baseline FHR variability:** moderate
- **Late or variable decelerations:** absent
- **Early decelerations:** present or absent
- **Accelerations:** present or absent

Interpretation: strongly predictive of normal fetal acid-base status at time of observation
Action: monitoring in a routine manner, with no specific action required

Category II: FHR tracings are indeterminate

These include all FHR tracings not categorized as category I or III, and may represent an appreciable fraction of those encountered in clinical care.

Interpretation: not predictive of abnormal fetal acid-base status
Action: evaluation and continued surveillance and reevaluation, taking into account the entire associated clinical circumstances

Category III: FHR tracings are abnormal

Criteria include absent baseline FHR variability and any of the following:

- Recurrent late decelerations
- Recurrent variable decelerations

- Bradycardia
- Sinusoidal pattern

Interpretation: associated with abnormal fetal acid-base status at time of observation; requires prompt evaluation

Action: expeditious intrauterine resuscitation to resolve the abnormal FHR pattern; if tracing does not resolve with these measures, prompt delivery should take place.

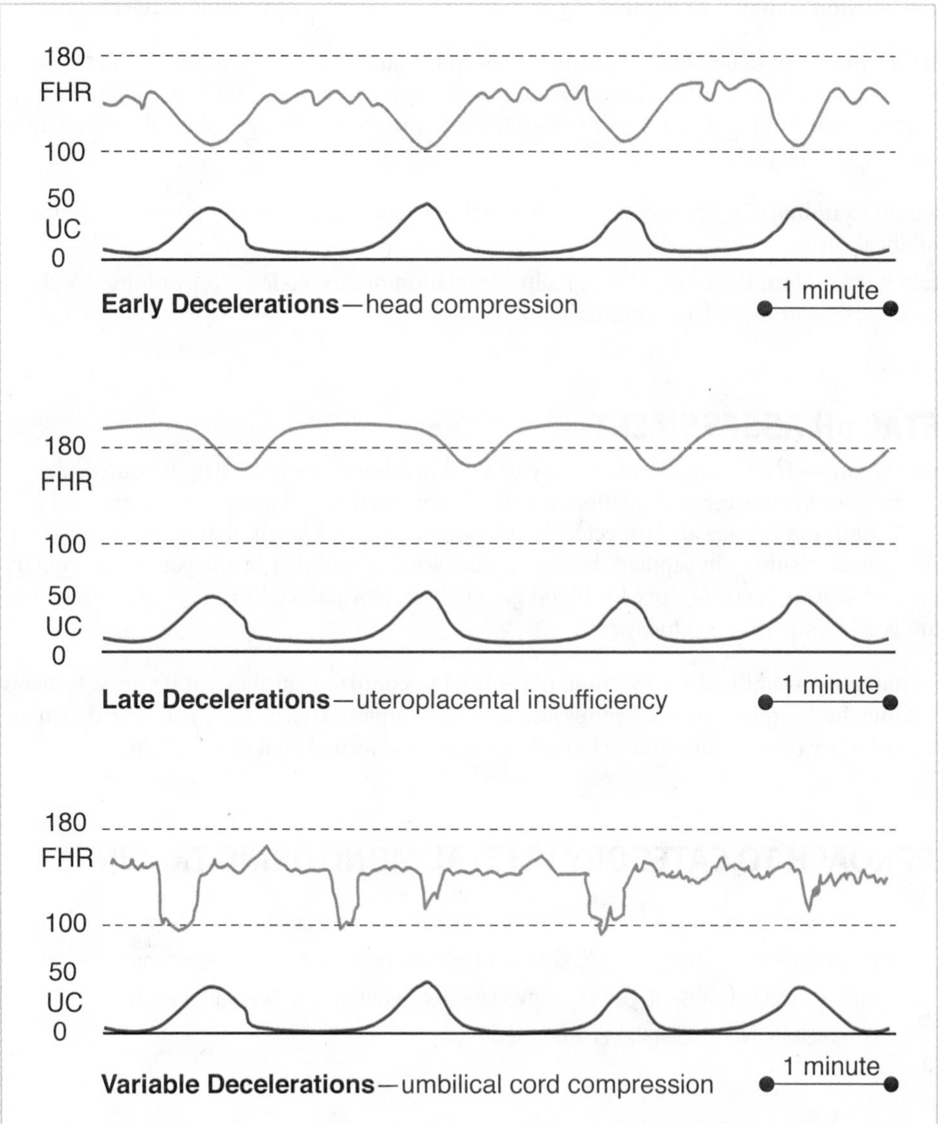

Figure I-16-3. Electronic Fetal Monitor Decelerations

INTRAUTERINE RESUSCITATION

Decrease uterine contractions: Turn off any IV oxytocin infusion or administer terbutaline 0.25 mg subcutaneously to enhance intervillous placental blood flow.

Augment IV fluid volume: Infuse the parturient with a 500 mL bolus of intravenous normal saline rapidly to enhance uteroplacental infusion.

Administer high-flow oxygen: Give the parturient 8–10 L of oxygen by facemask to increase delivery of maternal oxygen to the placenta.

Amniofusion is useful for eliminating or reducing the severity of variable decelerations.

Change position: Removing the parturient from the supine position decreases inferior vena cava compression and enhances cardiac return, thus cardiac output to the placenta. Turning the parturient from one lateral position to the other may relieve any umbilical cord compression that may be present.

Vaginal examination: Perform a digital vaginal examination to rule out possible prolapsed umbilical cord.

Scalp stimulation: Perform a digital scalp stimulation observing for accelerations, which would be reassuring of fetal condition.

FETAL pH ASSESSMENT

Intrapartum—fetal scalp blood pH may be used in labor if the EFM strip is equivocal. Prerequisites include cervical dilation, ruptured membranes, and adequate descent of the fetal head. Contraindications are suspected fetal blood dyscrasia. A small, shallow fetal scalp incision is made resulting in capillary bleeding. The blood is collected in a heparinized capillary tube and sent to the laboratory for blood gas analysis. Normal fetal pH is ≥7.20. This procedure is seldom performed today.

Postpartum—umbilical artery blood pH is used to confirm fetal status at delivery. It involves obtaining both umbilical cord venous and arterial samples. Arterial Pco_2 and base deficit values are higher than venous, but pH and Po_2 are lower. Normal fetal pH is ≥7.20.

APPROACH TO CATEGORY III FETAL MONITORING TRACINGS

A 20-year-old primigravida at 39 weeks' gestation is in active labor at 7 cm of cervical dilation. The EFM strip shows a baseline heart rate of 175 beats/min, and variability is absent, but repetitive late decelerations are seen after each contraction. No accelerations are noted.

Recognize that most abnormal tracings are not caused by fetal hypoxia. Ask whether the tracing has biologic plausibility.

- **Examine the EFM strip carefully** looking for baseline heart rate, degree of variability, and presence of periodic changes (accelerations, decelerations).
- **Confirm abnormal findings** using criteria discussed above (category II or III).
- **Identify nonhypoxic causes** present that could explain the abnormal findings.

- **Initiate the intrauterine resuscitation measures** described previously (Intrauterine Resuscitation) to enhance placental perfusion and fetal oxygenation.
- **Observe for normalization** of the EFM tracing.
- Prepare for delivery promptly if resuscitation measures do not normalize EFM tracing.

Specific Interventions If Immediate Delivery Is Indicated

- In stage 1 of labor, the only option is emergency cesarean section.
- In stage 2 of labor, an operative vaginal delivery (e.g., vacuum extractor assisted or obstetrical forceps) may be appropriate, or an emergency cesarean section must be performed.

Operative Obstetrics 17

Learning Objectives

- ❑ Describe the risks and indications for the use of obstetric forceps, vacuum extractor, emergency cesarean section, and elective cesarean section

Operative obstetrics refers to any method used to deliver the fetus other than uterine contractions and maternal pushing efforts. It may include vaginal or cesarean routes.

OBSTETRIC FORCEPS

Definition. These are metal instruments used to provide traction, rotation, or both to the fetal head.

- **Simpson:** used for traction only.
- **Kielland:** used for head rotation and traction.
- **Piper:** used for the after-coming head of a vaginal breech baby.
- **Barton:** used to deliver the head in occiput transverse position with a platypelloid pelvis.

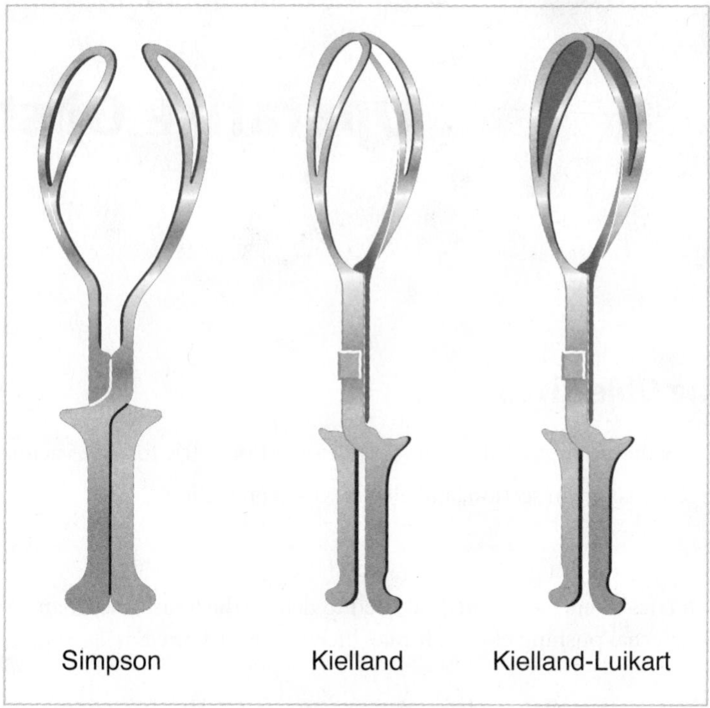

Figure I-17-1. Obstetric Forceps

Classification

- **Outlet:** fetal head is on the pelvic floor. Most forceps use is in this category.
- **Low:** fetal head is below +2 station, but has not reached the pelvic floor.
- **Mid:** fetal head is below 0 station, but has not reached +2 station. This is seldom used today.
- **High:** fetal head is unengaged, above 0 station. This is never appropriate in modern obstetrics because of the risk to both mother and fetus.

Indications

- **Prolonged second stage.** This may be because of dysfunctional labor or suboptimal fetal head orientation. This is the most common indication for forceps.
- **Category III EFM strip.** The fetal heart rate monitor pattern suggests the fetus is not tolerating labor.
- **Avoid maternal pushing.** These include a variety of conditions in which pushing efforts may be hazardous to the parturient, e.g., cardiac, pulmonary, or neurologic disorders.
- **Breech presentation.** Shorten the time to deliver the head of a vaginal breech fetus.

Prerequisites

- Clinically adequate pelvic dimensions
- Experienced operator
- Full cervical dilation
- Engaged fetal head
- Orientation of fetal head is certain.

Complications

- **Maternal:** lacerations to the vagina, cervix, perineum, and uterus.
- **Fetal-neonatal:** soft-tissue compression or cranial injury caused by incorrectly placed forceps blades.

VACUUM EXTRACTOR

Definition. These are cuplike instruments that are held against the fetal head with suction. Traction is thus applied to the fetal scalp, which along with maternal pushing efforts, results in descent of the head leading to vaginal delivery. The cups may be metal or plastic, rigid or soft.

Advantages Over Forceps

- **Fetal head orientation.** Precise knowledge of fetal head position and attitude is not essential.
- **Space required.** The vacuum extractor does not occupy space adjacent to the fetal head.
- **Perineal trauma.** Third- and fourth-degree lacerations are fewer.
- **Head rotation.** Fetal head rotation occurs spontaneously at the station best suited to fetal head configuration and maternal pelvis.

Disadvantages Over Forceps

- **Cup pop-offs.** Excessive traction can lead to sudden decompression as the cup suction is released.
- **Scalp trauma.** Scalp skin injury and lacerations are common.
- **Subgaleal hemorrhage and intracranial bleeding** are rare.
- **Neonatal jaundice** arises from scalp bleeding.

Indications Are Similar to Those of Forceps

- **Prolonged second stage.** This may be because of dysfunctional labor or suboptimal fetal head orientation.
- **Nonreassuring EFM strip.** The FHR monitor pattern suggests the fetus is not tolerating labor.
- **Avoid maternal pushing.** These include a variety of conditions in which pushing efforts may be hazardous to the parturient, e.g., cardiac, pulmonary, or neurologic disorders.

Prerequisites

- Clinically adequate pelvic dimension
- Experienced operator
- Full cervical dilation
- Engaged fetal head
- Gestational age is ≥34 weeks

Complications

- **Maternal:** vaginal lacerations from entrapment of vaginal mucosa between the suction cup and fetal head.
- **Neonatal:** neonatal **cephalohematoma** and scalp lacerations are common; life-threatening complications of **subgaleal hematoma** or **intracranial hemorrhage**, although uncommon, are associated with vacuum duration >10 min.

CESAREAN SECTION

Definition. This describes a procedure in which the fetus is delivered through incisions in the maternal anterior abdominal and uterine walls. The overall U.S. cesarean section rate in 2011 was approximately 33%, which includes both primary and repeat procedures.

Risks. Maternal mortality and morbidity is higher than with vaginal delivery, especially with emergency cesareans performed in labor. Maternal mortality is largely anesthetic related with overall mortality ratio of 25 per 100,000.

- **Hemorrhage:** Blood loss is twice that of a vaginal delivery with mean of 1,000 mL.
- **Infection:** Sites of infection include endometrium, abdominal wall wound, pelvis, urinary tract, or lungs. Prophylactic antibiotics can decrease infectious morbidity.
- **Visceral injury:** Surrounding structures can be injured (e.g., bowel, bladder, and ureters).
- **Thrombosis:** Deep venous thrombosis is increased in the pelvic and lower extremity veins.

Uterine Incisions

- **Low segment transverse.** This incision is made in the noncontractile portion of the uterus and is the one most commonly used. The bladder must be dissected off the lower uterine segment. It has a low chance of uterine rupture in subsequent labor (0.5%).
  - **Advantages** are trial of labor in a subsequent pregnancy is safe; the risk of bleeding and adhesions is less.
  - **Disadvantages** are the fetus(es) must be in longitudinal lie; the lower segment must be developed.

OB Triad

Low Transverse Uterine Incision

- Low risk of rupture (0.5% in labor)
- Less blood loss and adhesions
- Safe for subsequent labor trial

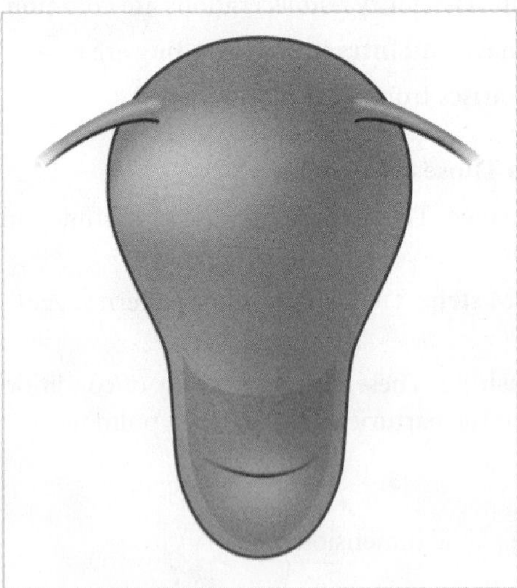

Figure I-17-2. Low Segment Transverse Incision

- **Classical.** This incision is made in the contractile fundus of the uterus and is less commonly performed. Technically it is easy to perform, and no bladder dissection is needed. Risk of uterine rupture both before labor as well as in subsequent labor is significant (5%). Repeat cesarean should be scheduled before labor onset.
  - **Advantages** are any fetus(es) regardless of intrauterine orientation can be delivered; lower segment varicosities or myomas can be bypassed.
  - **Disadvantages** are trial of labor in a subsequent pregnancy is unsafe; the risk of bleeding and adhesions is higher.

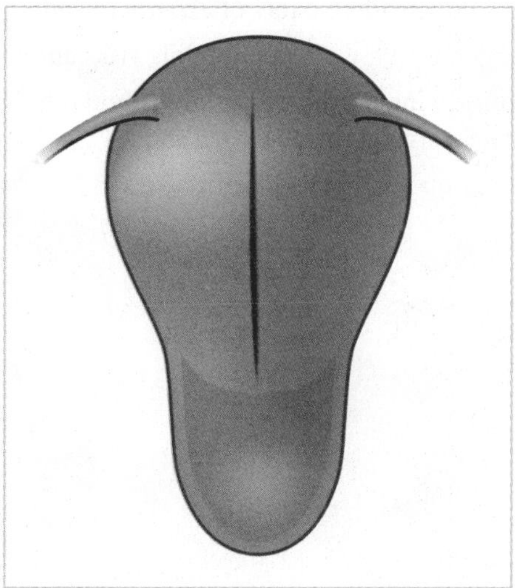

Figure I-17-3. Classical Uterine Incision

OB Triad

Classical Uterine Incision

- High risk of rupture (5% in labor)
- More blood loss and adhesions
- Risky for subsequent labor trial

Indications for Primary Cesarean Section

- **Cephalopelvic disproportion (CPD).** This is the **most common** indication for cesarean delivery. This term literally means the pelvis is too small for the fetal head. In actual practice, it most commonly indicates failure of the adequate progress in labor, which may be related to dysfunctional labor or suboptimal fetal head orientation.
- **Fetal malpresentation.** This refers most commonly to breech presentation, but also means any fetal orientation other than cephalic.
- **Category III EFM strip.** The FHR monitor pattern suggests the fetus may not be tolerating labor, but commonly this is a false-positive finding.

Vaginal Birth After Cesarean (VBAC)

- Successful vaginal delivery rate is up to 80% in carefully selected patients.
- Criteria for trial of labor include patient consent, nonrepetitive cesarean indication (e.g., breech, placenta previa), previous low segment transverse uterine incision, clinically adequate pelvis.

External Cephalic Version. This procedure consists of externally manipulating the gravid abdomen without anesthesia to turn the fetus from transverse lie or breech presentation. The optimum time for version is 37 weeks' gestation, and success rates are 60–70%. Potential hazards are umbilical cord compression or placental abruption requiring emergency cesarean section.

ELECTIVE CESAREAN

The U.S. National Institutes of Health (NIH) held a consensus conference in March 2006 to determine the scientific basis for maternal and fetal risks and benefits to cesarean delivery on maternal request (CDMR). After 2 days of presentations by experts in the field and input from the audience, the consensus was that "the available information comparing the risks and benefits of CDMR versus planned vaginal birth do not provide the basis for a recommendation in either direction."

Recommendations from the independent panel of experts include:

- Individual counseling for each woman regarding risks and benefits
- Women who are considering having >2 children should be aware that a cesarean section causes uterine scarring; these women should avoid a primary cesarean section.
- Women should not have a cesarean section prior to 39 weeks' gestation.

Postpartum Issues 18

Learning Objectives

- ❑ Describe the causes and management of postpartum hemorrhage and fever
- ❑ List the sequence of physiologic changes expected after delivery
- ❑ Provide and overview of the special considerations for immunizations and contraception postpartum

POSTPARTUM PHYSIOLOGIC ISSUES

Reproductive Tract Changes

Lochia. These are superficial layers of the endometrial decidua that are shed through the vagina during the first 3 postpartum weeks. For the first few days the color is red **(lochia rubra)**, changing during the next week to pinkish **(lochia serosa)**, ending with a whitish color **(lochia alba)** by the end of the second week.

Cramping. The myometrial contractions after delivery constrict the uterine venous sinuses, thus preventing hemorrhage. These lower midline cramps may be painful and are managed with mild analgesics.

Perineal Pain. Discomfort from an episiotomy or perineal lacerations can be minimized in the first 24 hours with ice packs to decrease the inflammatory response edema. A heat lamp or sitz bath is more helpful after the first day to help mobilize tissue fluids.

Urinary Tract Changes

Hypotonic Bladder. Intrapartum bladder trauma can result in increased postvoid residual volumes. If the residuals exceed 250 mL, the detrusor muscle can be stimulated to contract with bethanechol (Urecholine). Occasionally an indwelling Foley catheter may need to be placed for a few days.

Dysuria. Pain with urination may be seen from urethral irritation from frequent intrapartum catheterizations. **Conservative management** may be all that is necessary. A urinary analgesic may be required occasionally.

Gastrointestinal Tract Changes

Constipation. Decreased GI tract motility, because of perineal pain and fluid mobilization, can lead to constipation. Management is oral hydration and stool softeners.

Hemorrhoids. Prolonged second-stage pushing efforts can exaggerate preexisting hemorrhoids. **Management** is oral hydration and stool softeners.

Psychosocial Problems

Bonding. Impaired maternal–infant bonding is seen in the first few days postdelivery. Lack of interest or emotions for the newborn are noted. Risk is increased if contact with the baby is limited because of neonatal intensive care, as well as poor social support. **Management** is psychosocial evaluation and support.

Blues. Postpartum blues are very common within the first few weeks of delivery. Mood swings and tearfulness occur. Normal physical activity continues and care of self and baby is seen. **Management** is conservative with social support.

Depression. Postpartum depression is common but is frequently delayed up to a month after delivery. Feelings of despair and hopelessness occur. The patient often does not get out of bed with care of self and baby neglected. **Management** includes psychotherapy and antidepressants.

Psychosis. Postpartum psychosis is rare, developing within the first few weeks after delivery. Loss of reality and hallucinations occur. Behavior may be bizarre. **Management** requires hospitalization, antipsychotic medication, and psychotherapy.

OB Triad

Impaired Maternal–Infant Bonding

- Postpartum Day 1
- SVD: 1,900-g 31-week male in NICU
- Mom shows no interest in baby

OB Triad

Postpartum Blues

- Postpartum Day 2
- S/P SVD of term normal baby
- Mom cares for baby: tears

OB Triad

Postpartum Depression

- Postpartum Day 21
- S/P SVD of term normal baby
- Mom does not get out of bed, does not care for self or baby

OB Triad

Postpartum Psychosis

- Postpartum Day 21
- S/P SVD of term normal baby
- Mom exhibits bizarre behavior, hallucinations

POSTPARTUM CONTRACEPTION AND IMMUNIZATIONS

Contraception Planning

Breast feeding. Lactation is associated with temporary anovulation, so contraceptive use may be deferred for 3 months. A definitive method should be used after that time.

Diaphragm. Fitting for a vaginal diaphragm should be performed after involution of pregnancy changes, usually at the 6-week postpartum visit.

Intrauterine Device (IUD). Higher IUD retention rates, and decreased expulsions, are seen if IUD placement takes place at 6 weeks postpartum.

Combination Modalities. Combined estrogen-progestin formulations (e.g., pills, patch, vaginal ring) should not be used in breast-feeding women because of the estrogen effect of diminishing milk production. In nonlactating women, they should be started after 3 weeks postpartum to allow reversal of the hypercoagulable state of pregnancy and thus decrease the risk of deep venous thrombosis.

Progestin-only Contraception. Progestin steroids (e.g., mini-pill, Depo-Provera, Nexplanon) do not diminish milk production so can safely be used during lactation. They can be begun immediately after delivery.

Postpartum Immunizations

RhoGAM. If the mother is Rh(D) negative, and her baby is Rh(D) positive, she should be administered 300 μg of RhoGAM IM within 72 hours of delivery.

Rubella. If the mother is rubella IgG antibody negative, she should be administered active immunization with the live-attenuated rubella virus. She should avoid pregnancy for 1 month to avoid potential fetal infection.

POSTPARTUM HEMORRHAGE

Definition: vaginal delivery blood loss ≥500 mL **or** cesarean section blood loss ≥1,000 mL

Uterine Atony (80%)

This is the most common cause of excessive postpartum bleeding.

Risk Factors. Rapid or protracted labor (**most common**), chorioamnionitis, medications (e.g., $MgSO_4$, β-adrenergic agonists, halothane), and overdistended uterus.

Clinical Findings. A soft uterus (feels like dough) palpable above the umbilicus.

Management. Uterine massage and uterotonic agents (e.g., oxytocin, methylergonovine, or carboprost).

Lacerations (15%)

Risk Factors. Uncontrolled vaginal delivery (**most common**), difficult delivery, and operative vaginal delivery.

Clinical Findings. Identifiable lacerations (cervix, vagina, perineum) in the presence of a contracted uterus.

Management. Surgical repair.

Retained Placenta (5%)

Risk Factors. Accessory placental lobe (**most common**) and abnormal trophoblastic uterine invasion (e.g., cervix, vagina, perineum).

Clinical Findings. Missing placental cotyledons in the presence of a contracted uterus.

Management. Manual removal or uterine curettage under ultrasound guidance.

Disseminated Intravascular Coagulation (rare)

Risk Factors. Abruptio placenta (**most common**), severe preeclampsia, amniotic fluid embolism, and prolonged retention of a dead fetus.

Clinical Findings. Generalized oozing or bleeding from IV sites or lacerations in the presence of a contracted uterus.

Management. Removal of pregnancy tissues from the uterus, intensive care unit (ICU) support, and selective blood-product replacement.

Uterine Inversion (rare)

Risk Factors. Myometrial weakness (most common) and previous uterine inversion.

Clinical Findings. Beefy-appearing bleeding mass in the vagina and failure to palpate the uterus abdominally.

Management. Uterine replacement by elevating the vaginal fornices and lifting the uterus back into its normal anatomic position, followed by IV oxytocin.

Postpartum Hemorrhage

Clinical	Diagnosis	Management
Uterus not palpable	Inversion (rare)	Elevate vaginal fornices, IV oxytocin
Uterus like dough	Atony (80%)	Uterine massage, oxytocin, ergot, PG F2α
Tears vagina, cervix	Lacerations (15%)	Suture & repair
Placenta incomplete	Retain placenta (5%)	Manual removal or uterine curettage
Diffuse oozing	DIC (rare)	Remove POC, ICU care, blood products prn
Persistent bleeding	Unexplained (rare)	Ligate vessels or hysterectomy

Unexplained

If despite careful searching, no correctible cause of continuing hemorrhage is found, it may be necessary to perform a laparotomy and bilaterally surgically ligate the uterine or internal iliac arteries. Hysterectomy would be a last resort.

POSTPARTUM FEVER

Definition: Fever ≥100.4° F (38° C) on ≥2 occasions ≥6 hours apart, excluding first 24 hours post-partum

PP Day 0: Atelectasis

Risk Factors. General anesthesia with incisional pain (**most common**) and cigarette smoking.

Clinical Findings. Mild fever with mild rales on auscultation. Patient is unable to take deep breaths.

Management. Pulmonary exercises (e.g., deep breaths, incentive spirometry) and ambulation. Chest x-rays are unnecessary.

PP Day 1–2: Urinary Tract Infection

Risk Factors. Multiple intrapartum catheterizations and vaginal examinations due to prolonged labor.

Clinical Findings. High fever, costovertebral flank tenderness, positive urinalysis (e.g., WBC, bacteria) and urine culture.

Management. Single-agent intravenous antibiotics.

PP Day 2–3: Endometritis

Most common cause of postpartum fever.

Risk Factors. Emergency cesarean section after prolonged membrane rupture and prolonged labor.

Clinical Findings. Moderate-to-high fever with exquisite uterine tenderness. Peritoneal signs should be absent and peristalsis should be present.

Management. Multiple-agent intravenous antibiotics (e.g., gentamycin and clindamycin) to cover polymicrobial genital tract flora.

PP Day 4–5: Wound Infection

Risk Factors. Emergency cesarean section after prolonged membrane rupture and prolonged labor.

Clinical Findings. Persistent spiking fever despite antibiotics, along with wound erythema, fluctuance, or drainage.

Management. Intravenous antibiotics for cellulitis. Wound drainage with twice-daily, wet-to-dry wound packing used for an abscess, anticipating closure by secondary intention.

PP Day 5–6: Septic Thrombophlebitis

Risk Factors. Emergency cesarean section after prolonged membrane rupture and prolonged labor.

Clinical Findings. Persistent wide fever swings despite broad-spectrum antibiotics with normal pelvic and physical examination.

Management. Intravenous heparin for 7–10 days, keeping PTT values at 1.5 to 2.0 times baseline.

PP Day 7–21: Infectious Mastitis

Risk Factors. Lactational nipple trauma leading to nipple cracking and allowing Staphylococcus aureus bacteria to enter breast ducts and lobes.

Clinical Findings. Fever of variable degree with localized, unilateral breast tenderness, erythema, and edema.

Management. Oral cloxacillin. Breast feeding can be continued. Ultrasound imaging is needed to rule out an abscess if lactational mastitis does not respond to antibiotics.

Postpartum Fever

Physical Exam	Diagnosis	Management
Lung "crackles" PP Day 0	Atelectasis	Ambulation, pulmonary exercises
Flank pain, dysuria PP Day 1-2	Pyelonephritis	Single IV antibiotic
Tender uterus PP Day 2-3	Endometritis	IV gentamicin and clindamycin
Wound purulence PP Day 5-6	Wound infection	Wet-to-dry packs
Pelvic mass PP Day 5-6	Pelvic abscess	Percutaneous drainage
"Picket fence" fever PP Day 5-6	Septic thrombophlebitis	Full heparinization

SECTION II

Gynecology

Basic Principles of Gynecology 1

Learning Objectives

- ❑ Provide an overview of female reproductive anatomy
- ❑ List the Tanner stages of developed including expect changes and age of onset
- ❑ Describe the most common gynecologic procedures

FEMALE REPRODUCTIVE ANATOMY

Uterus

The embryologic origin of the uterus is from fusion of the two Müllerian ducts. **Major structures** include the corpus, cornu, isthmus and cervix. **Internal layers** of the uterus include the serosa, myometrium, and endometrium. **The ligaments** attached to the uterus include the broad ligament, round ligaments, cardinal ligaments, and uterosacral ligaments. **Anatomical positions** of the uterus include anteverted, retroverted, mid-position. Normal uterine position tips slightly anterior in the pelvis.

Oviducts

The oviducts extend from the uterus to the ovaries. **Segments** of the oviducts are the interstitium, isthmus, ampulla, and infundibulum. The oviducts function in facilitating sperm migration from the uterus to the ampulla and the transportation of the zygote toward the uterus. They are **attached** medially to the uterine corpus, laterally to the pelvic side wall, and inferiorly to the broad ligament.They receive dual **blood supply** from the ascending uterine artery and ovarian artery.

Ovaries

Functions of the ovaries include containment of oocytes within the ovarian follicles and **production of** reproductive and sexual hormones. The ovaries are **attached by the** ovarian ligament to the uterine fundus, by the suspensory ligaments to the pelvic side wall, and by the mesovarium to the broad ligament. **Lymphatic drainage** of the ovaries is through the pelvic and para-aortic lymph nodes.

Vagina

The vagina is a tubular structure, 8–9 cm in length that extends from the introitus to the cervix. The vagina traverses the urogenital diaphragm through the genital hiatus of the levator ani. It functions as the female copulatory organ, an outflow tract for menstrual flow, and birth canal in parturition.

TANNER STAGES OF DEVELOPMENT

The Tanner stages occur in a **predictable** sequence in the normal physical development of children, adolescents, and adults. The stages define physical measurements of development based on **external** primary and secondary sex characteristics, such as the size of breasts, genitalia, and development of pubic hair.

Pubic Hair

- **Tanner I:** none (prepubertal state)
- **Tanner II:** small amount of long, downy hair with slight pigmentation on the labia majora
- **Tanner III:** hair becomes more coarse and curly and begins to extend laterally
- **Tanner IV:** adult-like hair quality, extending across pubis but sparing medial thighs
- **Tanner V:** hair extends to medial surface of the thighs

Breasts

- **Tanner I:** no glandular tissue; areola follows the skin contours of the chest (prepubertal)
- **Tanner II:** breast bud forms with small area of surrounding glandular tissue; areola begins to widen
- **Tanner III:** breast begins to become more elevated and extends beyond the borders of the areola, which continues to widen but remains in contour with surrounding breast
- **Tanner IV:** increased breast size and elevation; areola and papilla form a secondary mound projecting from the contour of the surrounding breast
- **Tanner V:** breast reaches final adult size; areola returns to contour of the surrounding breast, with a projecting central papilla

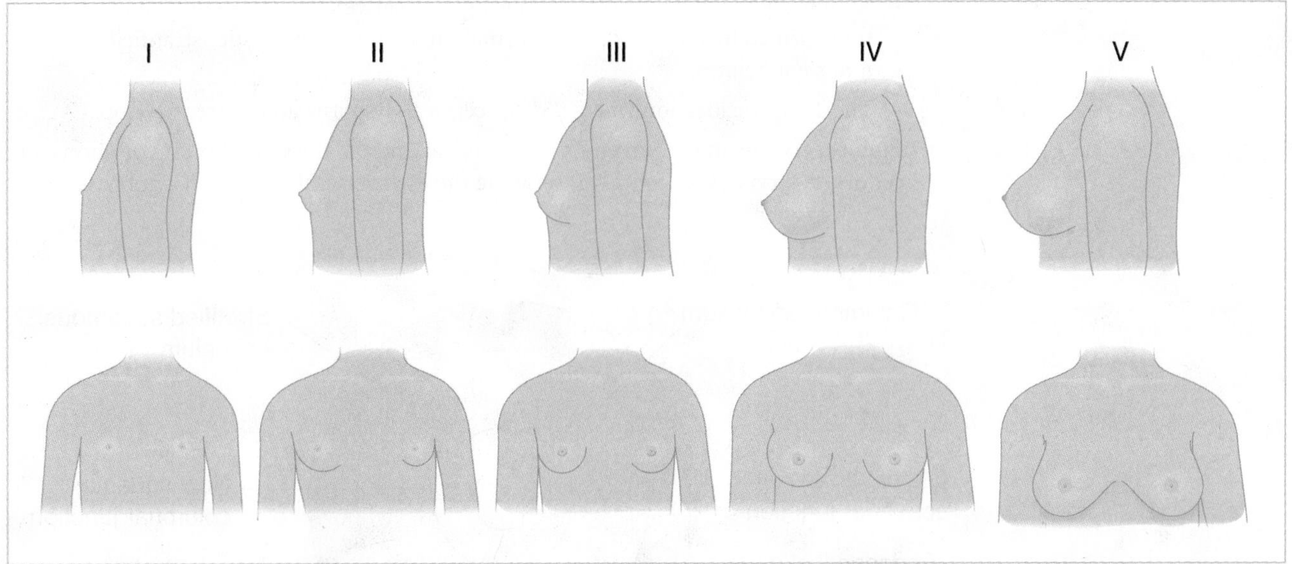

Figure II-1-1. Tanner Stages of the Maturing Female

GYNECOLOGIC PROCEDURES

Gynecologic Ultrasound

This imaging modality uses low-energy, high-frequency sound waves.

- **Transvaginal** transducers are utilized for lower pelvic masses, producing high-resolution images that are not influenced by the thickness of the maternal abdominal wall.
- **Transabdominal** transducers provide images throughout the entire pelvis as well as abdomen.
- Ultrasound works best when adjacent tissues have differing echodensities, particularly fluid/tissue interfaces.

Cervical Pap Smear

This is an outpatient office procedure. It is a screening, not diagnostic, test for premalignant cervical changes; it allows for early intervention, thus preventing cervical cancer.

The diagnostic test for cervical dysplasia or cancer requires a histologic assessment made on a tissue biopsy specimen.

Specimens required. Pap smear should include cytologic specimens from 2 areas: stratified squamous epithelium of transformation zone (TZ) of the ectocervix and columnar epithelium of the endocervical canal (EGG).

- **Ectocervix specimen.** Screening for squamous cell carcinoma, the most common cancer of the cervix (80%), involves scraping the TZ. The TZ is the area of the ectocervix between the old or "original" squamocolumnar junction (SCJ) and the new SCJ.

- At puberty the vaginal pH falls, causing the "native" columnar epithelium to be transformed by metaplasia into normal-appearing "metaplastic" stratified squamous epithelium.
- The TZ is the location where 95% of cervical dysplasia and cancer develop.

- **Endocervix specimen.** Screening for adenocarcinoma, the second most common cancer of the cervix (15%), involves scraping the endocervical canal with cytobrush.

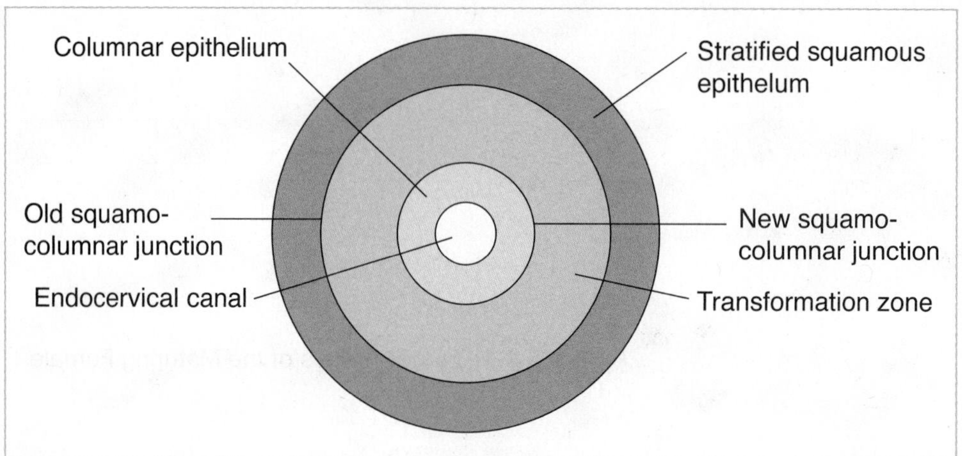

Figure II-1-2. Development of T-Zone

Specimen collection methods. Studies show that while the "liquid-based" methods, compared with the "traditional" method, reduces the percentage of unsatisfactory specimens, the 2 methods are equivalent in performance for detection of cervical dysplasia.

- **Traditional Pap smear**
  - Samples are obtained using a wooden **spatula** on the ectocervix and a **cyto-brush** for the endocervical canal rotating in one direction 360°. The cells from each area are then smeared evenly onto a glass slide, which is then fixed in formalin, then stained and examined under a microscope by a cytologist.
  - Potential problems include insufficient smearing of all abnormal cells onto the glass slide, air-drying artifacts if fixing is delayed, and clumping of cells, making cytology assessment difficult.
- **Liquid-based Pap smear**
  - Specimens can be collected using **cervical broom.** Long central bristles are placed into the endocervix and short outer bristles over the ectocervix. The broom is rotated 5 times in the same direction, collecting and sampling both endocervical cells and transformation zone. The cervical broom is placed in the preservative solution and rotated 10 times vigorously to release collected material into the solution.
  - Advantages include less chance of abnormal cells being discarded with the collecting instrument, less likelihood of air-drying artifacts, and cells spread more evenly on glass slide surface.

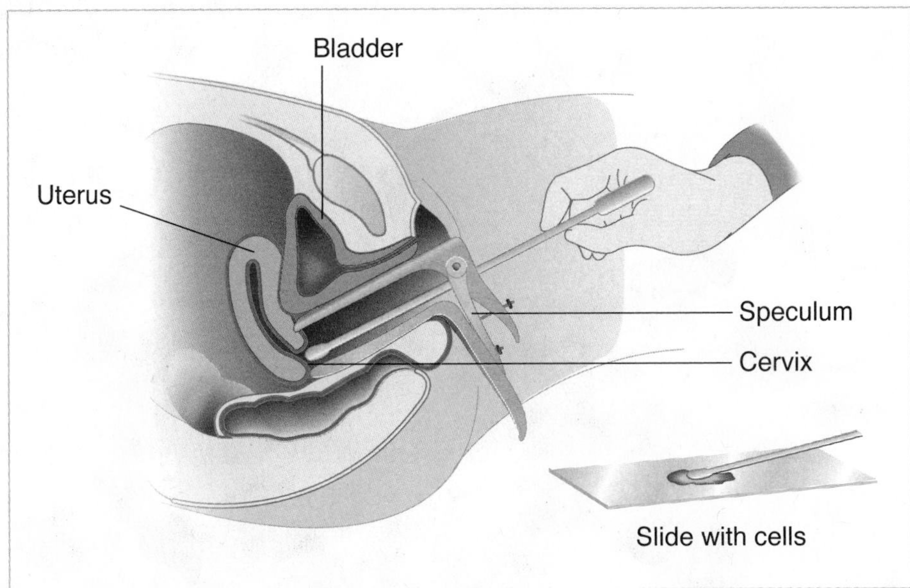

Figure II-1-3. Taking a Sample of Cells during Pap Smear

Colposcopy

Colposcopy is an outpatient office procedure. It uses a binocular, short focal-length instrument with a built-in light source to look at the cervix through a speculum. The purpose is to (1) visually identify where the abnormal Pap smear cells originated, and (2) biopsy that area to send for histologic diagnosis.

- The ectocervix is visually examined to localize areas of abnormal epithelium. Dilute acetic acid should be applied to the cervix to aid in the detection of dysplasia. Areas of abnormal-appearing tissue that are biopsied include **punctation**, **mosaicism**, **white epithelium**, and **abnormal vessels**. The specimens are sent to pathology for definitive diagnosis.

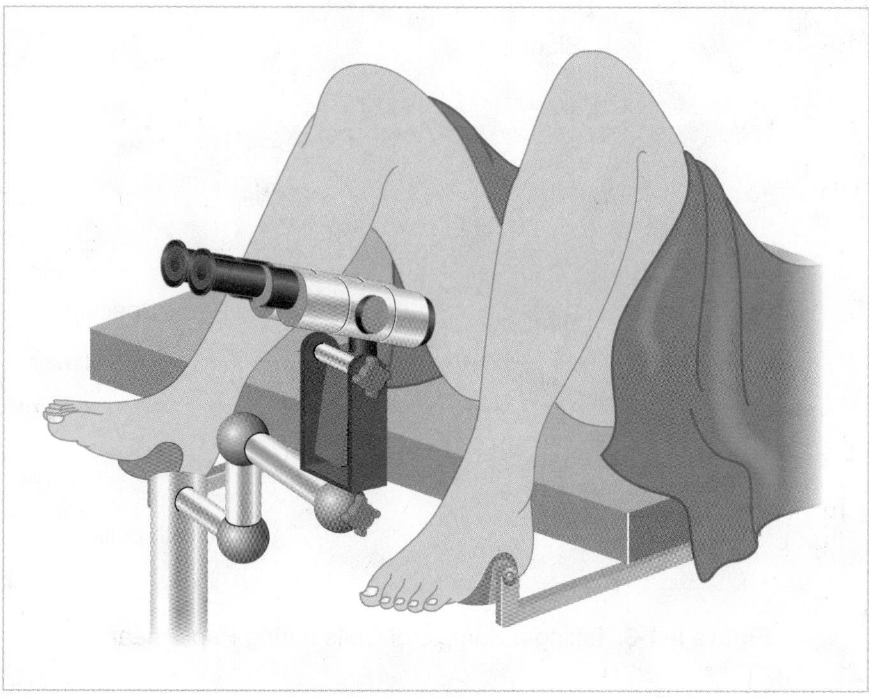

Figure II-1-4. Colposcopy

Cold Knife Cone Biopsy

Cold knife cone biopsy is a minor outpatient surgical procedure performed in the operating room under either local or general anesthesia. It is a diagnostic test that examines the histology of cervical lesions.

- A cone-shaped tissue specimen is obtained with a scalpel by performing a circumferential incision of the cervix with a diameter that is wider at the cervical os and narrower toward the endocervical canal. This tissue is sent to pathology for histologic diagnosis.
- **Wide-shallow cone** is performed if the Pap smear shows changes more severe than the colposcopically directed biopsy.
- **Narrow-deep cone** is performed if a lesion extends from the exocervix into the endocervical canal.
- Long-term risks include cervical **stenosis**, cervical **insufficiency**, and preterm birth.

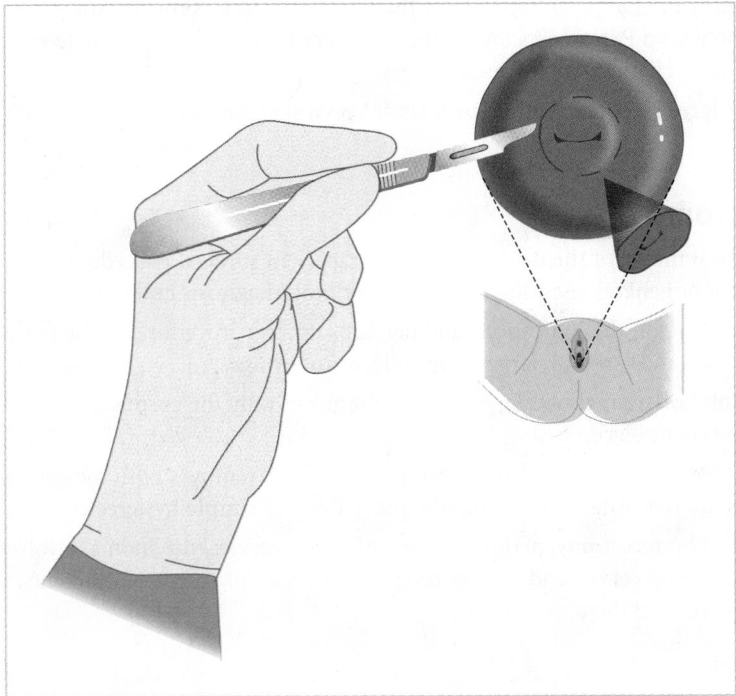

Figure II-1-5. Cold Knife Cone Biopsy

Loop Electrosurgical Excision Procedure (LEEP)

LEEP is a minor outpatient surgical procedure performed under local anesthesia. It is a diagnostic test that examines the histology of cervical lesions. Advantages are low cost, high success rate, and ease of use.

- This technique is used for diagnosing and treating cervical dysplasia. An electric current is passed through a thin wire loop to remove abnormal cervical tissues. The heated loop seals off blood vessels as it cuts.
- The tissue is sent to pathology. Followup Pap smears are performed every 6 months for 2 years to ensure that the dysplastic changes do not return.
- Long-term risks of LEEP include cervical stenosis and cervical insufficiency.

Cryotherapy

Cryotherapy is a minor outpatient procedure performed without anesthesia. It destroys dysplastic cervical tissue identified by colposcopy and cervical biopsy.

- A cryo probe is placed over the abnormal cervical epithelium. The probe temperature is lowered to –50°C with liquid nitrogen. This causes the metal cryo probe to freeze and destroy superficial abnormal cervical tissue. The freezing lasts for 3 minutes; the cervix is then allowed to thaw, and the freezing is repeated for another 3 minutes.

- A watery discharge will occur over the next few weeks as the destroyed tissue sloughs off. Followup Pap smears are performed every 6 months for 2 years to ensure that the dysplastic changes do not return.
- Long-term risks of cryotherapy include cervical **stenosis**.

Hysterectomy

Hysterectomy, removal of the uterus, is a major inpatient surgical procedure performed under either regional or general anesthesia. It is used for both diagnosis and therapy.

- Depending on the indications and pelvic exam, the procedure can be performed either vaginally, abdominally, laparoscopically, or robot-assisted.
- **Subtotal** or supracervical hysterectomy removes only the corpus of the uterus, leaving the cervix in place.
- **Total** hysterectomy, the most common procedure, removes both the corpus and cervix of the uterus. Total hysterectomy is also known as **simple** hysterectomy.
- **Radical hysterectomy**, performed for early-stage cervical carcinoma, involves removal of the uterus, cervix, and surrounding tissues, including cardinal ligaments, uterosacral ligaments, and the upper vagina.

Hysteroscopy

Hysteroscopy is a minor outpatient surgical procedure performed in the operating room under either local-intravenous or general anesthesia for diagnosis and possibly for therapy.

- A fiberoptic scope is placed through a previously dilated cervix to directly visualize the endometrial cavity. A clear fluid is infused through side ports of the scope to distend the uterine cavity, allowing visualization.
- Other side ports of the hysteroscope can be used in placing instruments to biopsy lesions or to resect submucous leiomyomas, polyps, or uterine septa.

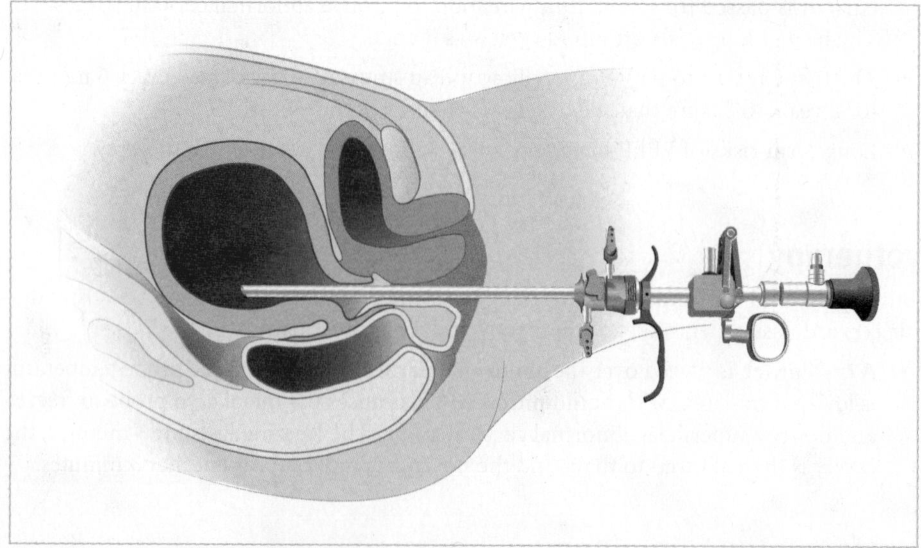

Figure II-1-6. Hysteroscopy

Laparoscopy

Laparoscopy is a minor outpatient surgical procedure performed in the operating room under general anesthesia for diagnosis and possibly for therapy.

- The pelvic-abdominal cavity is insufflated with pressured carbon dioxide to distend the abdomen and lift the abdominal wall away from the viscera. Through a port that is placed through the umbilicus, a fiberoptic scope is then inserted to visually examine the pelvis and abdomen.
- Common gynecologic indications for laparoscopy include diagnosing and treating causes of chronic pelvic pain (e.g., endometriosis or adhesions), resecting advanced ectopic pregnancies, and diagnosing and lysing tubal adhesions in infertility cases.

Hysterosalpingogram (HSG)

HSG is a diagnostic outpatient radiologic imaging procedure performed without anesthesia. A cannula is placed in the endocervical canal and radio-opaque fluid is injected, allowing assessment of uterine malformations (e.g., uterine septum, bicornuate uterus) and Asherman's syndrome.

Tubal pathology can also be assessed by observing internal tubal anatomy and seeing whether the dye spills into the pelvic cavity.

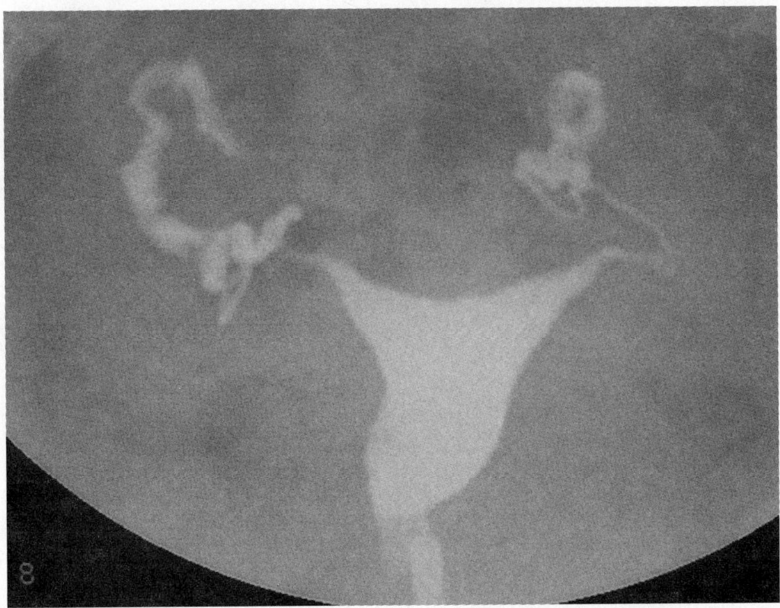

With permission, Medical Education Division of Brookside Associates, brooksidepress.org

Figure II-1-7. Normal HSG

Dilation and Curettage (D&C)

D&C is a minor outpatient surgical procedure performed under anesthesia in an operating room under either local-intravenous or general anesthesia. It is a diagnostic test that examines the histology of endometrial lesions.

D&C is performed similarly to an endometrial biopsy. However, the cervix frequently requires dilation with cervical dilators prior to introduction of the curette. The curette is used to scrape the endometrium, obtaining larger amounts of endometrial tissue that are then sent to pathology.

Endometrial Biopsy

Endometrial biopsy is an outpatient office procedure. It is a diagnostic test that examines the histology of endometrial lesions.

The direction of the cervical canal and endometrial cavity is identified by placing a uterine sound through the endocervical canal. A hollow suction cannula is then placed into the uterine cavity and suction is applied. As the cannula is rotated, endometrial tissue is aspirated into it. When the cannula is removed, the retrieved tissue is placed in formalin and sent to pathology.

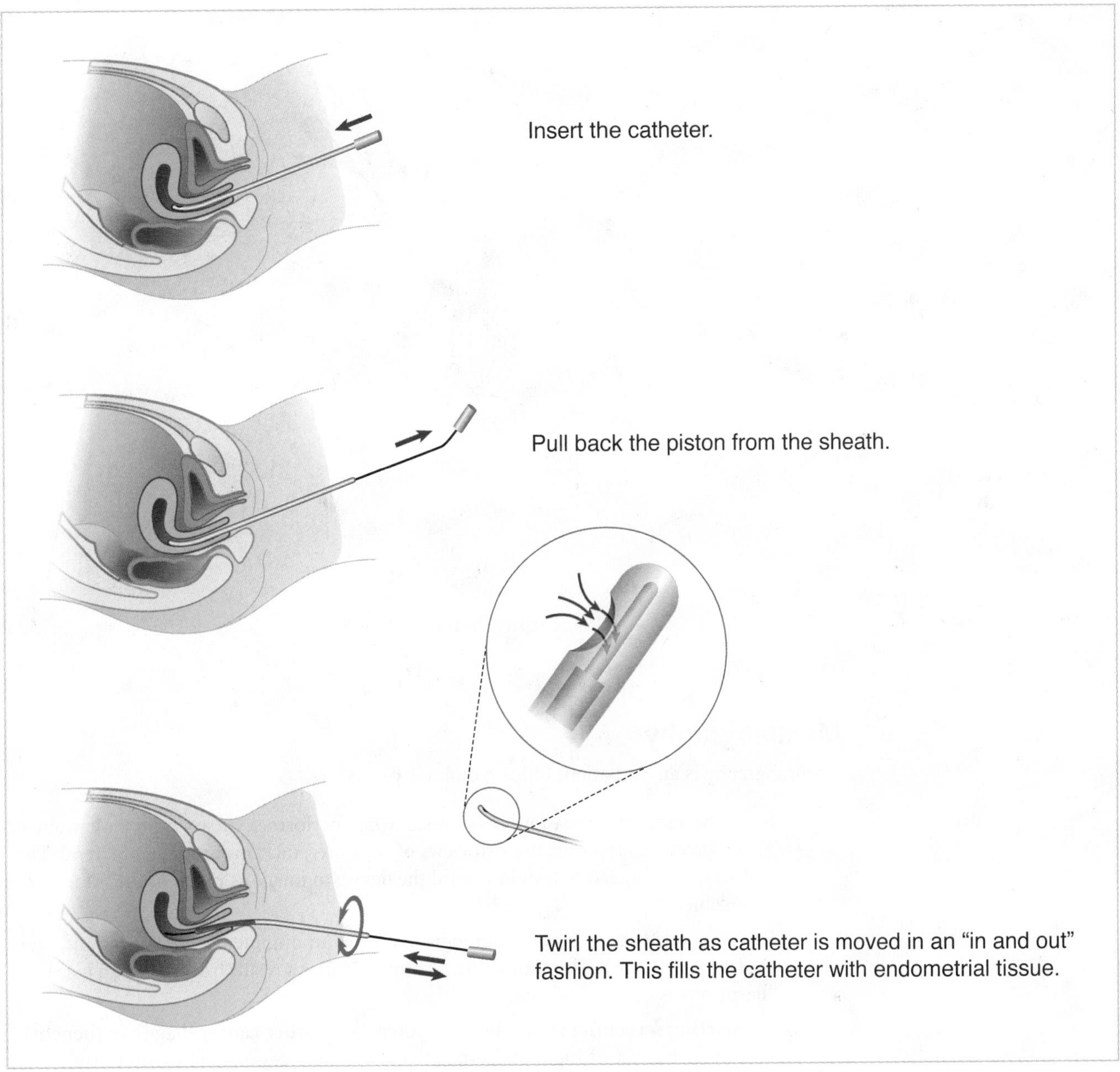

Figure II-1-8. Endometrial Biopsy

Vulvar Biopsy

This is a minor outpatient office procedure performed under local anesthesia. It is a diagnostic test that examines the histology of vulvar lesions.

- It can be performed using either a punch biopsy or a scalpel.

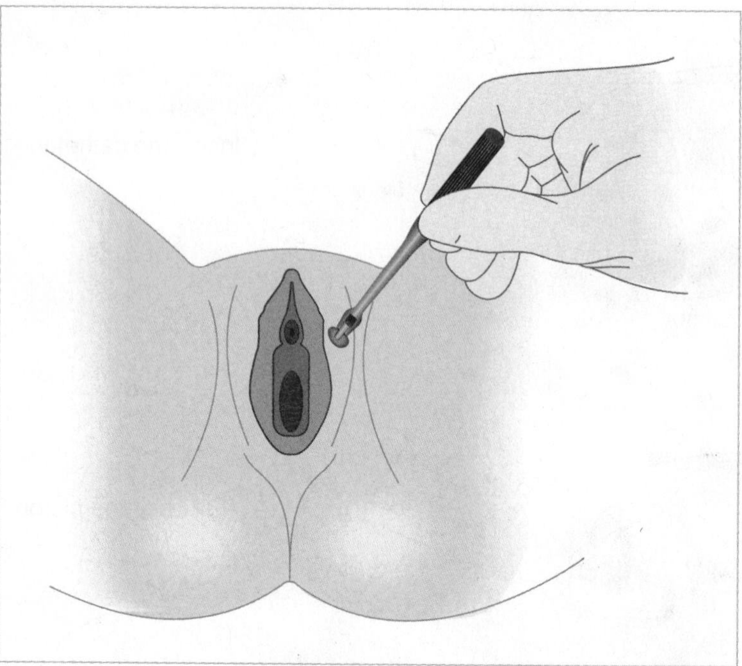

Figure II-1-9. Vulvar Biopsy

Mammography

Mammography is an outpatient office radiologic procedure.

- It may be a screening test for breast cancer when performed on asymptomatic women. These screenings typically use two views of each breast: **craniocaudal** and **lateral**. The patient is encouraged to lean in toward the device to image as much of the breast tissue as possible.
- Recommended **age to start mammograms** varies among medical organizations, ranging from age 40–50. The conflicting recommendations result from differing views of "harm versus benefit" studies.
  - **Starting screening at age 40** gives potentially earlier cancer diagnosis (benefit) but at the cost of higher false-positives with unnecessary follow-up testing and anxiety (harms). False-negatives occur more in younger women and those with denser breasts.
  - **Starting screening at age 50** gives fewer false negatives (benefit) but at a cost of potentially later diagnosis (harm).
  - The best strategy is for doctors to assess individual patient risk and engage in **shared decision-making** with the patient.
- If mammography is performed because of a breast complaint (e.g., breast mass, nipple discharge, abnormal screening mammogram), many images are taken, some under higher magnification to better visualize the target area.
- **Risks:** ionizing radiation exposure 0.7 mSv, which is about the same as the average person receives from background radiation in 3 months (1 Rad = 10 mSv).

2 Pelvic Relaxation

Learning Objectives

- ❑ Demonstrate the relation between uterine/vaginal prolapse and urinary incontinence
- ❑ Describe other expected complications

UTERINE AND VAGINAL PROLAPSE

A 62-year-old woman complains of low back pain and perineal pressure for 18 months. She had been recommended by another physician to wear a pessary, which she is reluctant to do. On pelvic examination a second-degree uterine prolapse with a cystocele and a rectocele is observed.

Anatomy. The pelvic floor is made up of the diaphragm and perineal membrane.

- **Pelvic diaphragm.** The pelvic diaphragm consists of the levator ani and coccygeus muscles. The levator ani consists of 3 muscles: puborectalis, pubococcygeus, and ileococcygeus.
- **Perineal membrane.** This is a triangular sheet of dense fibromuscular tissue that spans the anterior half of the pelvic outlet. The vagina and the urethra pass through the perineal membrane (urogenital diaphragm).
- **Uterine support.** The main structures that support the uterus are the cardinal ligaments, the uterosacral ligaments, and the endopelvic fascia.

Etiology. The etiology of pelvic relaxation is **most commonly** related to childbirth. The mechanical trauma of childbirth stresses and tears the supporting ligaments of the pelvic retroperitoneum in the pelvis whose main function is to support the pelvic viscera.

Classification. The components of pelvic relaxation include uterine prolapse, cystocele, rectocele, and enterocele. Lesser forms of pelvic relaxation include vaginal or vault prolapse.

- **Uterine prolapse.** The severity of prolapse is indicated by increase in grade from I to IV.
  - Grade I: Cervix descends half way to the introitus.
  - Grade II: Cervix descends to the introitus.
  - Grade III: Cervix extends outside the introitus.
  - Grade IV or procidentia: The entire uterus, as well as the anterior and posterior vaginal walls, extends outside the introitus.

GYN Triad

Cystocele

- Postmenopausal woman
- Anterior vaginal wall protrusion
- Urinary incontinence

- **Cystocele.** Herniation or bulging of the anterior vaginal wall and overlying bladder base into the vaginal lumen
- **Rectocele.** Herniation or bulging of the posterior vaginal wall and underlying rectum into the vaginal lumen
- **Enterocele.** Herniation of the pouch of Douglas containing small bowel into the vaginal lumen

Grade I: Uterine Prolapse

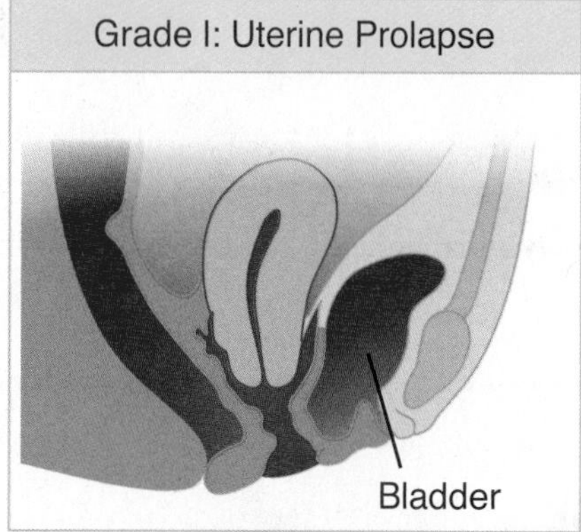

Grade II: Uterine Prolapse

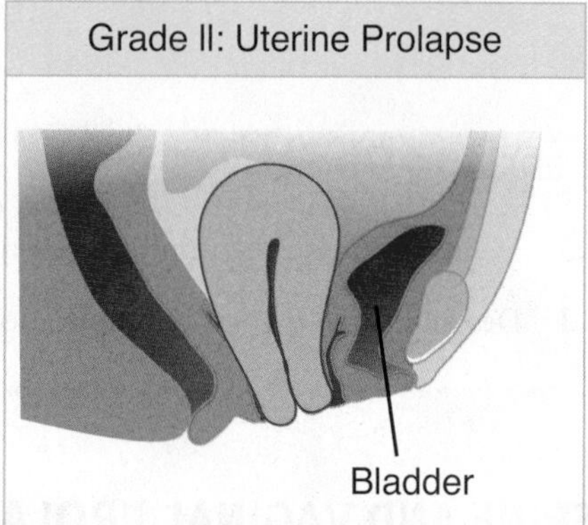

Grade III: Uterine Prolapse

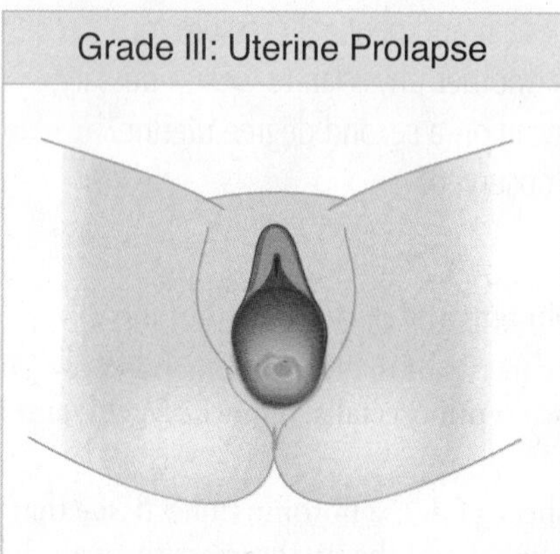

Complete Prolapse

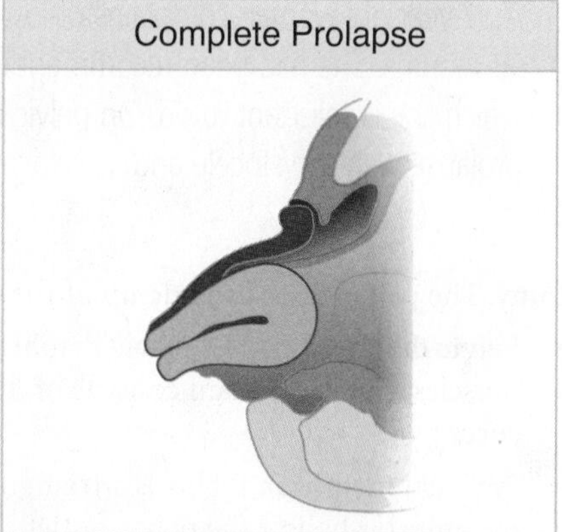

Figure II-2-1. Uterine Prolapse

GYN Triad

Rectocele

- Postmenopausal woman
- Posterior vaginal wall protrusion
- Digitally assisted removal of stool

Table II-2-1. Vaginal Prolapse

Anterior	Cystocele
Posterior	Rectocele
Pouch of Douglas	Enterocele

Diagnosis. The diagnosis of pelvic relaxation is mainly made through observation at the time of **pelvic examination**. The prolapsed vagina, rectum, and uterus are easily visualized particularly as the patient increases intraabdominal pressure by straining.

Management. The management of pelvic relaxation includes non-surgical and surgical treatment.

- **Non-surgical.** Used when there is a minor degree of relaxation. **Kegel** exercises involve voluntary contractions of the pubococcygeus muscle. **Estrogen** replacement may be useful in postmenopausal women. **Pessaries** are objects inserted into the vagina that elevate the pelvic structures into their more normal anatomic relationships.
- **Surgical.** Used when more conservative management has failed. The **vaginal hysterectomy** repairs the uterine prolapse, the anterior vaginal repair repairs the cystocele, and the posterior vaginal repair repairs the rectocele. The **anterior and posterior colporrhaphy** uses the endopelvic fascia that supports the bladder and the rectum, and a plication of this fascia restores normal anatomy to the bladder and to the rectum.

Follow-Up. Strenuous activity should be limited for about 3 months postoperatively to avoid recurrence of the relaxation.

URINARY INCONTINENCE

A 58-year-old woman complains of urinary leakage after exertion. She loses urine while coughing, sneezing, and playing golf. She underwent menopause 5 years ago and is not on estrogen therapy. On examination there is evidence of urethral detachment with a positive Q-tip test.

Definition. Urinary incontinence is the inability to hold urine, producing involuntary urinary leakage.

Physiology of Continence. Continence and micturition involve a balance between urethral closure and detrusor muscle activity. Urethral pressure normally exceeds bladder pressure, resulting in urine remaining in the bladder. The proximal urethra and bladder are normally both within the pelvis. Intraabdominal pressure increases (from coughing and sneezing) are transmitted to both urethra and bladder equally, leaving the pressure differential unchanged, resulting in continence. Normal voiding is the result of changes in both of these pressure factors: urethral pressure falls and bladder pressure rises. Spontaneous bladder muscle (detrusor) contractions are normally easily suppressed voluntarily.

Pharmacology of Incontinence

- **α-adrenergic receptors.** These are found primarily in the urethra and when stimulated cause contraction of urethral smooth muscle, preventing micturition. Drugs: ephedrine, imipramine (Tofranil), and estrogens. α-adrenergic blockers or antagonists relax the urethra, enhancing micturition. Drugs: phenoxybenzamine (Dibenzyline).
- **β-adrenergic receptors.** These are found primarily in the detrusor muscle and when stimulated cause relaxation of the bladder wall, preventing micturition. Drugs: flavoxate (Urispas) and progestins.
- **Cholinergic receptors.** These are found primarily in the detrusor muscle and when stimulated cause contraction of the bladder wall, enhancing micturition. Drugs: bethanecol (Urecholine) and neostigmine (Prostigmine). Anticholinergic medications block the receptors, inhibiting micturition. Drugs: oxybutynin (Ditropan) and propantheline (Pro-Banthine).

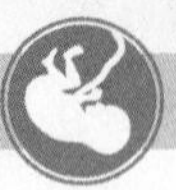

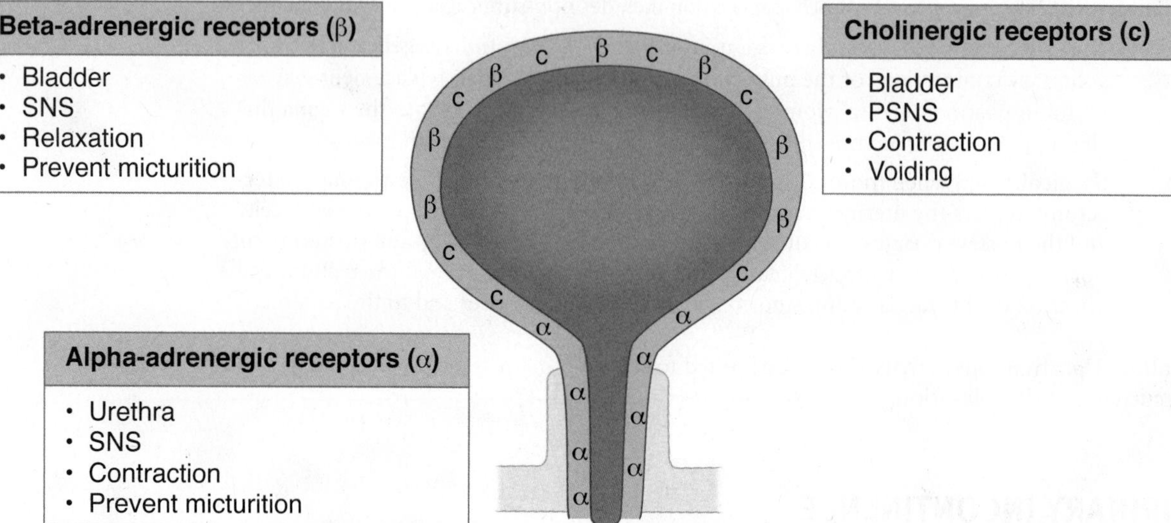

Figure II-2-2. Continence and Micturition

Cystometric studies. Basic office cystometry begins with the patient emptying her bladder as much as possible. A urinary catheter is first used to empty the bladder and then left in place to infuse saline by gravity, with a syringe into the bladder retrograde assessing the following:

- **Residual volume.** How much is left in the bladder? Normal is <50 mL.
- **Sensation-of-fullness volume.** How much infusion (in mL) until the patient senses fluid in her bladder? Normal is 200–225 mL.
- **Urge-to-void volume.** How much infusion (in mL) until the patient feels the need to empty her bladder? Normal is 400–500 mL.

Involuntary bladder contractions. By watching the saline level in the syringe rise or fall, involuntary detrusor contractions can be detected. The absence of contractions is normal.

Table II-2-2. Cystometric Volume Measurements

Post-void residual	<50 mL
Sensation of fullness	200–225 mL
Urge to void	400–500 mL

Classification of Incontinence

Most of the following types of incontinence result when bladder pressure rises in isolation of increases in urethral pressure.

Sensory Irritative Incontinence

- **Etiology.** Involuntary rises in bladder pressure occur owing to detrusor contractions stimulated by irritation from any of the following bladder conditions: infection, stone, tumor, or a foreign body.

- **History.** Loss of urine occurs with urgency, frequency, and dysuria. This can take place day or night.
- **Examination.** Suprapubic tenderness may be elicited, but otherwise the pelvic examination is unremarkable.
- **Investigative studies.** A urinalysis will show the following abnormalities: bacteria and white blood cells (suggest an infection) or red blood cells (suggest a stone, foreign body, or tumor). A urine culture is positive if an infection is present. Cystometric studies (which are usually unnecessary) would reveal normal residual volume with involuntary detrusor contractions present.
- **Management.** Infections are treated with antibiotics. Cytoscopy is used to diagnose and remove stones, foreign bodies, and tumors.

Genuine Stress Incontinence. This is the **most common** incontinence in **young women.**

- **Etiology.** Rises in bladder pressure because of intraabdominal pressure increases (e.g., coughing and sneezing) are not transmitted to the proximal urethra because it is no longer a pelvic structure owing to loss of support from pelvic relaxation.
- **History.** Loss of urine occurs in small spurts simultaneously with coughing or sneezing. **It does not take place when the patient is sleeping.**
- **Examination.** Pelvic examination may reveal a cystocele. Neurologic examination is normal. The Q-tip test is positive when a lubricated cotton-tip applicator is placed in the urethra and the patient increases intraabdominal pressure, the Q-tip will rotate >30 degrees.
- **Investigative studies.** Urinalysis and culture are normal. Cystometric studies are normal with no involuntary detrusor contractions seen.
- **Management.** Medical therapy includes Kegel exercises and estrogen replacement in postmenopausal women. Surgical therapy aims to elevate the urethral sphincter so that it is again an intraabdominal location (urethropexy). This is done by attachment of the sphincter to the symphysis pubis, using the Burch procedure as well as the Marshall-Marchetti-Kranz (MMK) procedure. The success rate of both of these procedures is 85–90%. A minimally invasive surgical procedure is the tension-free vaginal tape procedure in which a mesh tape is placed transcutaneously around and under the mid urethra. It does not elevate the urethra but forms a resistant platform against intraabdominal pressure.

GYN Triad

Stress Incontinence

- Involuntary loss of urine
- With coughing and sneezing
- No urine lost at night

Motor Urge (Hypertonic) Incontinence. This is the **most common** incontinence in **older women.**

- **Etiology.** Involuntary rises in bladder pressure occur from idiopathic detrusor contractions that cannot be voluntarily suppressed.
- **History.** Loss of urine occurs in large amounts often without warning. This can take place both day and night. The most common symptom is urgency.
- **Examination.** Pelvic examination shows normal anatomy. Neurologic examination is normal.
- **Investigative studies.** Urinalysis and culture are normal. Cystometric studies show normal residual volume, but involuntary detrusor contractions are present even with small volumes of urine in the bladder.
- **Management.** Anticholinergic medications (e.g., oxybutynin [Ditropan]); nonsteroidal antiinflammatory drugs (NSAIDs) to inhibit detrusor contractions; tricyclic antidepressants; calcium-channel blockers.

GYN Triad

Hypertonic Bladder

- Involuntary loss of urine
- Cannot suppress urge to void
- Urine loss day and night

GYN Triad

Hypotonic bladder
- Involuntary loss of urine
- Detrusor muscle not contracted
- Urine loss day and night

Overflow (Hypotonic) Incontinence

- **Etiology.** Rises in bladder pressure occur gradually from an overdistended, hypotonic bladder. When the bladder pressure exceeds the urethral pressure, involuntary urine loss occurs but only until the bladder pressure equals urethral pressure. The **bladder never empties**. Then the process begins all over. This may be caused by denervated bladder (e.g., diabetic neuropathy, multiple sclerosis) or systemic medications (e.g., ganglionic blockers, anticholinergics).
- **History.** Loss of urine occurs intermittently in small amounts. This can take place **both day and night**. The patient may complain of pelvic fullness.
- **Examination.** Pelvic examination may show normal anatomy; however, the neurologic examination will show decreased pudendal nerve sensation.
- **Investigative studies.** Urinalysis and culture are usually normal, but may show an infection. Cystometric studies show **markedly increased residual volume**, but involuntary detrusor contractions do not occur.
- **Management.** Intermittent self-catheterization may be necessary. Discontinue the offending systemic medications. Cholinergic medications to stimulate bladder contractions and α-adrenergic blocker to relax the bladder neck.

GYN Triad

Bypass Incontinence
- Involuntary loss of urine
- History: radical pelvic surgery or radiation
- Urine loss day and night continuously

Fistula

- **Etiology.** The normal urethral-bladder mechanism is intact, but is bypassed by urine leaking out through a fistula from the urinary tract.
- **History.** The patient usually has a history of radical pelvic surgery or pelvic radiation therapy. Loss of urine **occurs continually** in small amounts. This can take place **both day and night.**
- **Examination.** Pelvic examination may show normal anatomy and normal neurologic findings.
- **Investigative studies.** Urinalysis and culture are normal. An intravenous pyelogram (IVP) will demonstrate dye leakage from a urinary tract fistula. With a urinary tract-vaginal fistula, intravenous indigo carmine dye will leak onto a vaginal tampon.
- **Management.** Surgical repair of the fistula.

Table II-2-3. Inhibit/Promote Voiding

Inhibit Voiding	Promote Voiding
Bladder relaxants	**Bladder contraction**
Antispasmodics Oxybutynin (Ditropan) Flavoxate (Urispas)	**Cholinergics** Bethanechol (Urecholine) Neostigmine (Prostigmin)
Anticholinergics Pro-Banthine	
Tricyclics Imipramine (Tofranil)	
Vesical neck contraction	**Vesical neck relaxants**
Alpha adrenergics Ephedrine Imipramine	**Alpha antagonists** Methyldopa Phenothiazines
Estrogen stimulates alpha receptors	
Progesterone stimulates beta receptors	

Disorders of the Vagina and Vulva

3

Learning Objectives

- ❑ Describe the common causes, diagnosis, and treatment of vaginal discharge
- ❑ List the most common vulvar diseases

VAGINAL DISCHARGE

A 25-year-old woman complains of a whitish vaginal discharge. The patient states that this is the first time that she has this complaint, and it is associated with vaginal and vulvar pruritus. There is no significant medical history, and she is not on oral contraception.

Diagnostic Tests

- **Visual inspection.** The vulva and vagina should be examined for evidence of an inflammatory response as well as the gross characteristics of the vaginal discharge seen on speculum examination.
- **Vaginal pH.** Normal vaginal pH is an acidic <4.5. Identification of the pH is easily performed using pH-dependent Nitrazine paper. Normal vaginal discharge leaves the paper yellow, whereas an elevated pH turns the paper dark.
- **Microscopic examination.** Two drops of the vaginal discharge are placed on a glass slide with a drop of normal saline placed on one, and a drop of KOH placed on the other. The 2 sites are covered with cover slips and examined under the microscope for WBC, pseudohyphae, trichomonads, and clue cells.

Bacterial Vaginosis

Background. This is the **most common** (50%) cause of vaginal complaints in the United States. It is not a true infection but rather an alteration in concentrations of normal vaginal bacteria. The normal predominant lactobacilli are replaced by massive increases in concentrations of anaerobic species and facultative aerobes. It is frequently seen postmenopausally because of low levels of estrogen. It is not sexually transmitted, but it is associated with sexual activity.

Symptoms. The **most common** patient complaint is a fishy odor. Itching and burning are not present.

GYN Triad

Bacterial Vagino*sis*

- Vaginal discharge pH >4.5
- Fishy odor
- "Clue" cells

Speculum Examination. The vaginal discharge is typically thin, grayish-white. No vaginal inflammation is noted. The vaginal pH is elevated above 4.5. A positive **"whiff"** test is elicited when KOH is placed on the discharge, releasing a fishy odor.

Wet Mount. Microscopic examination reveals **"clue cells"** on a saline preparation. These are normal vaginal epithelial cells with the normally sharp cell borders obscured by increased numbers of anaerobic bacteria. WBCs are rarely seen.

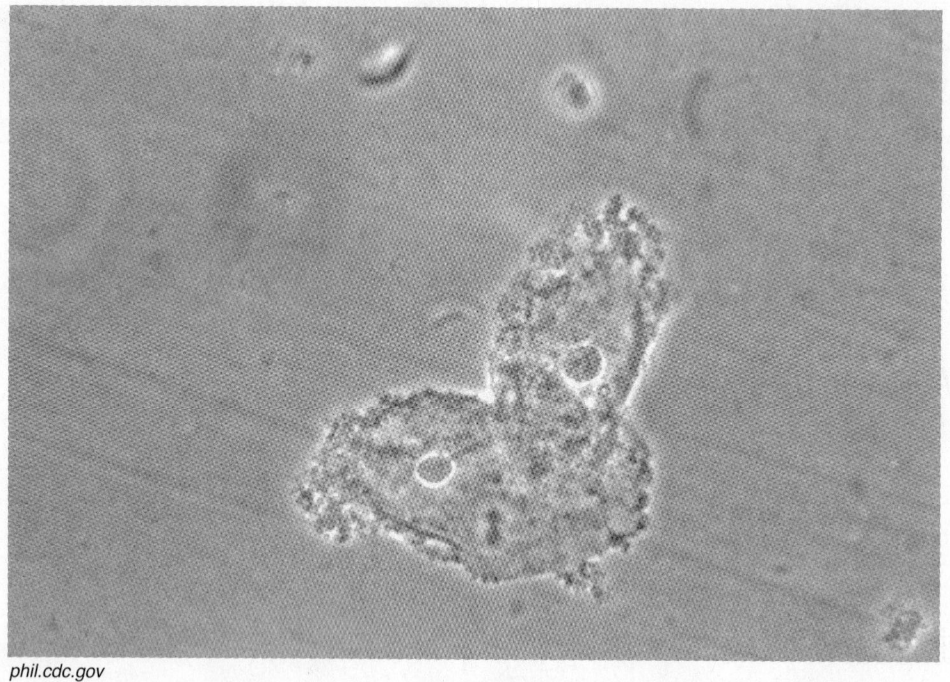

phil.cdc.gov

Figure II-3-1. Clue Cells on Wet Mount

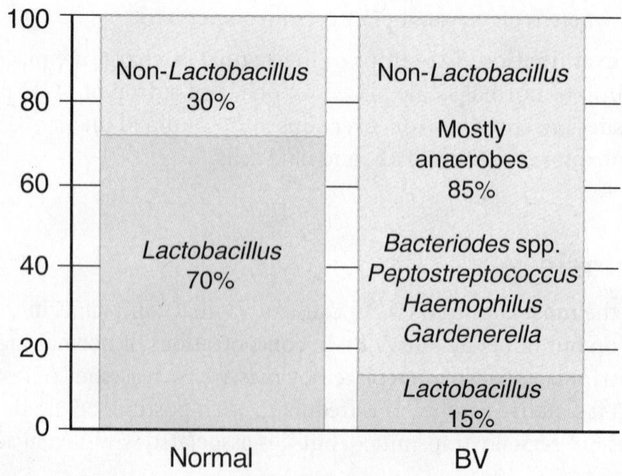

Figure II-3-2. Change in Vaginal Flora with Bacterial Vaginosis (BV)

Management. The treatment of choice is metronidazole or clindamycin administered either orally or vaginally. Metronidazole is safe to use during pregnancy, including the first trimester.

Trichomonas Vaginitis

Background. This is the **most common** cause of vaginal complaints worldwide and is the second most common sexually transmitted disease (**STD**) in the United States. It is caused by a flagellated pear-shaped protozoan that can reside asymptomatically in male seminal fluid.

Symptoms. The **most common** patient complaint is vaginal discharge associated with itching, burning, and pain with intercourse.

Speculum Examination. Vaginal discharge is typically frothy and green. The vaginal epithelium is frequently edematous and inflamed. The erythematous cervix may demonstrate the characteristic **"strawberry"** appearance. Vaginal pH is elevated >4.5.

Wet Mount. Microscopic examination reveals actively motile "trichomonads" on a saline preparation. WBCs are seen.

Management. The treatment of choice is oral metronidazole for both the patient and her sexual partner. Vaginal metronidazole gel has a 50% failure rate. Metronidazole is safe to use during pregnancy, including the first trimester.

GYN Triad

Trichomonas Vaginitis

- Vaginal discharge >4.5
- Itching and burning
- "Strawberry" cervix

Candida (Yeast) Vaginitis

Background. This is the second most common vaginal complaint in the United States. The **most common** organism is *Candida albicans.* It is not transmitted sexually.

Risk Factors. These include diabetes mellitus, systemic antibiotics, pregnancy, obesity, and decreased immunity.

Symptoms. The **most common** patient complaint is itching, burning, and pain with intercourse. *Candida* vaginitis is seen in non-sexually active patients as well.

Speculum Examination. Vaginal discharge is typically curdy and white. The vaginal epithelium is frequently edematous and inflamed. Vaginal pH is normal <4.5.

Wet Mount. Microscopic examination reveals **pseudohyphae** on a KOH prep. WBCs are frequently seen.

Management. The treatment of choice is either a single oral dose of fluconazole or vaginal "azole" creams. An asymptomatic sexual partner does not need to be treated.

GYN Triad

Yeast Vagin*itis*

- Vaginal discharge pH <4.5
- Itching and burning
- Pseudohyphae

Physiologic Discharge

Background. This condition is the result of the thin, watery cervical mucus discharge seen with estrogen dominance. It is a normal phenomenon and becomes a complaint with prolonged anovulation, particularly in patients with wide eversion of columnar epithelium.

Risk factors. These include chronic anovulatory conditions such as polycystic ovarian (PCOS) syndrome.

Symptoms. The **most common** patient complaint is increased watery vaginal discharge. There is no burning or itching.

Speculum Exam. The columnar epithelium of the endocervical canal extends over a wide area of the ectocervix, producing abundant mucus discharge. Vaginal discharge is typically thin and watery. The vaginal epithelium is normal appearing with no inflammation. Vaginal pH is normal (<4.5).

Wet Mount. Microscopic examination reveals an absence of WBCs, "clue cells," trichomonads, or pseudohyphae.

Management. The treatment of choice is steroid contraception with progestins, which will convert the thin, watery, estrogen-dominant cervical discharge to a thick, sticky progestin-dominant mucus.

VULVAR DISEASES

Vulvar Lesion with Pruritus/Neoplasia

A 70-year-old woman complains of vulvar itching for a year. She has been treated with multiple steroid medications with no relief. On pelvic examination there is a well-defined, 1-cm white lesion of the left labia minora. There are no other lesions in the vulva noted; however, there is a clinical enlargement of a left inguinal node.

Clinical Presentation. The **most common** symptom of both benign as well as malignant lesions is vulvar itching resulting in scratching.

Differential Diagnosis. This includes sexually transmitted diseases, benign vulvar dermatosis, or cancers.

Premalignant vulvar dermatosis

These are benign lesions with **malignant predisposition**. The most common symptom is vulvar itching, but most lesions are asymptomatic.

- **Squamous hyperplasia.** These lesions appear as whitish focal or diffuse areas that are firm and cartilaginous on palpation. Histologically, they show thickened keratin and epithelial proliferation. **Management** is fluorinated corticosteroid cream.
- **Lichen sclerosus.** This appears as bluish-white papula that can coalesce into white plaques. On palpation they feel thin and parchment-like. Histologically, they show epithelial thinning. **Management** is Clobetasol cream.
- **Squamous dysplasia.** These lesions appear as white, red, or pigmented, often multifocal in location. Histologically, they show cellular atypia restricted to the epithelium without breaking through the basement membrane. The appearance is almost identical to cervical dysplasia. **Management** is surgical excision.
- **CIS.** The appearance is indistinguishable from vulvar dysplasia. Histologically, the cellular atypia is full thickness but does not penetrate the basement membrane. **Management** is laser vaporization and vulvar wide local excision.

Note

Vulvar dystrophies must also be considered in patients presenting with vulvar itching.

Malignant vulvar lesions

Epidemiology. Vulvar carcinoma is an **uncommon** gynecologic malignancy, with a mean age at diagnosis of 65 years. It is the fourth most common gynecologic malignancy. Risk factors include older age, cigarette smoking, HIV, premalignant vulvar dermatosis.

- **Squamous cell** (90%). The **most common** type of invasive vulvar cancer is squamous cell carcinoma, which has been associated with HPV. Pathogenesis is chronic inflammation (for older women) and HPV infection (for younger women). The **most common** stage at diagnosis is Stage 1.
- **Melanoma** (5%). The **second most common** histologic type of vulvar cancer is melanoma of the vulva, and the most important prognostic factor for this type of tumor is the depth of invasion. Any dark or black lesion in the vulva should be biopsied and considered for melanoma.
- **Paget disease.** An uncommon histologic lesion is Paget disease of the vulva. Paget disease is characteristically a **red lesion**, which is **most common** in postmenopausal white women. Any patient with a red vulvar lesion must be considered for the possibility of Paget disease. Most of the time Paget disease is an intraepithelial process; however, in approximately 18–20% of cases invasion of the basement membrane has been identified. Patients with Paget disease of the vulva have a higher association of other cancers mainly from the GI tract, the genitourinary system, and breast.

Diagnosis. Biopsy. All vulvar lesions of uncertain etiology should be biopsied. Patients with vulvar pruritus should be considered for the possibility of preinvasive or invasive vulvar carcinomas if there is a vulvar lesion. A biopsy of this patient's lesion reveals invasive squamous cell carcinoma of the vulva.

Pattern of spread. It starts with local growth and extension that embolizes to inguinal lymph nodes and finally, hematogenous spread to distant sites.

Staging. Staging is **surgical.**

Stage 0: CIS (basement membrane is intact)

Stage I: Tumor confined to the vulva with size ≤2 cm; nodes not palpable

- IA. Invasion ≤1 mm deep
- IB. Invasion >1 mm deep

Stage II: Tumor confined to the vulva with size >2 cm; nodes not palpable

Stage III: Tumor any size with spread to lower urethra, vagina, or anus; unilateral nodes

Stage IV: Widespread metastases

- IVA. Involves upper urethra, bladder or rectum, pelvic bone, bilateral nodes
- IVB. Distant metastasis

Management

- **Wide local excision only:** used only for stage IA; risk of metastasis is negligible so no lymphadenectomy is needed
- **Modified radical vulvectomy:** involves radical local excision
  - Ipsilateral inguinal dissection is used only if stage is IB & unifocal lesion >1 cm from midline AND no palpable nodes
  - Bilateral inguinal dissection is used if at least stage IB or a centrally located lesion OR palpable inguinal nodes or positive ipsilateral nodes

- **Radical vulvectomy:** involves removal of labia minora & majora, clitoris, perineum, perineal body, mons pubis; seldom performed due to high morbidity
- **Pelvic exenteration**. In addition to radical vulvectomy, it involves removal of cervix, vagina and ovaries in addition to lower colon, rectum and bladder (with creation of appropriate stomas); seldom indicated or performed due to high morbidity.
- **Radiation therapy:** used for patients who cannot undergo surgery

Table II-3-1. Management of Vulvar Carcinoma

Radical vulvectomy	Removes entire vulva (subcutaneous and fatty tissue, labia minora and majora, perineal skin, clitoris)	Sexual dysfunction
Modified radical vulvectomy	Wide local excision (for **unilateral** labial lesions that do not cross the midline)	Less sexual morbidity
Lymphadenectomy	Inguinal node dissection (**bilateral** if midline lesions >1 mm invasion; **unilateral** selectively)	Lower-extremity edema

Benign Vulvar Lesions

- ***Mulluscom contagiosum.*** A common benign, viral skin infection. Most commonly seen in children, sexually active adults, and immunodeficient patients. The mollusci-pox virus causes spontaneously regressing, umbilicated tumors of the skin rather than poxlike vesicular lesions. Mulluscom contagiosum is transmitted primarily through direct skin contact with an infected individual. **Management** includes observation, curettage, and cryotherapy.
- **Condylomata acuminata.** These are benign cauliflowerlike vulvar lesions due to HPV types 6 & 11. They have no malignant predisposition. Condylomata are discussed in detail in chapter 7. **Management** is to treat clinical lesions only.
- **Bartholin cyst.** Obstruction of the Bartholins gland duct may occur due to infection mostly due to *E. coli* and anaerobic *Bacteroides* species, and seldom due to gonococcus. After immune defenses overcome the infection the duct remains obstructed resulting in cystic dilation of the gland. Aspiration of the cyst yields sterile fluid. **Management** is conservative unless pressure symptoms due to size. Bartholin cyst is discussed in chapter 7.

Disorders of the Cervix and Uterus 4

Learning Objectives

- ❑ Explain the use of vaccination to prevent cervical dysplasia
- ❑ List the common findings and their significance when diagnosing cervical lesions
- ❑ Give an overview of the epidemiology and management of cervical neoplasia
- ❑ Describe Müllerian anomalies
- ❑ Give a differential diagnosis for enlarged uterus and describe the treatment and prognosis of endometrial neoplasia

CERVICAL LESIONS

Cervical Polyps

Description. Cervical polyps are fingerlike growths that start on the surface of the cervix or endocervical canal. These small, fragile growths hang from a stalk and push through the cervical opening.

- The cause of cervical polyps is not completely understood. They may be associated with chronic inflammation, an abnormal response to increased levels of estrogen, or thrombosed cervical blood vessels.
- Cervical polyps are relatively common, especially in older multiparous women. Only a single polyp is present in most cases, but sometimes two or three are found.

Findings

- The history is usually positive for vaginal bleeding, often after intercourse. This bleeding occurs between normal menstrual periods.
- Speculum examination reveals smooth, red or purple, fingerlike projections from the cervical canal.
- A cervical biopsy typically reveals mildly atypical cells and signs of infection.

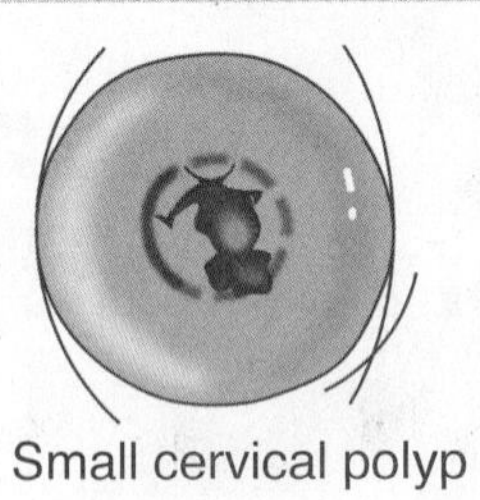

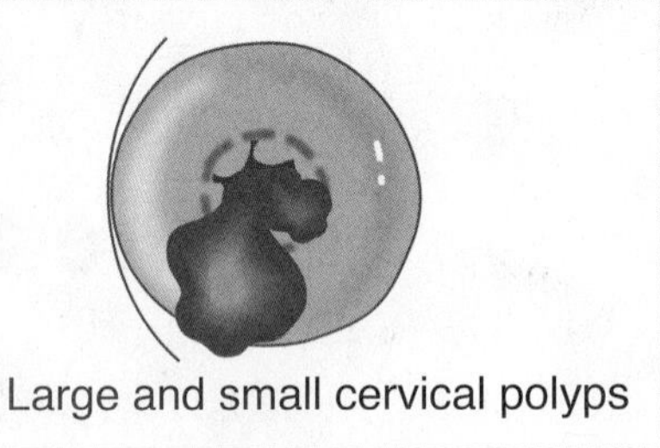

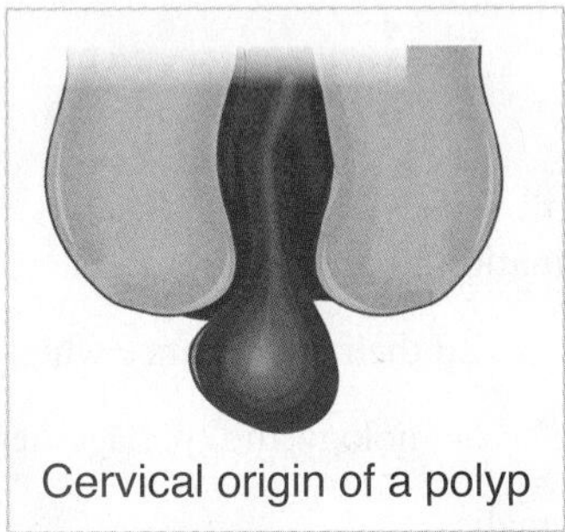

Figure II-4-1. Cervical Polyps

Management

- Polyps can be removed by gentle twisting or by tying a surgical string around the base and cutting it off. Removal of the polyp's base is done by electrocautery or with a laser.
- Because many polyps are infected, an antibiotic may be given after the removal even if there are no or few signs of infection. Although most cervical polyps are benign, the removed tissue should be sent to pathology. Regrowth of polyps is uncommon.

Nabothian Cysts

A nabothian cyst is a mucus-filled cyst on the surface of the uterine cervix. The cervical canal is lined by glandular cells that normally secrete mucus. These endocervical glands can become covered by squamous epithelium through metaplasia.

This is a benign condition. Rarely, cysts may become so numerous or enlarged that the cervix becomes clinically enlarged.

- These nests of glandular cells (nabothian glands) on the cervix may become filled with secretions. As secretions accumulate, a smooth, rounded lump may form just under the surface of the cervix and become large enough to be seen or felt upon examination.
- Each cyst appears as a small, white, pimple-like elevation. The cysts can occur singly or in groups, and they are not a threat to health. The cysts are more common in women of reproductive age, especially women who have already had children. There are no observable symptoms.

Findings. Pelvic examination reveals a small, smooth, rounded lump (or collection of lumps) on the surface of the cervix. Rarely, a colposcopic exam is necessary to distinguish nabothian cysts from other types of cervical lesions.

Management. No treatment is necessary. However, nabothian cysts do not clear spontaneously. They can be easily cured through electrocautery or cryotherapy. Both procedures can be done in the doctor's office.

Cervicitis

Symptoms. Often, there are no symptoms, except vaginal discharge.

Examination. The **most common** finding is mucopurulent cervical discharge and a friable cervix. This diagnostic finding is confirmed by endocervical bleeding easily induced by passage of a cotton swab through the cervical os. No pelvic tenderness is noted. Patient is afebrile.

Investigative Findings. Routine cervical cultures are positive for chlamydia or gonorrhea. WBC and ESR are normal.

Management. Oral azithromycin in a single dose or oral doxycycline BID for 7 days.

CERVICAL NEOPLASIA

Abnormal Pap Smear

> A 24-year-old woman is referred because of a Pap smear showing HSIL (high-grade squamous intraepithelial lesion). The patient, states that her Pap smear 3 years ago was negative. She has been on combination steroid vaginal ring contraception for the past 4 years. Her cervix appears unremarkable on gross visual inspection.

Presentation. Premalignant lesions of the cervix are usually **asymptomatic**. The progression from premalignant to invasive cancer has been reported to be approximately 8–10 years. Most lesions will spontaneously regress; others remain static, with only a minority progressing to cancer.

Etiology. The **most common** etiology of cervical cancer is the human papilloma virus (HPV). Over 75 subtypes of HPV have been identified. HPV **16, 18, 31, 33,** and **35** are the **most common** HPV types associated with premalignant and cancerous lesions of the cervix. HPV **6** and **11** are the **most common** HPV types associated with benign condyloma acuminata.

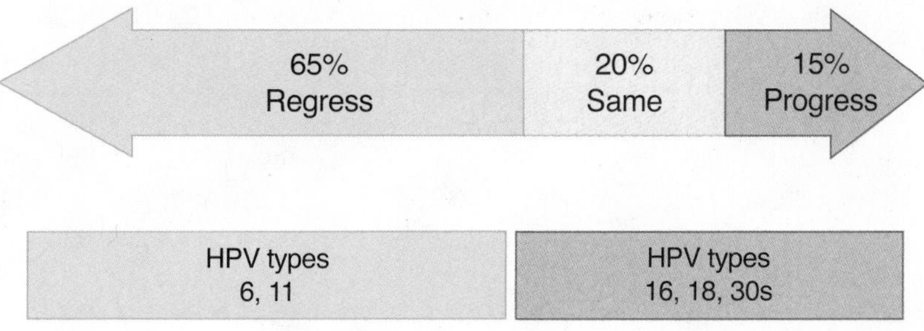

Figure II-4-2. Natural History of Cervical Dysplasia: Response to HPV types

Risk Factors. These include early age of intercourse, multiple sexual partners, cigarette smoking, and immunosuppression. The mediating factor for all these conditions is probably HPV.

Screening and Performing a Pap Smear

The best screening test for premalignant lesions is **cytology**. Cytologic screening uses the **Pap test**. The **most common** site for cervical dysplasia is the transformation zone (T-zone).

- **How is it performed?** Two specimens are obtained with the Pap smear: an ectocervical sample performed by scraping the T-zone with a spatula, and an endocervical sample obtained with a cytobrush in the nonpregnant woman or a cotton-tip applicator in a pregnant woman.
- **What cytologic screening methods can be used?**
  - With the **conventional method**, the specimens are smeared onto a glass slide, which is placed in fixative and then microscopically examined.
  - With the **thin-layer, liquid-based cytology**, the specimens are rinsed into a preserving solution and are then deposited on a slide as a thin layer of processed cells.
  - Both methods are equivalent for cancer screening but the liquid-based method has the advantage of doing reflex HPV-DNA typing.

Pap smear should be started at the following ages:

- **Age <21**: no Pap test or screening for HPV, regardless of sexual activity
- **Age 21**: Start Pap test with cytology alone without HPV testing; the recommendation is the same whether HPV vaccinated or not

The frequency of recommended Pap smear is as follows:

- **Age 21–29**: repeat Pap every 3 years with cytology alone; do not perform HPV testing in this age group
- **Age 30–65**: repeat Pap every 3 years with cytology but no HPV testing **OR** repeat Pap every 5 years if both cytology and HPV testing (the recommended option in this age group)

Pap smears should be discontinued:

- **After age 65** if negative cytology and/or HPV tests for past 10 years **AND** no history of CIN 2, CIN 3 or cervical carcinoma
- **Any age** if total hysterectomy **AND** no history of cervical neoplasia

Pap Smear Classification

The **Bethesda system** is the current classification used in the United States.

- **Negative** for intraepithelial lesion or malignancy; comments may report trichomoniasis, candida, BV, HSV, or atrophy
- **Abnormal squamous cells** (99% of abnormal Pap smears)
  - **ASC-US (atypical squamous cells of undetermined significance):** changes suggestive of but not adequate to label LSIL
  - **LSIL (low-grade squamous intraepithelial lesion):** biopsy is expected to show histologic findings of HPV, mild dysplasia, or CIN 1
  - **ASC-H (atypical squamous cells can't rule out HSIL):** changes suggestive of but not adequate to label HSIL
  - **HSIL (high-grade squamous intraepithelial lesion):** biopsy is expected to show histologic findings of moderate–severe dysplasia, CIN 2, CIN 3, or CIS
  - **Squamous cell carcinoma:** biopsy is expected to show histologic findings of invasive cancer
- **Abnormal endocervical cells** (1% of abnormal Pap smears)
  - **AGC-NOS (atypical glandular cells, not otherwise specified)**
  - **AGC-neoplastic (atypical glandular cells, can't rule out neoplasia):** changes suggestive of but not adequate to call AIS or cancer
  - **AIS (adenocarcinoma in situ)**
  - **Adenocarcinoma**

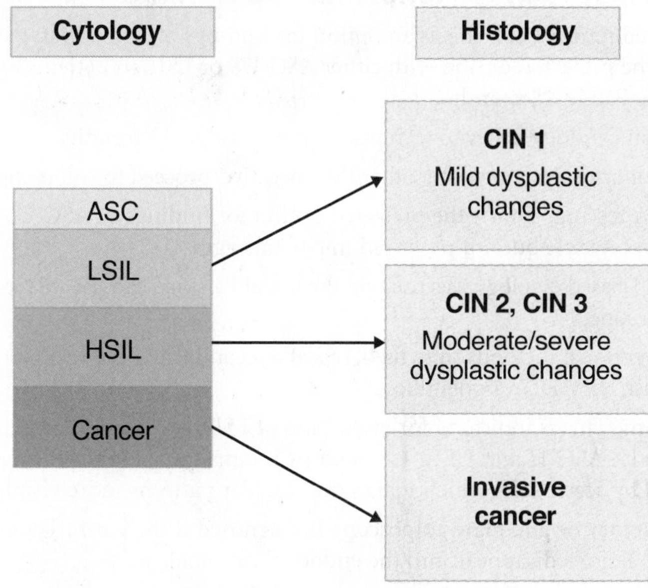

Figure II-4-4. Classification of Cervical Dysplasias

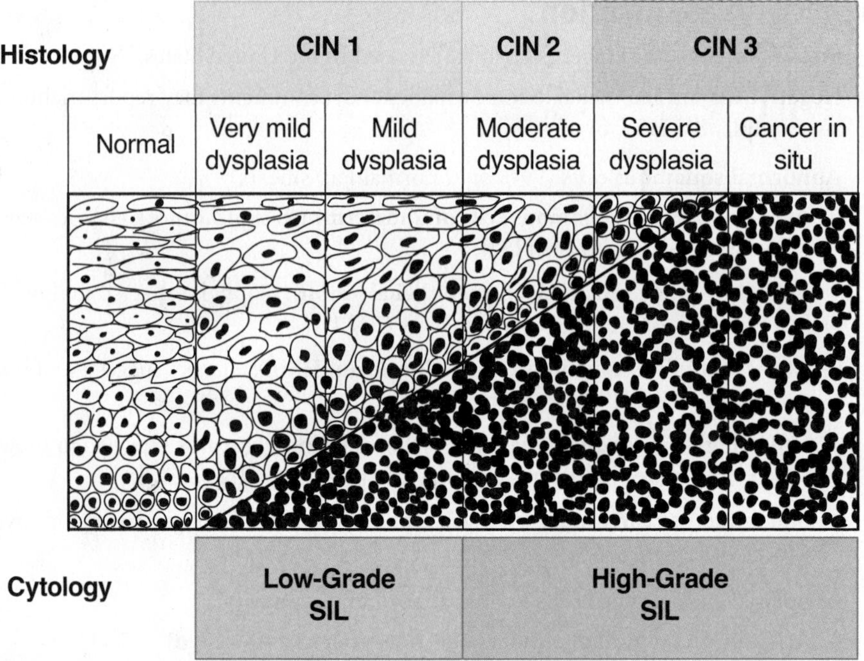

Figure II-4-5. Histologic Appearance of Cervical Dysplasia with Progressive Severity

Diagnostic Approach to Abnormal Pap Smears

- **Accelerated repeat Pap.** This is an option for findings of ASC-US in patients of any age, and the preferred option with either ASC-US or LSIL in patients ages 21-24. Repeat the Pap in 12 months.
  - If repeat cytology is negative, repeat Pap in another 12 months.
  - If repeat cytology is anything other than negative, proceed to colposcopy and biopsies.
- **HPV DNA testing.** This is the preferred option for findings of ASC-US in patients age ≥25.It is acceptable but not preferred in patients ages 21-24.
  - If liquid-based cytology was used on the initial Pap, one can use this specimen for DNA testing.
  - If conventional methods were used, repeat a second Pap. Perform colposcopy only if high-risk HPV DNA is identified.
- **Colposcopy.** This is indicated for evaluation of LSIL in patients age ≥25, and all patients with ASC-H and HSIL. Colposcopy is a magnification of the cervix (10–12x); it is aided by acetic acid, which makes the vascular patterns more visible.
  - **Satisfactory or adequate** colposcopy is diagnosed if the entire T-zone is visualized and no lesions disappear into the endocervical canal.
  - **Unsatisfactory or inadequate** colposcopy is diagnosed if the entire T-zone cannot be fully visualized.
- **Endocervical curettage (ECC).** All nonpregnant patients undergoing colposcopy which shows metaplastic epithelium entering the endocervical canal will undergo an ECC to rule out endocervical lesions.

- **Ectocervical biopsy.** Lesions identified on the ectocervix by colposcopy (e.g., mosaicism, punctation, white lesions, abnormal vessels) are biopsied and sent for histology.
- **Compare Pap smear and biopsy.** When the biopsy histology is complete, it is compared with the level of Pap smear abnormality to ensure the level of severity is comparable.
- **Cone biopsy.** If the Pap smear is worse than the histology (suggesting the site of abnormal Pap smear cells was not biopsied), then a cone biopsy is performed. Other indications for conization of the cervix include abnormal ECC histology, a lesion seen entering the endocervical canal, and a biopsy showing microinvasive carcinoma of the cervix. Deep cone biopsies can result in an **incompetent cervix.** Another risk of cone biopsy is **cervical stenosis.**

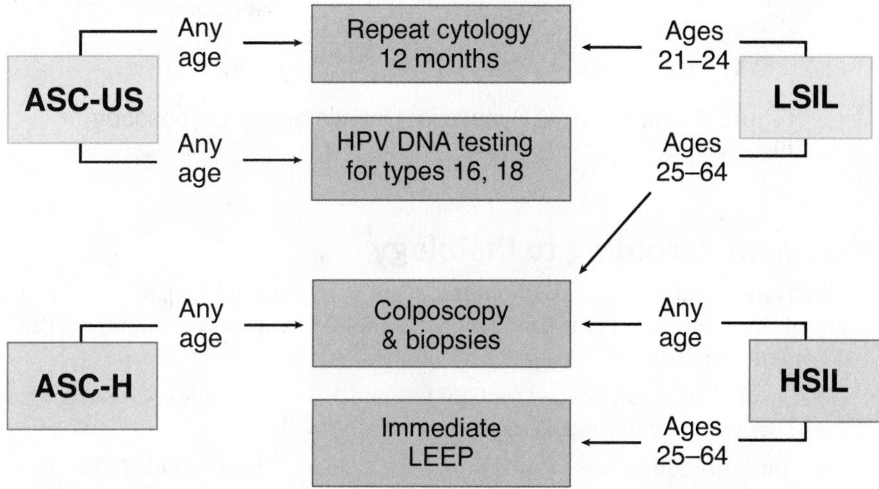

Figure II-4-7. Diagnostic Options for Abnormal Pap Smear (2013)

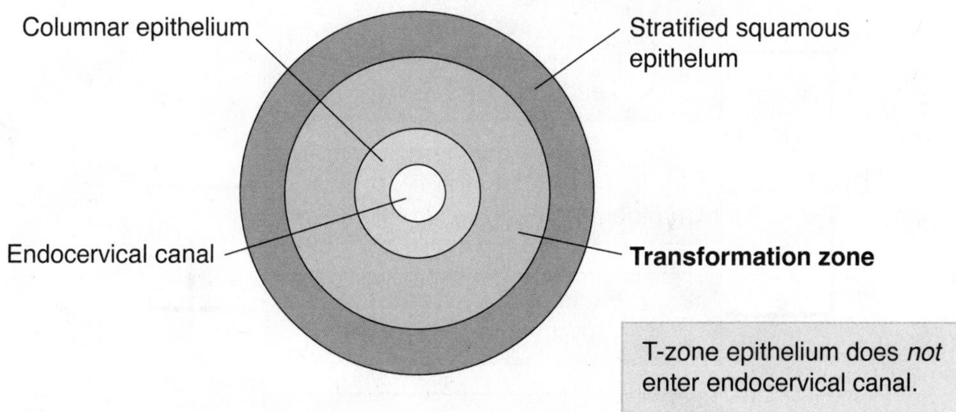

Figure II-4-8. Cervical Dysplasia: Satisfactory Colposcopy

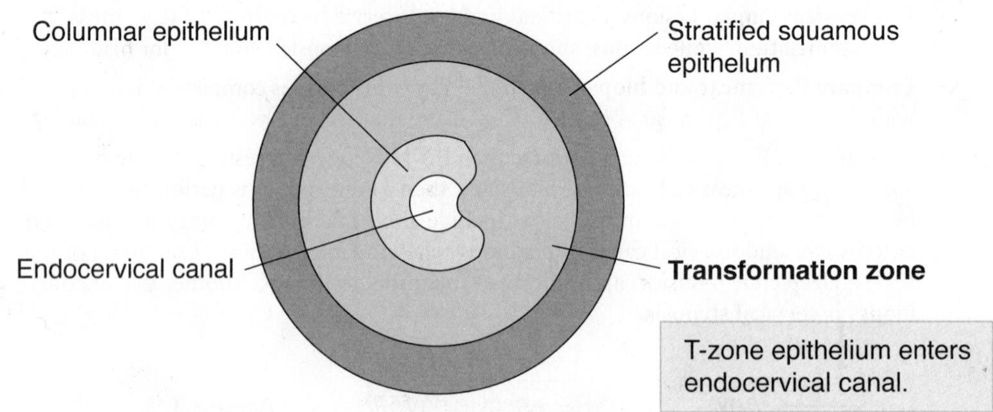

Figure II-4-9. Cervical Dysplasia: Unsatisfactory Colposcopy

Management According to Histology

- Observation and follow-up without treatment is appropriate for CIN 1 and includes any of the following: repeat Pap in 6 and 12 months; colposcopy and repeat Pap in 12 months; or HPV DNA testing in 12 months.
- Ablative modalities can be used for CIN 1, 2, and 3. These include cryotherapy (freezing), laser vaporization, and electrofulguration.
- Excisional procedures can be used for CIN 1, 2, and 3. These include LEEP (loop electrosurgical excision procedure) or cold-knife conization.
- Hysterectomy is only acceptable with biopsy-confirmed, recurrent CIN 2 or 3.

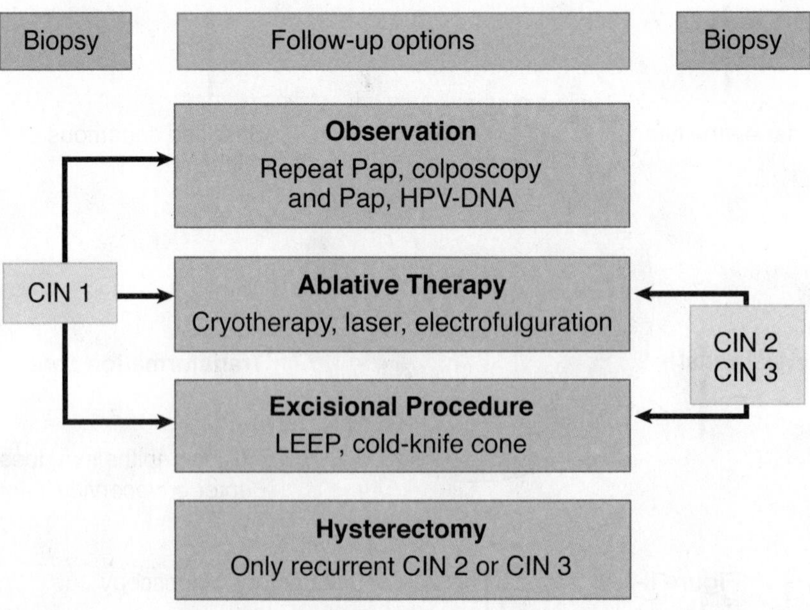

Figure II-4-10. Cervical Dysplasia: Management According to Histology

Follow-Up. Patients treated with either ablative or excisional procedures require follow-up repeat Pap smears, colposcopy and Pap smear, or HPV DNA testing every 4 to 6 months for 2 years.

Invasive Cervical Cancer

A 43-year-old woman complains of intermenstrual postcoital bleeding for the past 6 months between regular menstrual cycles that occur every 28 days. On pelvic examination a 3-cm exophytic mass is seen from the anterior lip of the cervix. The rest of the pelvic examination, including a rectovaginal examination, is normal.

Definition. Cervical neoplasia that has penetrated through the basement membrane.

Presentation. Patients with invasive cervical cancer can present with postcoital vaginal bleeding. Other symptoms of cervical cancer include irregular vaginal bleeding and, in advanced stage, lower extremity pain and edema.

Epidemiology. Cervical carcinoma is the **third most common** gynecologic malignancy with a mean age at diagnosis of **45 years**.

Diagnostic Tests/Findings

- **Cervical biopsy.** The initial diagnostic test should be a cervical biopsy, in which the most common diagnosis is squamous cell carcinoma.
- **Metastatic workup.** Once a tissue diagnosis of invasive carcinoma is made, a metastatic workup should be done that includes pelvic examination, chest x-ray, intravenous pyelogram, cystoscopy, and sigmoidoscopy.
- **Imaging studies.** Invasive cervical cancer is the only gynecologic cancer that is staged clinically; an abdominal pelvic CT scan or MRI cannot be used for clinical staging.

Staging. Staging is **clinical** based on pelvic examination and may include an intravenous pyelogram (IVP).

Stage 0: Carcinoma in-situ (CIS). The basement membrane is intact.

Stage I: Spread **limited** to the cervix. This is the **most common** stage at diagnosis.
- Ia1. Invasion is ≤3 mm deep (minimally invasive)
- Ia2. Invasion is >3 but ≤5 mm deep (microinvasion)
- IB. Invasion is >5 mm deep (frank invasion)

Stage II: Spread **adjacent** to the cervix
- IIa. Involves upper two thirds of vagina
- IIb. Invasion of the parametria

Stage III: Spread **further** from the cervix
- IIIA. Involves lower one third of vagina
- IIIB. Extends to pelvic side wall or hydronephrosis

Stage IV: Spread **furthest** from the cervix
- IVA. Involves bladder or rectum or beyond true pelvis
- IVB. Distant metastasis

Management. Patients treated surgically are evaluated for risk factors for metastatic disease and tumor recurrence. These include metastatic disease to the lymph nodes, tumor size >4 cm, poorly differentiated lesions, or positive margins. Patients with these findings are offered adjuvant therapy (radiation therapy and chemotherapy).

- **Specific by stage:**

  Stage Ia1: Total simple hysterectomy, either vaginal or abdominal

  Stage Ia2: Modified radical hysterectomy

  Stage IB or IIA: Either radical hysterectomy with pelvic and paraaortic lymphadenectomy (if premenopausal) and peritoneal washings or pelvic radiation (if postmenopausal). In patients who can tolerate surgery, a radical hysterectomy is preferred; however, studies have demonstrated equal cure rates with radiation or surgical treatment.

  Stage IIB, III, or IV: Radiation therapy and chemotherapy for all ages.

Table II-4-1. Stage I—Most Common (Spread Limited to Cervix)

Ia1	• ≤3 mm • Minimal invasion	Total simple hysterectomy
Ia2	• >3 mm but ≤5 mm • Microinvasion	Modified radical hysterectomy
IB	• >5 mm • Frank invasion	Radical hysterectomy

Follow-Up. All patients with invasive cervical cancer should be followed up with Pap smear every 3 months for 2 years after treatment, and then every 6 months for the subsequent 3 years.

- Patients who have a **local recurrence** can be treated with radiation therapy; if they had received radiation previously, they might be considered candidates for a pelvic exenteration.
- Patients with **distant metastases** should be considered for chemotherapy treatment. The most active chemotherapeutic agent for cervical cancer is cisplatinum.

Cervical Neoplasia in Pregnancy

A 25-year-old woman with intrauterine pregnancy at 14 weeks by dates is referred because of a Pap smear showing as HSIL (high-grade squamous intraepithelial lesion). On pelvic examination there is a gravid uterus consistent with 14 weeks size, and the cervix is grossly normal to visual inspection.

Diagnostic Tests/Findings

- **Effect of pregnancy.** Pregnancy per se does not predispose to abnormal cytology and does not accelerate precancerous lesion progression into invasive carcinoma.

- **Colposcopy and biopsy.** A patient who is pregnant with an abnormal Pap smear should be evaluated in the same fashion as when in a nonpregnant state. An abnormal Pap smear is followed with colposcopy with the aid of acetic acid for better visualization of the cervix. Any abnormal lesions of the ectocervix are biopsied.
- **Perform an ECC?** Owing to increased cervical vascularity, ECC is not performed during pregnancy.

Management

- **CIN.** Patients with intraepithelial neoplasia or dysplasia should be followed with Pap smear and colposcopy every 3 months during the pregnancy. At 6–8 weeks postpartum the patient should be reevaluated with repeat colposcopy and Pap smear. Any persistent lesions can be definitively treated postpartum.
- **Microinvasion.** Patients with microinvasive cervical cancer on biopsy during pregnancy should be evaluated with cone biopsy to ensure no frank invasion. If the cone biopsy specimen shows microinvasive carcinoma during pregnancy, these patients can also be followed conservatively, delivered vaginally, reevaluated, and treated 2 months postpartum.
- **Invasive cancer.** If the punch biopsy of the cervix reveals frankly invasive carcinoma, then treatment is based on the gestational age.
  - In general, if a diagnosis of invasive carcinoma is made **before 24 weeks** of pregnancy, the patient should receive definitive treatment (e.g., radical hysterectomy or radiation therapy).
  - If the diagnosis is made **after 24 weeks** of pregnancy, then conservative management up to about 32–33 weeks can be done to allow for fetal maturity to be achieved, at which time cesarean delivery is performed and definite treatment begun.

Prevention of Cervical Dysplasia by Vaccination

The quadrivalent HPV recombinant vaccine (**Gardasil**) is recommended for all females 8–26 years of age, with a target age of 11–12.

- The vaccine uses noninfectious particles to protect against the 4 HPV types (6, 11, 16, 18) that cause 70% of cervical cancer and 90% of genital warts.
- Three doses are given: initial, then 2 months later, then 6 months later, for an approximate cost of $300.

Recommendations

- Administer to all females age 9–26, with a target age of 11–12. Efficacy is highest before the patient's immune system has been presented with HPV.
- Testing for HPV is not recommended before vaccination. No easy method of identifying all HPV types is currently available.
- Continue regular Pap smears according to current guidelines because the vaccine does not prevent against all HPV types that can cause genital warts or cervical cancer.
- Sexually active women can receive the vaccine. Women with previous abnormal cervical cytology or genital warts also can receive the vaccine, but it may be less effective. It can be given to patients with previous CIN, but benefits may be limited.
- The vaccine is not recommended for pregnant, lactating, or immunosuppressed women.

MÜLLERIAN ANOMALIES

Uterine anomalies have been divided into 7 types by the American Fertility Society (1988). This classification is based on the developmental problem responsible for the irregular shape. Uterine anomalies may result from 3 mechanisms:

Stage 1: failure of one or both of the 2 müllerian ducts to form

Stage 2: failure of the 2 ducts to fuse completely

Stage 3: failure of the 2 fused mullerian ducts to dissolve the septum that results from fusion

Failure to Form

Hypoplasia/Agenesis

- A woman may lack a vagina, a cervix (the bottom one-third of the uterus that opens into the vagina), the fallopian tubes, or the entire vagina and body of the uterus (except for the fundus). This occurs from a developmental problem with a section of both of the müllerian ducts.
- These anomalies are commonly associated with urinary tract anomalies because the structures that give rise to the urinary tract lie close to the müllerian ducts and are affected by the same injurious insult.

Unicornuate Uterus

- When one of the müllerian ducts fails to form, a single-horn (banana-shaped) uterus develops from the healthy müllerian duct. This single-horn uterus may stand alone. However, in 65% of women with a unicornuate uterus, the remaining müllerian duct may form an incomplete (rudimentary) horn.
- There may be no cavity in this rudimentary horn, or it may have a small space within it, but there is no opening that communicates with the unicornuate uterus and vagina.
- In the latter case, a girl may have monthly pain during adolescence because there is no outlet for the menses from this rudimentary horn. This pain would lead to identification of this problem. In some cases, the rudimentary horn contains a cavity that is continuous with the healthy single-horn uterus, but is much smaller than the cavity within the healthy uterus.
- There is a risk that a pregnancy will implant in this rudimentary horn, but because of space limitations, 90% of such pregnancies rupture.

Failure to Fuse

Didelphys Uterus

- A double uterus results from the complete failure of the 2 Müllerian ducts to fuse together (stage 1 of development). So each duct develops into a separate uterus, each of which is narrower than a normal uterus and has only a single horn.
- These 2 uteri may each have a cervix or they may share a cervix. In 67% of cases, a didelphys uterus is associated with 2 vaginas separated by a thin wall. Preterm delivery is common if pregnancy occurs in these patients.

Bicornuate Uterus

- This is the most common congenital uterine anomaly (45%). It results from failure of fusion between the müllerian ducts at the "top." This failure may be "complete," which results in 2 separate single-horn uterine bodies sharing one cervix.
- Alternatively, in a "partial" bicornuate uterus, fusion between the müllerian ducts had occurred at the "bottom" but not the "top." Thus, there is a single uterine cavity at the bottom with a single cervix, but it branches into 2 distinct horns at the top. Because the ducts never fused at the top, these 2 horns are separate structures when seen from the outside of the uterus.
- Preterm delivery and malpresentation are common with pregnancy.

Failure to Dissolve Septum

Septate Uterus

- A septate uterus results from a problem in stage 2 or 3 of uterine development. The two müllerian ducts fused normally; however, there was a failure in degeneration of the median septum.
- If this failure was "complete," a median septum persists in the entire uterus, separating the uterine cavity into two single-horned uteri that share one cervix.
- If this failure was "partial," resorption of the lower part of the median septum occurred in stage 2 but the top of the septum failed to dissolve in stage 3. Thus, there is a single cervix and uterine cavity at the bottom, but at the top that cavity divides into two distinct horns.
- Because this uterine anomaly occurs later in uterine development, after complete duct fusion, the external shape of the uterus is a normal-appearing single unit. This is distinct from the bicornuate uterus, which can be seen branching into two distinct horns when viewed from the outside.
- Preterm delivery and malpresentation are common with pregnancy.

Arcuate Uterus

This type of uterus is essentially normal in shape with a small midline indentation in the uterine fundus, which results from failure to dissolve the median septum completely.

- It is given a distinct classification because it does not seem to have any negative effects on pregnancy in regard to preterm labor or malpresentation.

DES Uterus

The daughters of mothers exposed to diethylstilbestrol (DES) during pregnancy are predisposed to uterine abnormalities and clear cell carcinoma of the vagina.

- Two-thirds have abnormalities, including a small, incompletely formed uterus ("hypoplastic") and/or a T-shaped cavity; and 50% have cervical defects, for example, an incompletely formed cervix that predisposes to cervical insufficiency. The mechanism by which DES disrupts normal uterine development is not known.

ENLARGED UTERUS

Leiomyoma Uteri

Location. It is a benign smooth muscle growth of the myometrium. It is the **most common** benign uterine tumor. It is 5 times more common in black women than white women. It can develop in a number of anatomic locations.

- **Intramural.** The **most common** location of a leiomyoma is within the wall of the uterus. When small it is usually asymptomatic and cannot be felt on examination unless it enlarges to where the normal uterine external contour is altered.
- **Submucosal.** These myomas are located beneath the endometrium and can distort the uterine cavity. The distorted overlying endometrium may not respond appropriately to the normal hormonal fluctuations, resulting in unpredictable, often intermenstrual, bleeding. Abnormal vaginal bleeding is the **most common** symptom of a submucosal myoma and can result in anemia. Menorrhagia is defined as heavy menses and metrorrhagia is defined as irregular bleeding in between menses. Menometrorrhagia consists of both heavy menses and bleeding in between the menses.
- **Subserosal.** These are located beneath the uterine serosa. As they grow they distort the external contour of the uterus causing the firm, nontender asymmetry. Depending on their location they can put pressure on the bladder, rectum or ureters. If they are pedunculated, attached to the uterus by a stalk, they can become parasitic fibroids. They break away from the uterus and receive their blood supply from another abdominal organ (such as the omentum or the mesentery of the intestine).

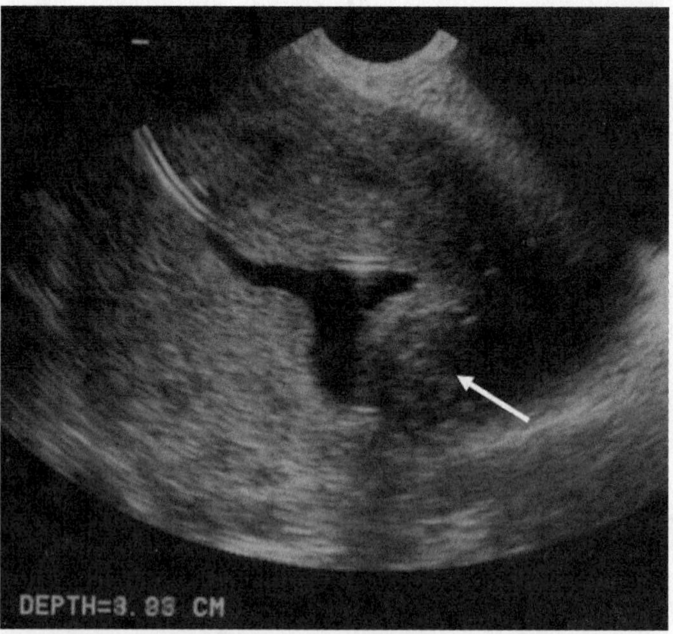

With permission Lyndon M. Hill, M.D., Magee Women's Hospital, iame.com

Figure II-4-11. Submucosal Leiomyoma

Natural History. Changes in size are dependent on the reproductive life stage of the woman.

- **Slow growth.** Most leiomyomas are small, grow slowly, and cause no symptoms. Only when massive in size do they cause pelvic pressure symptoms.
- **Rapid growth.** Estrogen receptors are increased in leiomyomas resulting in rapid enlargement during times of high estrogen levels, such as pregnancy.
- **Degeneration.** During times of rapid growth, myomas may outgrow their blood supply, resulting in ischemic degeneration of a fibroid. Common degenerations that are seen include hyaline, calcific, and red degeneration. The latter, also known as carneous degeneration, can cause such extreme, acute pain that the patient requires hospitalization and narcotics. This is **most common** during pregnancy.
- **Shrinkage.** When estrogen levels fall, with estrogen receptors no longer stimulated, leiomyomas will typically decrease in size. This predictably occurs after menopause but can also occur when estrogen levels are medically reduced through gonadotropin releasing hormone (GnRH) agonist suppression of follicle-stimulating hormone (FSH).

Diagnosis

- **Pelvic examination.** In most cases the diagnosis is made clinically by identifying an enlarged, asymmetric, nontender uterus in the absence of pregnancy. The size of the fibroid is compared with the size of a pregnant uterus. A pregnant uterus that reaches the umbilicus is approximately 20 weeks in gestation; if the pregnant uterus reaches the symphysis pubis, it is approximately 12 weeks in gestation.
- **Sonography.** Traditional abdominal or vaginal ultrasound can image large intramural or subserosal myomas. Saline infusion sonography is helpful for identifying submucosal myomas by instilling 5–10 mL of saline into the uterine cavity before visualizing the uterine cavity with an endovaginal sonogram probe.

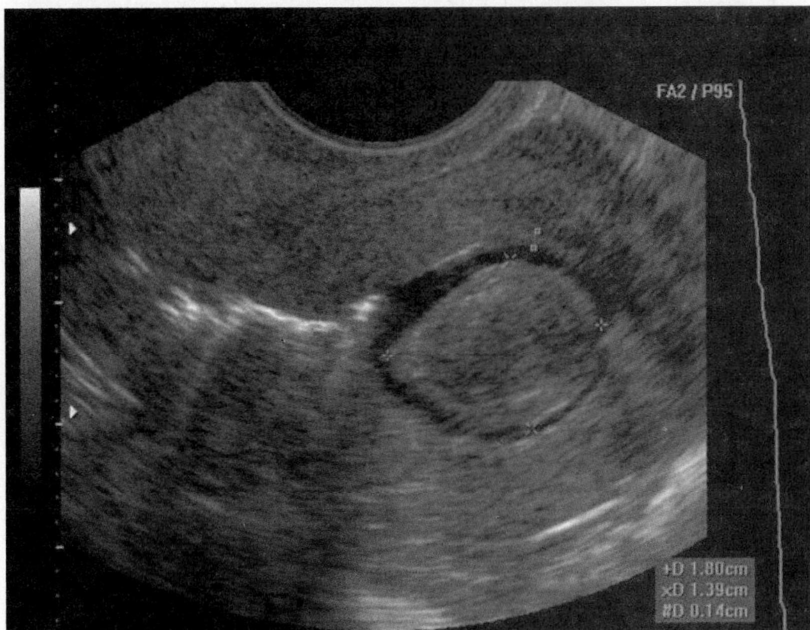

With permission Lyndon M. Hill, M.D., Magee Women's Hospital, iame.com

Figure II-4-12. Saline Ultrasonography Demonstrating an Intracavitary Leiomyoma

- **Hysteroscopy.** Submucosal myomas may be identified by visualizing them directly with hysteroscopy.
- **Histology.** The only definitive diagnosis is by surgical confirmation of excised tissue.

Management

- **Observation.** Most leiomyomas can be managed conservatively and followed expectantly with regular pelvic examinations.
- **Presurgical shrinkage.** After 3–6 months of GnRH analog therapy, with resultant hypoestrogenic state, a 60–70% reduction in size of the fibroids can be expected. However, once the leuprolide (Lupron) is terminated, there will be a regrowth of the fibroid within 6 months. Thus, GnRH analogs cannot be used for definitive cure, but they can be used in the adjuvant setting with surgical therapy. If a myomectomy is done, a decrease in size will be associated with a decrease in blood loss, and if a hysterectomy is planned, then perhaps a vaginal instead of an abdominal hysterectomy can be performed.
- **Myomectomy.** This is a surgical procedure performed if the patient desires to maintain fertility. The uterus is incised and the myoma removed through either a laparoscopic or laparotomy approach. If the myomectomy incision entered the endometrial cavity, delivery of any subsequent pregnancy should be by cesarean section because of increased risk of scar rupture in labor.
- **Embolization.** This is an invasive radiology procedure in which a catheter is placed into the vessels supplying the myoma. Microspheres are injected, causing ischemia and necrosis of the myoma.
- **Hysterectomy.** If the patient has completed her childbearing, definitive therapy is an abdominal or vaginal hysterectomy.

Table II-4-2. Management of Leiomyomas

Management	Clinical effect/Method of Treatment
Observation	Most Serial pelvic exams
Presurgical shrinkage	↓ size by 70% GnRH analog 3–6 months; regrowth after stopping
Myomectomy	Preserves fertility Laparotomy, laparoscopy
Embolization	Preserves uterus Invasive radiology
Hysterectomy	Fertility completed Total abdominal hysterectomy, total vaginal hysterectomy

Adenomyosis

A 42-year-old woman complains of increasing pain with her menstrual periods for the past 8 months. She also states her periods are getting heavier, leaving her tired and weak. She underwent a postpartum tubal ligation after her last child 10 years ago. She has been treated for chronic hypertension for the past 3 years. On pelvic examination her uterus is 12-week size, globular, soft, and tender. Rectovaginal examination is unremarkable.

Definition. Ectopic endometrial glands and stroma are located within the myometrium of the uterine wall. The **most common** presentation is diffuse involvement of the myometrium. The lesion is known as an **adenomyoma** if the involvement is focal, surrounded by a pseudocapsule.

Diagnosis. In most cases the diagnosis is made clinically by identifying an enlarged, symmetric, tender uterus in the absence of pregnancy. The only definitive diagnosis is by histologic confirmation of the surgically excised tissue.

Table II-4-3. Differential Diagnosis for Enlarged Non-pregnant Uterus

Leiomyoma	Adenomyosis
Asymmetric	Symmetric
Firm	Soft
Nontender	Tender

Symptoms. The majority of women are asymptomatic. The most common symptoms are secondary dysmenorrhea and menorrhagia.

Examination. The uterus is globular and diffusely up to 2–3 times the normal size. Tenderness is most common immediately before and during menses.

Imaging. Ultrasound study or MRI imaging shows a diffusely enlarged uterus with cystic areas found within the myometrial wall.

Management. Medical treatment includes the levonorgestrel (LNG) intrauterine system (IUS), which may decrease heavy menstrual bleeding. Surgery, in the form of hysterectomy, is the definitive treatment.

ENDOMETRIAL NEOPLASIA

Postmenopausal Bleeding

A 65-year-old patient complains of vaginal bleeding for 3 months. Her last menstrual period was at age 52. She has not taken any hormone replacement. She was diagnosed with type 2 diabetes 20 years ago and was treated with oral hypoglycemic agents. She has chronic hypertension, for which she is treated with oral antihypertensives. Her height is 62 inches and weight 200 lb. Physical examination is normal with a normal-sized uterus and no vulvar, vaginal, or cervical lesions.

Definition. A patient is considered to be in menopause after 3 continuous months of cessation of menses and elevated gonadotropins. Menopause usually occurs at approximately 52 years of age. Postmenopausal bleeding is any bleeding that occurs after menopause.

Epidemiology. Endometrial carcinoma is the **most common** gynecologic malignancy, occurring in 1% of women. The mean age at diagnosis is 61 years.

Differential Diagnosis. The differential diagnosis of postmenopausal bleeding includes endometrial carcinoma, vaginal or endometrial atrophy, and postmenopausal hormonal replacement therapy. Although the **most common** cause of postmenopausal bleeding is vaginal or endometrial atrophy, the most important diagnosis to rule out is endometrial carcinoma.

Pathophysiology. The mediating factor for most endometrial carcinomas appears to be unopposed estrogen. This results from excessive hyperstimulation of the endometrium without the stabilizing effect of progesterone.

Risk Factors. These include **obesity**, **hypertension**, and **diabetes mellitus**. Other risk factors include nulliparity, late menopause, and chronic anovulation conditions, such as PCO disease.

Diagnostic Tests: Either endometrial biopsy or transvaginal U/S can be used as an initial test for evaluating the endometrium.

- **Endometrial sampling.** This office procedure has historically been the initial diagnostic test for postmenopausal bleeding, due its high sensitivity, low complication rate, and low cost. It is ideal for global lesions but not very sensitive for diagnosing localized structural lesions such as polyps or submucus leiomyomas.
- **Transvaginal sonogram.** This is an acceptable alternative initial test for non-persistent minimal bleeding in women who are not on hormone replacement. A thin, homogenous endometrial stripe <5 mm can reasonably exclude endometrial carcinoma. A thicker endometrial stripe warrants further assessment with an endometrial sampling.
- **Hysteroscopy.** This procedure allows direct visualization of the endocervical canal and endometrial cavity. Endocervical or endometrial polyps, or submucus leiomyomas, can be removed at the time of the hysteroscopy.

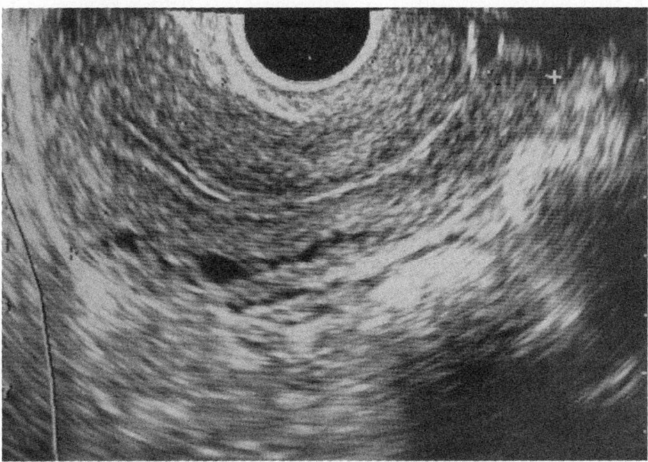

With permission, Brookside Associates, brooksidepress.org

Figure II-4-13. Ultrasonography Demonstrating Normal Endometrial Stripe (<5 mm)

Staging

Staging is done after an evaluation of the pathology report. Staging is surgical.

- Stage I: Spread **limited** to the uterus (**most common** stage at diagnosis)
  - IA. Limited to the endometrium or invasion less than half of myometrium
  - IB. Invasion more than half of myometrium
- Stage II: Extension to the cervix but not outside the uterus
- Stage III: Spread **adjacent** to the uterus
  - IIIA. Invades serosa or adnexa or positive cytology
  - IIIB. Invasion of vagina
  - IIIC. Invasion of pelvic or para-aortic nodes
- Stage IV: Spread **further** from the uterus
  - IVA. Involves bladder or rectum
  - IVB. Distant metastasis

Management. If the endometrial histology sampling reveals atrophy and no evidence of cancer, it can be assumed the patient is bleeding from atrophy and can be treated with hormone replacement therapy. With hormone replacement therapy, estrogen and progesterone should be given to the patient. If estrogen is given alone, the risk of endometrial cancer increases.

If the endometrial sampling reveals adenocarcinoma, the patient should be treated surgically.

- **Surgical therapy.** The mainstay of treatment of endometrial carcinoma is a total abdominal hysterectomy (TAH) and bilateral salpingo-oophorectomy (BSO), pelvic and para-aortic lymphadenectomy, and peritoneal washings.
- **Radiation therapy.** An evaluation of the postoperative pathology report will classify patients into poor or good prognosis. Patients with poor prognosis should be considered for radiation therapy. Poor prognostic factors include metastasis to lymph nodes, >50% myometrial invasion, positive surgical margins, or poorly differentiated histology.
- **Chemotherapy.** Medical treatment is used for metastatic disease and involves **progestins** and cytotoxic agents.

Table II-4-4. Endometrial Carcinoma Management

TAH-BSO: Basic Treatment for All Stages		
Stage I	TAH BSO Lymph node dissection	—
Stage II		Radiation
Stage III		Radiation, chemotherapy
Stage IV		

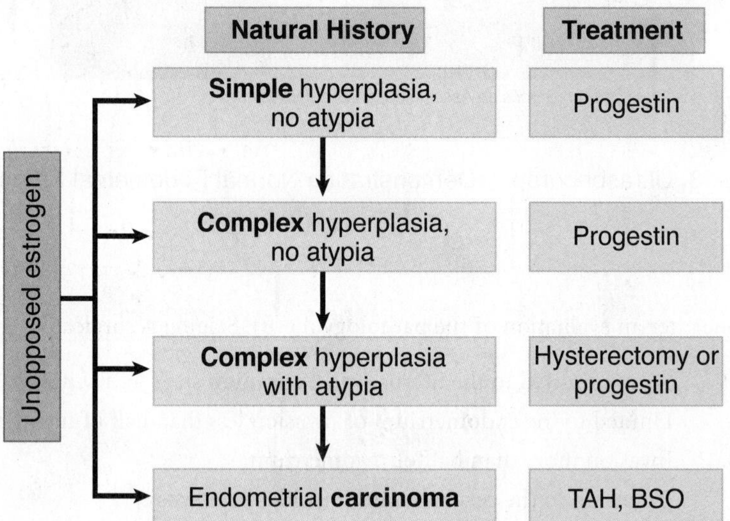

Figure II-4-14. Management of Endometrial Hyperplasia

Prevention

Postmenopausal patients taking estrogen replacement therapy must be also treated with progestins to prevent unopposed estrogen stimulation, which may lead to endometrial cancer.

Reproductive age women who have chronic anovulation, such as PCO syndrome, should also be treated with progestins to avoid endometrial hyperplasia from unopposed estrogen.

Disorders of the Ovaries and Oviducts

5

Learning Objectives

- ❑ Differentiate between physiologic enlargement of the adnexa and abnormal enlargement or painful adnexal mass
- ❑ List the causes of pelvic mass found prepubertal, premenopausal, and postmenopausal

PHYSIOLOGIC ENLARGEMENT

Functional Cysts

A 22-year-old woman comes for annual examination and requests oral contraceptives pills. On pelvic examination, a 6-cm mobile, smooth, soft, left adnexal mass is palpable. An endovaginal pelvic ultrasound shows a 6-cm, round, fluid-filled, simple ovarian cyst without septations or calcifications. She has no other significant personal or family history.

Definition. The **most common** cause of a simple cystic mass in the reproductive age years is a physiologic cyst (luteal or follicular cyst). During the reproductive years the ovaries are functionally active, producing a dominant follicle in the first half of the cycle and a corpus luteum after ovulation in the second half of the menstrual cycle. Either of these structures, the follicle or the corpus luteum, can become fluid-filled and enlarged, producing a functional cyst.

Differential Diagnosis

- **Pregnancy.** The **most common** cause of a pelvic mass in the reproductive years is pregnancy.
- **Complex mass.** The **most common** complex adnexal mass in young women is a dermoid cyst or benign cystic teratoma. Other diagnoses include endometrioma, tubo-ovarian abscess, and ovarian cancer.

Diagnosis

- **Qualitative b-human chorionic gonadotropin (β-hCG) test.** If negative, this will rule out pregnancy.
- **Sonogram.** A complex mass on ultrasound appearance is incompatible with a functional cyst.

GYN Triad

Functional Ovarian Cyst

- Pelvic mass in reproductive years
- β-hCG (–)
- Sonogram: fluid-filled ovarian simple cyst

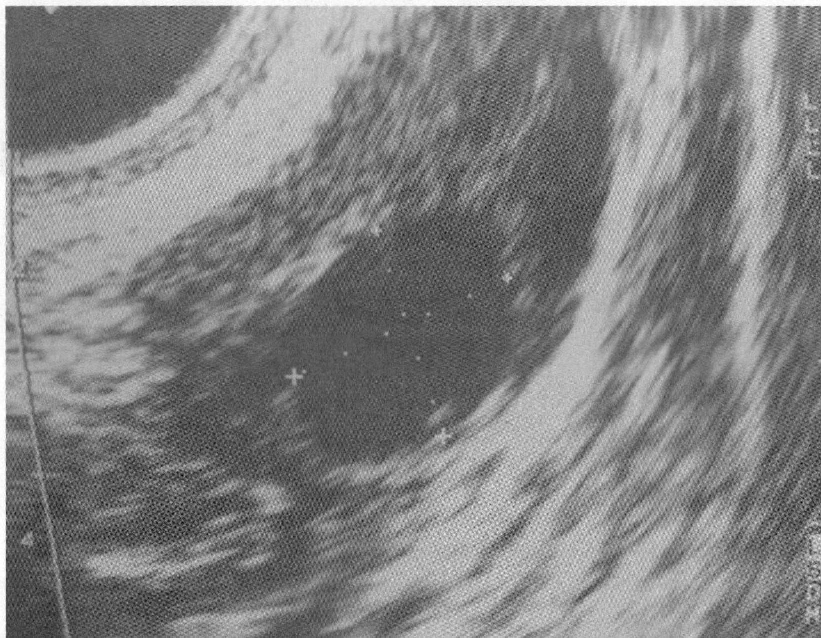

With permission, Brookside Associates, brooksidepress.org

Figure II-5-1. Ultrasonographic Appearance of a Functional Cyst

Management. Most functional cysts can be managed expectantly, but surgery is indicated if certain characteristics are present.

- **Observation.** If the sonogram shows a simple cyst it is probably benign but careful follow-up is needed. Follow-up examination should be in 6–8 weeks, at which time the functional cyst should have spontaneously resolved. During this period of observation the patient should be alerted to the possibility of acute onset of pain, which may be indicative of torsion of the adnexal cyst. Oral contraceptive medication can be used to help prevent further functional cysts from forming.
- **Laparoscopy.** Even if the cyst is simple in appearance, surgical evaluation should be performed if the cyst is >7 cm or if patient had been on prior steroid contraception. Physiologic cysts do not usually get larger than 7 cm in diameter. Functional cysts should not form if the patient has been on oral contraception for at least 2 months because gonadotropins should have been suppressed.

Polycystic Ovarian Syndrome

The ovaries are bilaterally enlarged with multiple peripheral cysts (20-100 in each ovary). This is due to high circulating androgens and high circulating insulin levels causing arrest of follicular development in various stages. This along with stromal hyperplasia and a thickened ovarian capsule results in enlarged ovaries bilaterally. PCOS is associated with **valproic acid** use. Management is conservative regarding ovaries. For further discussion of PCOS pathophysiology and treatment, refer to chapter 12, Hormonal Disorders.

Ovarian Hyperthecosis

Definition. Ovarian hyperthecosis refers to the presence of nests of luteinized theca cells in the ovarian stroma that may be steroidogenically active. These nests, or islands, of luteinized theca cells are scattered throughout the stroma of the ovary, rather than being confined to areas around cystic follicles, as in polycystic ovary syndrome (PCOS). The result is greater production of androgens.

- Why hyperthecosis occurs is not known.
- The ovarian secretion of large amounts of androgen in women with hyperthecosis means that peripheral estrogen production is increased. As a result, the risks of endometrial hyperplasia and endometrial carcinoma are increased, especially in postmenopausal women.

Findings. The clinical features of hyperthecosis are similar to PCOS, and most patients are obese. However, women with ovarian hyperthecosis have more severe hirsutism, with shaving being common. Virilization is frequent, with clitoral enlargement, temporal balding, deepening of the voice, and a male habitus.

- Most patients have amenorrhea, and the remainder have irregular and anovulatory cycles. Most patients will have severe insulin resistance with high risk of type 2 diabetes mellitus and cardiovascular disease.
- Unlike PCOS, which occurs only during the reproductive years, hyperthecosis of the ovaries can occur in postmenopausal women. Severe hirsutism and virilization in postmenopausal women are more often due to ovarian hyperthecosis than to virilizing ovarian tumors.

Management. Treatment is similar to that for hirsutism, using oral contraceptive pills both to suppress androgen production (by reducing LH stimulation of the theca cells) and to decrease free androgens (by stimulating sex hormone binding globulin).

Luteoma of Pregnancy

Luteoma of pregnancy is a rare, **non-neoplastic tumor-like mass** of the ovary that emerges during pregnancy and **regresses spontaneously** after delivery. It is usually **asymptomatic** and is found **incidentally** during a cesarean section or postpartum tubal ligation. It can be **hormonally active** and produce **androgens** resulting in maternal and fetal hirsutism and virilization.

Theca Lutein Cysts

These are benign neoplasms stimulated by **high levels of FSH and β-hCG**. They are **associated with twins** and **molar** pregnancies but they are only rarely associated with a normal singleton pregnancy. The **natural course** of these tumors is postpartum **spontaneous regression and require only conservative managment**.

PREPUBERTAL PELVIC MASS

> An 8-year-old girl is evaluated in the emergency department for sudden onset of severe lower abdominal pain. A general surgery consult was obtained, and appendicitis is ruled out. Pelvic ultrasound reveals a 7-cm solid and irregular right adnexal mass. Pelvic examination is consistent with a 7-cm right adnexal mass, and there is lower abdominal tenderness but no rebound present.

Etiology. An adnexal mass in the prepubertal age group is abnormal. During the prepubertal and the postmenopausal years, functional ovarian cysts are not possible because ovarian follicles are not functioning. Therefore any ovarian enlargement is suspicious for neoplasm.

Differential Diagnosis. If sonography shows a complex adnexal mass in a girl or teenager, the possibility of **germ cell** tumors of the ovary has to be considered. The following serum **tumor markers** should be obtained: lactate dehydrogenase (LDH) for dysgerminoma, β-hCG for choriocarcinoma, and α-fetoprotein for endodermal sinus tumor.

Presentation. Sudden onset of acute abdominal pain is a typical presentation of germ cell tumors of the ovary. These tumors characteristically grow rapidly and give early symptomatology as opposed to the epithelial cancers of the ovary that are diagnosed in advanced stages. Germ cell tumors of the ovary are **most common** in young women and present in early stage disease.

Diagnosis. Surgical exploration. In a prepubertal patient who is symptomatic and has ultrasound evidence of an adnexal mass, a surgical evaluation is recommended.

- **Simple mass.** If the ultrasound shows the consistency of the mass to be simple (no septations or solid components), this mass can be evaluated through a laparoscopic approach.
- **Complex mass.** If the mass has septations or solid components, a laparoscopy or laparotomy should be performed, depending on the experience of the surgeon.

Table II-5-1. Prepubertal Pelvic Mass

Surgical diagnosis	Simple cyst	Laparoscopy
	Complex mass	Laparotomy
Management	Benign	Cystectomy Annual followup
	Malignant	Unilateral S&O Staging, chemotherapy
Prognosis	95% survival with chemotherapy	

Definition of abbreviations: S&O, Salpingo-oophorectomy.

Management

- **Benign histology.** A cystectomy should be performed instead of a salpingo-oophorectomy. Because of the patient's age the surgical goal should be toward conservation of both ovaries. If the frozen section pathology analysis is benign, no further surgery is needed. **Follow-up** is on an annual basis.

- **Germ cell tumor.** A unilateral salpingo-oophorectomy and surgical staging (peritoneal and diaphragmatic biopsies, peritoneal cytology, pelvic and para-aortic lymphadenectomy, and omentectomy) should be done. All patients with germ cell tumors require postoperative chemotherapy. The most active regimen used is vinblastine, bleomycin, and cisplatin. Follow-up after conservative surgery is every 3 months with pelvic examination and tumor marker measurements.

Prognosis. The current survival is >95% in patients with germ cell tumors managed with conservative management and chemotherapy. Before the chemotherapy age the majority of these patients succumbed to their disease.

PREMENOPAUSAL PELVIC MASS

Complex Mass

A 28-year-old woman is in the emergency department complaining of lower abdominal discomfort the last 5 days. She has no history of steroid contraceptive use. A year ago, her pelvic exam and Pap smear were negative. Pelvic exam today shows a 7-cm, mobile, painless right adnexal mass. An endovaginal sonogram in the emergency department confirms a 7-cm, mobile, irregular complex mass with prominent calcifications.

GYN Triad

Dysgerminoma

- **Solid** pelvic mass in reproductive years
- β-hCG (–)
- ↑ LDH level

Definition. The **most common** complex adnexal mass in young women is a dermoid cyst or benign cystic teratoma (discussed below). Other diagnoses include endometrioma, tubo-ovarian abscess, and ovarian cancer.

Differential Diagnosis

- Pregnancy
- Functional cysts

Diagnosis.

- **Qualitative β-human chorionic gonadotropin (β-hCG)** test to rule out pregnancy.
- The appearance of a complex mass on ultrasound will rule out a functional cyst.

Management. Patients in the reproductive age group with a complex adnexal mass should be treated surgically. The surgery can be done by a laparoscopy or a laparotomy according to the experience of the surgeon.

- **Cystectomy.** At the time of surgery an ovarian cystectomy should be attempted to preserve ovarian function in the reproductive age. Careful evaluation of the opposite adnexa should be performed, as dermoid cysts can occur bilaterally in 10–15% of cases.
- **Oophorectomy.** If an ovarian cystectomy cannot be done because of the size of the dermoid cyst, then an oophorectomy is performed, but conservative management should always be attempted before an oophorectomy is done.

GYN Triad

Benign Cystic Teratoma

- Pelvic mass: reproductive years
- β-hCG (–)
- Sonogram: complex mass, calcifications

Benign cystic teratoma

Dermoid cysts are benign tumors. They can contain cellular tissue from all 3 germ layers. The most common histology seen is ectodermal skin appendages (hair, sebaceous glands), and therefore the name "dermoid." Gastrointestinal histology can be identified, and carcinoid syndrome has been described originating from a dermoid cyst. Thyroid tissue can also be identified, and if it comprises more than 50% of the dermoid, then the condition of struma ovarii is identified. Rarely, a malignancy can originate from a dermoid cyst, in which case the most common histology would be squamous cell carcinoma, which can metastasize.

PAINFUL ADNEXAL MASS

> A 31-year-old woman is taken to the emergency department complaining of severe sudden lower abdominal pain for approximately 3 h. She was at work when she suddenly developed lower abdominal discomfort and pain, which got progressively worse. On examination the abdomen is tender, although no rebound tenderness is present, and there is a suggestion of an adnexal mass in the cul-de-sac area. Ultrasound shows an 8-cm left adnexal mass with a suggestion of torsion of the ovary.

GYN Triad

Ovarian Torsion

- Abrupt **unilateral** pelvic pain
- β-hCG (–)
- Sonogram: >7 cm adnexal mass

Diagnosis. Sudden onset of severe lower abdominal pain in the presence of an adnexal mass is presumptive evidence of ovarian torsion.

Management. The management of the torsion should be to untwist the ovary and observe the ovary for a few minutes in the operating room to assure revitalization. This can be performed with laparoscopy or laparotomy.

- **Cystectomy.** If revitalization occurs, an ovarian cystectomy can be performed with preservation of the ovary.
- **Oophorectomy.** If the ovary is necrotic, a unilateral salpingo-oophorectomy is performed.

Follow-Up. Patients should have routine examination 4 weeks after the operation and then should be seen on a yearly basis. The pathology report should be checked carefully to make sure that it is benign, and if this is the case, then they go to routine follow-up.

POSTMENOPAUSAL PELVIC MASS

> A 70-year-old woman comes for annual examination. She complains of lower abdominal discomfort; however, there is no weight loss or abdominal distention. On pelvic examination a nontender, 6-cm, solid, irregular, fixed, left adnexal mass is found. Her last examination was 1 year ago, which was normal.

Definition. A pelvic mass identified after menopause. Ovaries in the postmenopausal age group should be atrophic; anytime they are enlarged, the suspicion of **ovarian cancer** arises.

Diagnostic Tests

- **GI tract lesions.** Abdominal pelvic CT scan or a pelvic ultrasound, and GI studies (barium enema) to rule out any intestinal pathology such as diverticular disease
- **Urinary tract lesions.** IVP to identify any impingement of the urinary tract

Screening Test. There is no current screening test for ovarian cancer. Pelvic ultrasound is excellent for finding pelvic masses, but is not specific for identifying which are benign and which are malignant. Only 3% of patients undergoing laparotomy for sonographically detected pelvic masses actually have ovarian cancer.

Epidemiology. Ovarian carcinoma is the **second most common** gynecologic malignancy, with a mean age at diagnosis of 69 years. One percent of women die of ovarian cancer. It is the **most common** gynecologic cancer leading to death.

Risk Factors. These include **BRCA1 gene**, positive family history, high number of lifetime ovulations, infertility, and use of perineal talc powder.

Protective Factors. These are conditions that decrease the total number of lifetime ovulations: oral contraceptive pills, chronic anovulation, breast-feeding, and short reproductive life.

Classification of Ovarian Cancer

- **Epithelial tumors—80%.** The **most common** type of histologic ovarian carcinoma is epithelial cancer, which predominantly occurs in postmenopausal women. These include serous, mucinous, Brenner, endometrioid, and clear cell tumors. The **most common** malignant epithelial cell type is **serous.**
- **Germ cell tumors—15%.** Another histologic type of ovarian cancer is the germ cell tumor, which predominantly occurs in teenagers. Examples are dysgerminoma, endodermal sinus tumors, teratomas, and choriocarcinoma. The **most common** malignant germ cell type is **dysgerminoma.** It is uniquely x-ray sensitive.
- **Stromal tumors—5%.** The third type of ovarian tumor is the stromal tumor, which is functionally active. These include granulosa-theca cell tumors, which secrete estrogen and can cause bleeding from endometrial hyperplasia and Sertoli-Leydig cell tumors, which secrete testosterone and can produce masculinization syndromes. Patients with stromal tumors usually present with early stage disease and are treated either with removal of the involved adnexa (for patients who desire further fertility) or a TAH and BSO (if their family has been completed). They metastasize infrequently, and then they require chemotherapy (vincristine, actinomycin, and Cytoxan).
- **Metastatic tumor.** These are cancers from a primary site other than the ovary. The **most common** sources are the endometrium, GI tract, and breast. **Krukenberg tumors** are mucin-producing tumors from the stomach or breast metastatic to the ovary.

GYN Triad

Serous Carcinoma

- Postmenopausal woman
- Pelvic mass
- ↑ CEA or CA-125 level

GYN Triad

Choriocarcinoma

- Postmenopausal woman
- Pelvic mass
- ↑ hCG level

GYN Triad

Sertoli-Leydig Tumor

- Postmenopausal pelvic mass
- Masculinization
- ↑ testosterone level

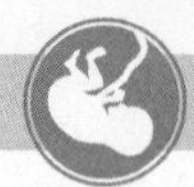

GYN Triad

Endometrial Carcinoma Metastatic to Ovaries

- Postmenopausal woman with **bilateral** pelvic masses
- Postmenopausal bleeding
- Enlarged uterus

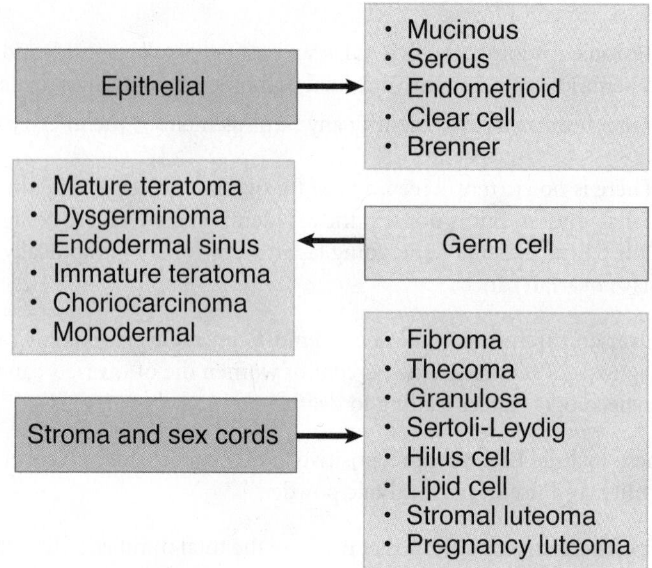

Figure II-5-2. Overview of Ovarian Oncology

Table II-5-2. Classic Histology Types of Ovarian Cancer

Type	Percentage	Age Group
Epithelial	80%	Older
Germ cell	15%	Young
Stromal	5%	All

Tumor Markers

- **CA-125** (cancer antigen 125) and **CEA** (carcinoembryonic antigen) should also be drawn for the possibility of ovarian epithelial cancer.
- **LDH, hCG,** and **α-fetoprotein** should be drawn for the possibility of germ cell tumors.
- **Estrogen** and **testosterone** should be drawn for the possibility of stromal tumors.

Staging. Staging is surgical.

Stage I: Spread limited to the **ovaries**
- IA. Limited to one ovary, capsule intact, negative cytology
- IB. Limited to both ovaries, capsules intact, negative cytology
- IC. One or both ovaries but ruptured capsule, positive cytology

Stage II: Extension to the **pelvis**
- IIA. Extension to uterus or tubes
- IIB. Extension to other pelvic structures
- IIC. Extension to pelvis with positive cytology

Stage III: **Peritoneal** metastases or positive nodes. This is the **most common** stage at diagnosis.

- IIIA. Microscopic peritoneal metastases
- IIIB. Macroscopic peritoneal metastases ≤2 cm
- IIIC. Macroscopic peritoneal metastases >2 cm

Stage IV: **Distant** metastases

- IVA. Involves bladder or rectum
- IVB. Distant metastasis

Management. A surgical exploration should follow preoperative studies and medical evaluation. If abdominal or pelvic CT scan shows no evidence of ascites or spread to the abdominal cavity, and if the surgeon is an experienced laparoscopist, then the evaluation could be performed laparoscopically. At the time of surgery, a unilateral salpingo-oophorectomy (USO) is done and sent for frozen section.

Benign Histology. If the patient is not a good surgical candidate or the patient desires to maintain her uterus and contralateral ovary, a USO is sufficient treatment. If the USO by frozen section is benign and the patient is a good surgical candidate, then a TAH and BSO may be performed even though it is benign disease because the uterus and ovaries are not unusual sites of pathology in a woman.

Malignant Histology. In this case, a debulking procedure (cytoreduction) should be performed. This procedure consists of a TAH and BSO, omentectomy, and bowel resection, if necessary. Postoperative chemotherapy (carboplatin and Taxol) should be administered.

Follow-Up. If the final pathology report of the enlarged adnexa was benign, the patient can be followed up in the office on a yearly basis for regular examination. If the pathology report was carcinoma, then she would be followed up every 3 months for the first 2 years and then every 6 months for the next 2 years with follow-up of the CA-125 tumor marker.

Borderline Cancers. Another entity of ovarian cancer is the borderline tumors also known as tumors of low malignant potential. These are characterized by no invasion of the basement membrane and can also be treated conservatively.

- **Conservative surgery.** A patient who desires further fertility with a unilateral borderline cancer of the ovary can be treated with a USO with preservation of the uterus and the opposite adnexa.
- **Aggressive surgery.** If the patient has completed her family then the most acceptable treatment would be a TAH and BSO.
- **Chemotherapy.** Patients with borderline cancer of the ovary do not require chemotherapy unless they have metastasis, and this is a rare occurrence.

Adnexal Mass With Ascites

A 65-year-old woman is referred for evaluation of abdominal distention and ascites and an adnexal mass. The patient has noted abdominal distention for the past 6 months, and on pelvic examination there is a 7-cm irregular and solid mass in the cul-de-sac, which is palpable by rectovaginal examination.

GYN Triad

Ovarian Carcinoma with Peritoneal Metastasis

- Postmenopausal bilateral pelvic masses
- Weight gain, anorexia
- Abdominal "shifting dullness"

Definition. Ascites is an abdominal accumulation of fluid in the peritoneal cavity, which usually causes abdominal distention.

Differential Diagnosis. The etiology of ascites can be multifactorial and includes heart, kidney, and liver disease and ovarian cancer. In a female patient with ascites, ovarian carcinoma must always be considered. Although the etiology of ovarian carcinoma is not known, ovulation inhibition, as occurs with OCPs or pregnancy, does decrease the risk of epithelial ovarian cancer. **Meigs syndrome** is the triad of ascites, pleural effusion, and benign ovarian fibroma.

Laboratory Abnormalities/Diagnostic Criteria. In a patient with an adnexal mass and ascites, an abdominal pelvic CT scan should be ordered for evaluation of the upper abdomen. The **most common** method of ovarian carcinoma spread is by peritoneal dissemination (exfoliation) and is commonly seen metastatic to the omentum and to the GI tract. The cause of death of patients with advanced ovarian carcinoma is bowel obstruction.

Management Steps

- **Surgical staging.** After an abdominal pelvic CT scan confirms the presence of ascites and the adnexal mass, an exploratory laparotomy and surgical staging should be performed. A salpingo-oophorectomy of the enlarged ovary should be done and sent for frozen section evaluation.
- **Debulking surgery.** If ovarian carcinoma is confirmed, then a debulking (cytoreductive) surgical procedure should be performed. This procedure usually includes a TAH, BSO, omentectomy, and, frequently, bowel resection.
- **Chemotherapy.** Postoperatively patients should be treated with 6 courses of a standard chemotherapy regimen, which includes Taxol and carboplatin. Patients are followed with the tumor marker CA-125.

Gestational Trophoblastic Neoplasia 6

Learning Objectives

❏ Explain origin of gestational trophoblastic neoplasia

GESTATIONAL TROPHOBLASTIC NEOPLASIA (GTN)

A 24-year-old Filipino nurse is 14 weeks pregnant by dates. She complains of vaginal bleeding as well as severe nausea and vomiting. Her uterus extends to her umbilicus but no fetal heart tones can be heard. Her blood pressure is 150/95. A dipstick urine shows 2+ proteinuria.

GYN Triad

Molar Pregnancy

- Pregnancy <20 weeks
- HTN and proteinuria
- No fetal heart tones (FHT)

Definition. GTN, or **molar pregnancy**, is an abnormal proliferation of placental tissue involving both the cytotrophoblast and/or syncytiotrophoblast. It can be benign or malignant. Malignant GTN can be characterized as either localized or metastatic as well as classified into either **Good Prognosis** or **Poor Prognosis**.

GYN Triad

Molar Pregnancy

- Pregnancy <20 weeks
- HTN and proteinuria
- Vaginal passage of vesicles

Classification

- **Benign GTN** is the classic hydatidiform mole (H-mole). Incidence is 1:1200 in the US, but 1:120 in the Far East.
  - **Complete mole** is the most common benign GTN. It results from fertilization of an empty egg with a single X sperm resulting in paternally derived (androgenetic) **normal 46,XX** karyotype. No fetus, umbilical cord or amniotic fluid is seen. The uterus is filled with grape-like vesicles composed of edematous avascular villi. Progression to malignancy is 20%.
  - **Incomplete mole** is the less common benign GTN. It results from fertilization of a normal egg with two sperm resulting in **triploid 69,XXY** karyotype. A fetus, umbilical cord and amniotic fluid is seen which results ultimately in fetal demise. Progression to malignancy is 10%.
- **Malignant GTN** is the gestational trophoblastic tumor (**GTT**) which can develop in 3 categories.
  - **Non-metastatic disease** is localized only to the uterus.
  - **Good Prognosis metastatic disease** has distant metastasis with the most common location being the pelvis or lung. Cure rate is >95%.
  - **Poor Prognosis metastatic disease** has distant metastasis with the most common location being the brain or the liver. Other poor prognosis factors are serum β-hCG levels >40,000, >4 months from the antecedent pregnancy, and following a term pregnancy. Cure rate is 65%.

Table II-6-1. Benign Gestational Trophoblastic Neoplasia—H Mole

Complete	Incomplete
Empty egg	Normal egg
Paternal X's only	Maternal and paternal X's
46,XX (**di**ploidy)	69,XXY (**tri**ploidy)
Fetus absent	Fetus nonviable
20% → malignancy	10% → malignancy
No chemotherapy; serial β-hCG titers until (–); follow-up 1 year on oral contraceptive pill	

Table II-6-2. Malignant Gestational Trophoblastic Neoplasia

Nonmetastatic	Good Prognosis	Poor Prognosis
Uterus only	Pelvis or lung	Brain or liver
100% cure	>95% cure	65% cure
Single-agent chemotherapy		Multiple agent chemotherapy
1 year follow-up on oral contraceptive pill after β-hCG (–)		5 year follow-up on oral contraceptive pill

Risk Factors. Increased prevalence **geographically** is most common in **Taiwan** and the **Philippines**. Other risk factors are maternal age extremes (<20 years old, >35 years old) and folate deficiency.

Clinical Findings

- **The most common** symptom is bleeding prior to 16 weeks' gestation and passage of vesicles from the vagina. Other symptoms of a molar pregnancy include hypertension, hyperthyroidism, and hyperemesis gravidarum, and no fetal heart tones appreciated.
- The **most common** sign is fundus larger than dates, absence of fetal heart tones, bilateral cystic enlargements of the ovary known as **theca-lutein cysts.**
- The **most common site of distant metastasis** is the **lungs.**

Diagnosis. "Snowstorm" ultrasound. The diagnosis is confirmed with sonogram showing homogenous intrauterine echoes without a gestational sac or fetal parts.

Management

- Baseline quantitative β-hCG titer
- Chest X-ray to rule out lung metastasis
- Suction D&C to evacuate the uterine contents

Place the patient on effective contraception (oral contraceptive pills) for the duration of the follow-up period to ensure no confusion between rising β-hCG titers from recurrent disease and normal pregnancy.

Table II-6-3. Gestational Trophoblastic Neoplasia—Basic Approach

β-hCG titer	Baseline for future comparison
Chest x-ray	Lung metastasis is ruled out
Suction D&C	Empty uterus contents
Oral contraceptive pills for 1 year	Prevent confusion: recurrent disease and normal pregnancy

- Treatment is then based on histology and location of metastasis.
  - **Benign GTN:** Weekly serial β-hCG titers until negative for 3 weeks, then monthly titers until negative for 12 months. **Follow-up is for 1 year.** If serial β-hCG titers plateau or rise and normal intrauterine pregnancy is ruled out by vaginal sonogram, the patients are diagnosed with persistent gestational trophoblastic disease. They should undergo a metastatic workup (CT scans of the brain, the thorax, the abdomen and the pelvis) and be managed as below.
  - **Non-metastatic or Good Prognosis metastatic disease: Single agent** (**methotrexate** or actinomycin D) until weekly β-hCG titers become negative for 3 weeks, then monthly titers until negative for 12 months. **Follow-up is for 1 year.**
  - **Poor Prognosis metastatic disease: Multiple agent** chemotherapy (which includes methotrexate, actinomycin-D and cytoxan) until weekly β-hCG titers become negative for 3 weeks, then monthly titers for 2 years, then every 3 months for another 3 years. F**ollow-up is for 5 years.**

Table II-6-4. Gynecologic Malignancy

Clinical staging	Cervical cancer
Surgical staging	Endometrial, ovarian, vulvar, and trophoblastic cancer

Sexually Transmitted Diseases 7

Learning Objectives

- ❑ Give an overview of the organisms involved in STDs
- ❑ Differentiate between STDs with and without ulcers
- ❑ Explain the role of azithromycin in treating STDs
- ❑ Describe what is known about the sexual transmission of hepatitis B and HIV

SPECTRUM OF ORGANISMS

Bacterial. These include chancroid, lymphogranuloma venereum, granuloma inguinale, chlamydia, gonorrhea, syphilis.

Viral. These include condyloma acuminatum, herpes simplex, hepatitis B virus, and human immunodeficiency virus.

Protozoan. This includes trichomoniasis.

STDs WITH ULCERS

Herpes Simplex Virus (HSV)

Refer to Obstetrics, Chapter 7, Perinatal Infections.

Syphilis

Refer to Obstetrics, Chapter 7, Perinatal Infections.

Chancroid

Chancroid is caused by *Haemophilus ducreyi*, a Gram-negative bacterium. It is uncommon in the United States. It is a cofactor for HIV transmission.

Symptoms. This is one of the two STDs that presents with a **painful** ulcer. A pustule, usually on the vulva, becomes a painful ulcer within 72 hours, with a typically "ragged edge."

Diagnosis. A positive culture confirms the diagnosis, although a diagnosis is often made clinically after excluding syphilis and genital herpes.

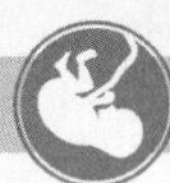

Management. CDC-recommended treatment includes a single oral dose of azithromycin, a single IM dose of ceftriaxone, or oral erythromycin base for 7 days.

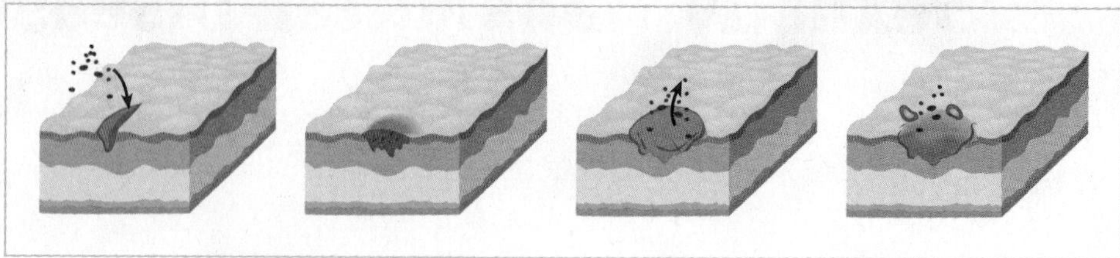

Figure II-7-1. Pathophysiology of Chancroids

Lymphogranuloma Venereum (LGV)

LGV is caused by the L serotype of *Chlamydia trachomatis.* It is uncommon in the United States.

Symptoms. The initial lesion is a **painless** ulcer.

Examination. A painless vesiculopustular eruption, usually on the vulva, spontaneously heals. This is replaced within a few weeks by perirectal adenopathy that can lead to abscesses and fistula formation. The classic clinical lesion is a double genitocrural fold, the "groove sign."

Diagnosis. A positive culture of pus aspirated from a lymph node confirms the diagnosis.

Management. CDC-recommended treatment includes oral doxycycline or erythromycin for 3 weeks.

Granuloma Inguinale (Donovanosis)

This disease is caused by *Calymmatobacterium granulomatis*, a Gram-negative intracellular bacterium. It is uncommon in the United States.

Symptoms. The initial lesion is a **painless** ulcer.

Examination. A vulvar nodule breaks down, forming a painless, beefy red, highly vascular ulcer with fresh granulation tissue without regional lymphadenopathy. Lymphatic obstruction can result in marked vulvar enlargement. Chronic scarring can lead to lymphatic obstruction.

Diagnosis. Culture of the organism is difficult but microscopic examination of an ulcer smear will reveal Donovan bodies.

Management. CDC-recommended treatment includes oral doxycycline or azithromycin for 3 weeks.

AZITHROMYCIN

Table II-7-1. Comparison of STDs

With Ulcers	No Ulcers	Painful Ulcers
Chancroid Granuloma inguinale Genital herpes LGV Syphilis	Chlamydia HPV Gonorrhea Hepatitis B HIV	Chancroid Genital herpes

Table II-7-2. Comparison of STDs with Ulcers

Chancroid (painful)	Ragged, soft edge inflamed
LGV	Groove sign
Granuloma inguinale	Beefy red; Donovan bodies
Syphilis	Rolled, hard edge
Herpes (painful)	Smooth edge inflamed

STDs WITHOUT ULCERS

Condyloma Acuminatum

Background. This disease is caused by the **human papilloma virus** (HPV). It is the **most common** overall STD in women, as well as the most common viral STD. Transmission can occur with subclinical lesions. HPV subtypes 16 and 18 are associated with cervical and vulvar carcinoma whereas condyloma is associated with HPV types 6 and 11. Predisposing factors include immunosuppression, diabetes, and pregnancy.

Symptoms. HPV is subclinical in most infected women. Symptoms of pain, odor, or bleeding occur only when lesions become large or infected.

Examination. Clinical lesions are found in only 30% of infected women. The characteristic appearance of a condyloma is a pedunculated, soft papule that progresses into a cauliflower-like mass. The most common site of lesions is the cervix.

Diagnosis. The lesions have an appearance so characteristic that biopsy is seldom necessary.

Management: is topical or local. Systemic therapy is not available.

- **Patient-applied topical treatment:** podofilox [Condylox] solution or gel (antimitotic drug); imiquimod [Aldara] cream (topically active immune-enhancer); or sinecatechins ointment (green-tea extract)
- **Provider-administered local treatment:** cryotherapy (liquid nitrogen or cryoprobe); podophyllin resin (not used in pregnancy); trichoroacetic acid [TCA] or biochloroacetic acid [BCA] (caustic agents); or surgical removal

Trichomonas Vaginitis

Refer to Gynecology, Chapter 3, Disorders of the Vagina and Vulva.

Chlamydia

Background. This disease is caused by *Chlamydia trachomatis*, an obligatory intracellular bacterium. It is the **most common** bacterial STD in women, occurring up to 5 times more frequently than gonorrhea. The long-term sequelae arise from pelvic adhesions, causing chronic pain and infertility. When the active infection ascends to the upper genital tract and becomes symptomatic, it is known as acute pelvic inflammatory disease (**acute PID**). Transmission from an infected gravida to her newborn may take place at delivery, causing conjunctivitis and otitis media.

Symptoms. Most chlamydial cervical infections, and even salpingo-oophoritis, are asymptomatic.

Examination. The classic cervical finding is mucopurulent cervical discharge. Urethral and cervical motion tenderness may or may not be noted.

Diagnosis. Nucleic acid amplification tests (NAAT) of either cervical discharge or urine is used.

Management. The CDC-recommended treatment includes a single oral dose of azithromycin or oral doxycycline for 7 days. Patients should avoid coitus for 7 days after therapy. A test-of-cure (repeat testing 3–4 weeks after completing therapy) is recommended for pregnant women.

Gonorrhea

Background. This disease is caused by *Neisseria gonorrhoeae*, a Gram-negative diplococcus. The long-term sequelae arise from pelvic adhesions, causing chronic pain and infertility. When the active infection becomes symptomatic, it is known as acute pelvic inflammatory disease (**acute PID**). Systemic infection can occur.

Symptoms. Lower genital tract infection may lead only to vulvovaginal discharge, itching, and burning with dysuria or rectal discomfort. Upper genital tract infection leads to bilateral abdominal-pelvic pain. Disseminated gonorrhea is characterized by dermatitis, polyarthralgia, and tenosynovitis.

Examination. Vulvovaginitis is seen on inspection. Mucopurulent cervical discharge is seen on speculum exam. Cervical motion tenderness is common with bimanual pelvic exam. A Bartholin abscess may be found if the gland duct becomes obstructed due to an acute infection. Petechial skin lesions, septic arthritis, and rarely, endocarditis or meningitis, may demonstrate with disseminated gonorrhea.

Diagnosis. Same as for chlamydia, above.

Management. Dual therapy for gonococcus and chlamydia is recommended by the CDC because of the frequency of coinfection. The CDC-treatment recommendations include a single dose of IM ceftriaxone plus a single oral dose of azithromycin. A Bartholin abscess needs to undergo incision and drainage with a Word catheter.

Bartholin Abscess/Cyst

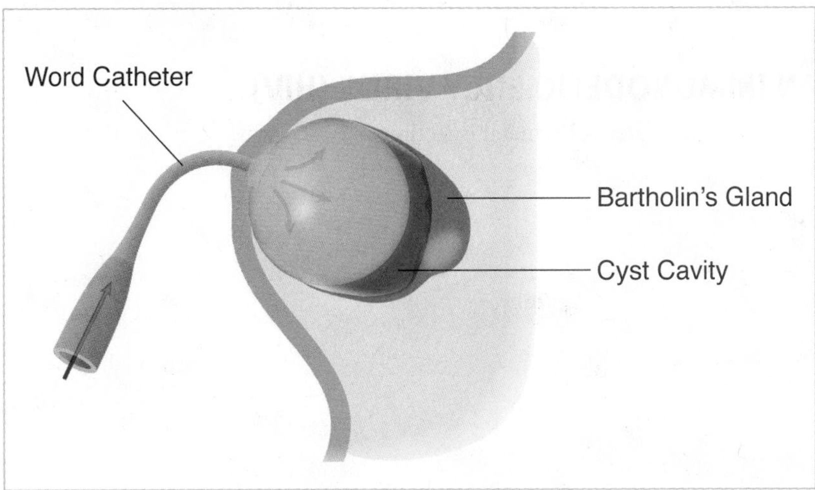

Figure II-7-2. Use of Word Catheter

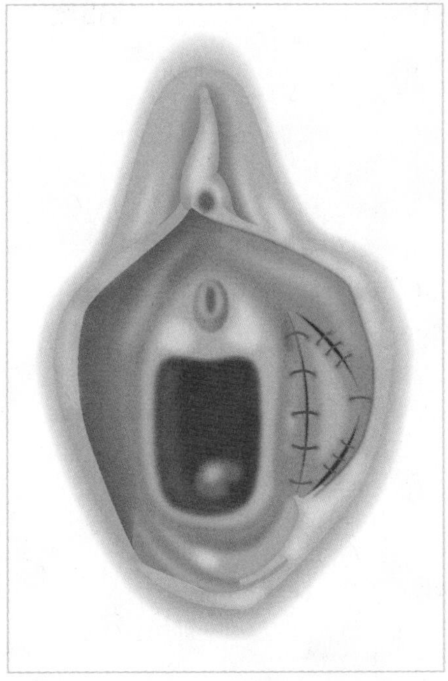

Figure II-7-3. Marsupialization

HEPATITIS B (HBV)

Refer to Obstetrics, Chapter 7, Perinatal Infections.

HUMAN IMMUNODEFICIENCY VIRUS (HIV)

Refer to Obstetrics, Chapter 7, Perinatal Infections.

Pelvic Pain 8

Learning Objectives

- ❑ Differentiate primary and secondary dysmenorrhea
- ❑ Provide an overview of the diagnosis and treatment of pelvic inflammatory disease

PELVIC INFLAMMATORY DISEASE (PID)

A 19-year-old nulligravida presents to the emergency department with bilateral lower abdominal pelvic pain. The onset was 24 hours ago after she had just finished her menstrual period. She is sexually active but using no contraception. Speculum examination reveals mucopurulent cervical discharge. Bimanual pelvic examination shows bilateral adnexal tenderness and cervical motion tenderness. She is afebrile. Qualitative urinary β-hCG test is negative. Complete blood cell count shows WBC 14,000. ESR is elevated.

Definition. PID is a nonspecific term for a **spectrum** of upper genital tract conditions ranging from acute bacterial infection to massive adhesions from old inflammatory scarring.

The **most common** initial organisms are **chlamydia** and **gonorrhea.** With persistent infection, secondary bacterial invaders include anaerobes and gram-negative organisms.

Pathophysiology

- **Cervicitis.** The initial infection starts with invasion of endocervical glands with chlamydia and gonorrhea. A mucopurulent cervical discharge or friable cervix may be noted. Cervical cultures will be positive, but symptoms are usually absent.
- **Acute salpingo-oophoritis.** Usually after a menstrual period with breakdown of the cervical mucus barrier, the pathogenic organisms ascend through the uterus, causing an endometritis, and then the bacteria enter the oviduct where acute salpingo-oophoritis develops.
- **Chronic PID.** If the salpingo-oophoritis is not appropriately treated, the body's immune defenses will often overcome the infection but at the expense of persistent adhesions and scarring.
- **Tubo-ovarian abscess (TOA).** If the body's immune defenses cannot overcome the infection, the process worsens, producing an inflammatory mass involving the oviducts, ovaries, uterus, bowel, and omentum.

Risk Factors. The **most common** risk factor is female sexual activity in adolescence, with multiple partners. PID is increased in the month after insertion of an IUD, but this is probably exacerbation of preexisting subclinical infection.

Cervicitis

Symptoms. Often there are no symptoms except vaginal discharge.

Examination. The **most common** finding is mucopurulent cervical discharge or a friable cervix. No pelvic tenderness is noted. The patient is afebrile.

Investigative Findings. This can be either a laboratory diagnosis or a clinical diagnosis. See Diagnosis section for chlamydia. WBC and ESR are normal.

Management. Single dose orally of cefixime and azithromycin.

Acute salpingo-oophoritis

Symptoms. Bilateral lower abdominal-pelvic pain may be variable ranging from minimal to severe. Onset may be gradual to sudden, often after menses. Nausea and vomiting may be found if abdominal involvement is present.

Examination. Mucopurulent cervical discharge, cervical-motion tenderness, and bilateral adnexal tenderness are present. Fever, tachycardia, abdominal tenderness, peritoneal signs, and guarding may be found depending on the extent of infection progression.

Investigative Findings. WBC and ESR are both elevated. Pelvic sonography is usually unremarkable. Laparoscopy will show erythematous, edematous, purulent oviducts. Cervical cultures will come back positive for chlamydia or gonorrhea.

Differential Diagnosis. Adnexal torsion, ectopic pregnancy, endometriosis, appendicitis, diverticulitis, Crohn disease, and ulcerative colitis.

Diagnosis. This is a made on **clinical grounds** using the following:

- **Minimal criteria:**
  - Sexually active young woman
  - Pelvic or lower abdominal pain
  - Tenderness: cervical motion or uterine or adnexal
- **Supportive criteria (but not necessary for diagnosis):**
  - Oral temperature >101°F (>38.3°C)
  - Abnormal cervical or vaginal mucopurulent discharge
  - Presence of abundant WBC on vaginal fluid saline microscopy
  - Elevated erythrocyte sedimentation rate
  - Positive lab findings of cervical *N. gonorrhoeae* or *C. trachomatis*
  - Most specific criteria for diagnosis:
  - Endometrial biopsy showing endometritis
  - Vaginal sono or MRI imaging showing abnormal adnexae
  - Laparoscopic abnormalities consistent with PID

GYN Triad

Acute Salpingo-Oophoritis

- **Bilateral** abdominal/pelvic pain
- Mucopurulent cervical discharge
- Cervical motion tenderness

Management is often based on a presumptive diagnosis. Empiric broad spectrum coverage need to include *N. gonorrhoeae* or *C. trachomatis* as well as anaerobes (e.g., *B. fragilis*).

- **Outpatient treatment** is equivalent to inpatient in mild to moderate cases.
  - **Criteria:** absence of inpatient criteria
  - **Antibiotics:** Ceftriaxone IM x 1 plus doxycycline po bid for 14 days with/without metronidazole po bid for 14 days
- **Inpatient treatment** is essential with severe cases
  - **Criteria:** Appendicitis cannot be ruled out; failed outpatient therapy; unable to tolerate oral medications; severe illness, high fever, nausea/vomiting; tubo-ovarian abscess or pregnancy
  - **Antibiotics:** (1) Cefotetan IV 12 h plus doxycycline po or IV q 12 h or (2) clindamycin plus gentamicin IV q 8 h

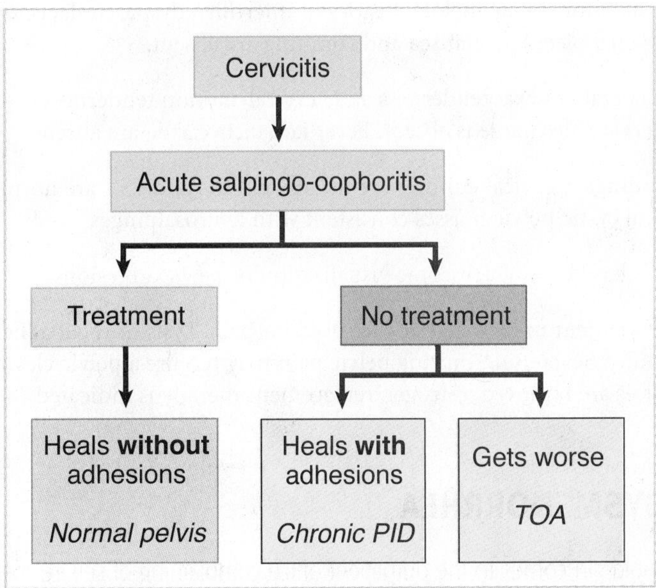

Figure II-8-1. Pelvic Inflammatory Disease

Tubo-ovarian abscess (TOA)

TOA is the accumulation of pus in the adnexae forming an inflammatory mass involving the oviducts, ovaries, uterus, or omentum.

Symptoms. The patient looks septic. Lower abdominal-pelvic pain is severe. Often the patient has severe back pain, rectal pain, and pain with bowel movements. Nausea and vomiting are present.

Examination. The patient appears gravely sick. She has high fever with tachycardia. She may be in septic shock with hypotension. Abdominal examination shows peritoneal signs, guarding, and rigidity. Pelvic examination may show such severe pain that a rectal examination must be performed. Bilateral adnexal masses may be palpated.

Investigative Findings. Cervical cultures are positive for chlamydia or gonorrhea. Blood cultures may be positive for gram-negative bacteria and anaerobic organisms such as *Bacteroides fragilis*. Culdocentesis may yield pus. WBC and ESR are markedly elevated. Sonography or CT scan will show bilateral complex pelvic masses.

Differential Diagnosis. Septic abortion, diverticular or appendiceal abscess, and adnexal torsion.

Management. Inpatient IV clindamycin and gentamicin should result in fever defervescence within 72 hours. If the patient does not respond or there is rupture of the abscess exposing free pus into the peritoneal cavity, significant mortality can occur. Exploratory laparotomy with possible TAH and BSO or percutaneous drainage through a colpotomy incision may be required.

GYN Triad

Chronic Salpingo-Oophoritis

- **Bilateral** abdominal/pelvic pain
- No cervical discharge
- Cervical motion tenderness

Chronic PID

Symptoms. Chronic bilateral lower abdominal-pelvic pain is present, varying from minimal to severe. Other symptoms may include history of infertility, dyspareunia, ectopic pregnancy, and abnormal vaginal bleeding. Nausea and vomiting are absent.

Examination. Bilateral adnexal tenderness and cervical-motion tenderness is present, but mucopurulent cervical discharge is absent. Fever and tachycardia are absent.

Investigative Findings. Cervical cultures are negative. WBC and ESR are normal. Sonography may show bilateral cystic pelvic masses consistent with hydrosalpinges.

Diagnosis. This is based on laparoscopic visualization of pelvic adhesions.

Management. Outpatient mild analgesics are used for pain. Lysis of tubal adhesions may be helpful for infertility. Severe unremitting pelvic pain may require a pelvic clean-out (TAH, BSO). If the ovaries are removed, estrogen replacement therapy is indicated.

PRIMARY DYSMENORRHEA

> A 15-year-old girl comes to the outpatient office complaining of severe menstrual-period pain that started 6 months ago. Onset of menarche was age 13. The pain can be so severe that she is unable to attend school or carry on normal activities. She describes it as cramping in nature, and it is associated with nausea, vomiting, and diarrhea. When her menses are completed, the pain is gone. She is not sexually active. General exam is normal for age. Pelvic exam is unremarkable.

Definition. Primary dysmenorrhea refers to recurrent, crampy lower abdominal pain, along with nausea, vomiting, and diarrhea, that occurs during menstruation in the absence of pelvic pathology.

It is the **most common** gynecologic complaint among adolescent females. (Secondary dysmenorrhea refers to painful menstruation in the presence of pelvic pathology. It is more common among women in the fourth and fifth decades of life.)

Findings

- Onset of pain generally does not occur until ovulatory menstrual cycles are established. Maturation of the hypothalamic-pituitary-gonadal axis leading to ovulation occurs in half of teenagers within 2 years postmenarche, and the majority of the remainder by 5 years postmenarche.
- The symptoms typically begin several hours prior to the onset of menstruation and continue for 1 to 3 days.
- The severity of the disorder can be categorized by a grading system based on the degree of menstrual pain, presence of systemic symptoms, and impact on daily activities.

Pathogenesis

- Symptoms appear to be caused by excess production of endometrial **prostaglandin** $F_{2\alpha}$ resulting from the spiral arteriolar constriction and necrosis that follow progesterone withdrawal as the corpus luteum involutes. The prostaglandins cause dysrhythmic uterine contractions, hypercontractility, and increased uterine muscle tone, leading to **uterine ischemia**.
- The effect of the prostaglandins on the gastrointestinal smooth muscle also can account for nausea, vomiting, and diarrhea via stimulation of the gastrointestinal tract.

Management. Suppression of prostaglandins is the objective of treatment. Nonsteroidal anti-inflammatory drugs (**NSAIDs**, i.e., prostaglandin synthetase inhibitors) are the first choice in treatment.

- Continuous combination estrogen-progesterone steroid agents (e.g., oral contraceptives) are the second choice for suppressing prostaglandin release.

GYN Triad

Endometriosis

- Chronic pelvic pain
- Painful intercourse
- Painful bowel movements

SECONDARY DYSMENORRHEA

Endometriosis

A 34-year-old woman complains of painful periods, painful sex, painful bowel movements, and infertility for 2 years. She had used combination oral contraceptive pills from age 25 to 30. Pelvic examination reveals a tender, 5-cm cul-de-sac mass, along with tenderness and nodularity of the uterosacral ligaments.

Definition. Endometriosis is a benign condition in which endometrial glands and stroma are seen outside the uterus. This is not a premalignant condition.

Pathophysiology. Although the etiology of endometriosis is not known, the most accepted theory of explanation is that of Sampson, which is **retrograde menstruation**.

- The **most common** site of endometriosis is the ovary, and because this is functioning endometrium, it bleeds on a monthly basis and can create adnexal enlargements known as endometriomas, also known as a **chocolate cyst**.
- The **second most common** site of endometriosis is the **cul-de-sac**, and in this area the endometriotic nodules grow on the uterosacral ligaments, giving the characteristic **uterosacral ligament nodularity** and tenderness appreciated by rectovaginal examination. Menstruation into the cul-de-sac creates fibrosis and adhesions of bowel to the pelvic organs and a rigid cul-de-sac, which accounts for **dyspareunia**.

Clinical Findings

- **Symptoms.** Pelvic-abdominal pain is not necessarily related to the extent of disease. Painful intercourse (**dyspareunia**) is often experienced along with painful bowel movements (dyschezia). Infertility of endometriosis is not necessarily related to the extent of disease.
- **Examination.** Pelvic tenderness is common. A fixed, retroverted uterus is often caused by cul-de-sac adhesions. Uterosacral ligament nodularity is characteristic. Enlarged adnexa may be found if an endometrioma is present.
- **Investigative findings.** WBC and erythrocyte sedimentation rate (ESR) are normal. CA-125 may be elevated. Sonogram will show an endometrioma if present.

Diagnosis. The diagnosis of endometriosis is made by laparoscopy. There is a suspicion of the disease based on history and physical examination; however, laparoscopic identification of endometriotic nodules or endometriomas is the definitive way of making the diagnosis.

Medical therapy of endometriosis seeks to prevent shedding of the ectopic endometrial tissue, thus decreasing adhesion formation and pain.

- **Pregnancy** can be helpful to endometriosis because during pregnancy there is no menstruation and also the dominant hormone throughout pregnancy is progesterone, which causes atrophic changes in the endometrium. However, infertility may make this impossible.
- **Pseudopregnancy** achieves this goal through preventing progesterone withdrawal bleeding. Continuous oral medroxyprogesterone acetate (MPA [Provera]), subcutaneous medroxyprogesterone acetate (SQ-DMPA [Depo Provera]), or combination oral contraceptive pills (OCPs) can mimic the atrophic changes of pregnancy.
- **Pseudomenopause** achieves this goal by making the ectopic endometrium atrophic. The treatment is based on inhibition of the hypothalamic–pituitary–ovarian axis to decrease the estrogen stimulation of the ectopic endometrium. Several medications can be used to achieve inhibition of the axis.
  - Testosterone derivative (danazol or Danocrine)
  - Gonadotropin-releasing hormone (GnRH) analog (leuprolide or Lupron)

The best inhibition of the hypothalamic–pituitary–ovarian axis is achieved by GnRH analogs. GnRH stimulates the pituitary in a pulsatile fashion, and GnRH analogs stimulate by continuous stimulation, which produces a condition known as down-regulation of the pituitary.

Although regression of the endometriotic nodules can be achieved, the patient can become symptomatic with menopausal complaints. Patients on Lupron therapy for >3–6 months can complain of menopausal symptoms, such as hot flashes, sweats, vaginal dryness, and personality changes. Lupron medication is continued for 3–6 months' duration, and then a more acceptable medication for the inhibition of the axis can be used, such as birth control pill medication. An alternative to Lupron is DMPA (Depo Provera), which also suppresses FSH and LH but does not result in vasomotor symptoms.

Surgical management may be conservative or aggressive.

- **Conservative.** If preservation of fertility is desired, the procedures can be performed in many cases through laparoscopic approach. Lysis of paratubal adhesions may allow adherent fimbria to function and achieve pregnancy. Ovarian cystectomies as well as oophorectomies can be treatment for endometriomas. Laser vaporization of visible lesions is also performed laparoscopically.

- **Aggressive.** If fertility is not desired, particularly if severe pain is present because of diffuse adhesions, definitive surgical therapy may be carried out through a total abdominal hysterectomy (TAH) and bilateral salpingo-oophorectomy (BSO). Estrogen replacement therapy is then necessary.

Follow-Up. Endometriosis is not a malignant condition but is associated with higher risk of ovarian carcinoma; mechanism unclear.

Adenomyosis

Refer to Chapter 4, Disorders of the Cervix and Uterus.

Ectopic Pregnancy

Refer to Obstetrics, Chapter 2, Failed Pregnancy.

Fertility Control 9

Learning Objectives

- ❏ List the advantages and disadvantages of different forms of contraception including barrier-spermicidal methods, steroid contraception, intrauterine contraception, coitus interruptus, natural family planning, lactation, vaginal douche, and sterilization

OVERVIEW OF FERTILITY CONTROL

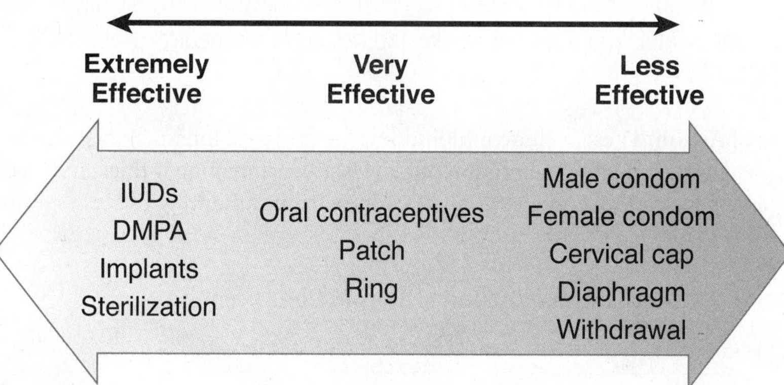

Figure II-9-1. Contraception

BARRIER-SPERMICIDAL METHODS

A 16-year-old adolescent comes to the family planning clinic requesting contraception. She has heard about the diaphragm and wonders if it would be appropriate for her.

Mechanisms of Action. These are locally active devices preventing entry of sperm in through the cervix, thus preventing pregnancy.

Advantages. Barrier methods become increasingly effective with advancing age and the associated natural decline in fertility. They do protect against some STDs. They do not have systemic side effects.

Disadvantages. Failure rate approaches 20%. They are coitally dependent, requiring a decision for each use, thus decreasing spontaneity. Barrier methods have no impact on excessive menstrual flow or excessively painful menses.

Specific Types

- **Condoms.** These are penile sheaths that must be placed on the erect penis. No individual fitting is required. They are the **most common** barrier contraceptive method used.
- **Vaginal diaphragm.** This is a dome-shaped device placed in the anterior and posterior vaginal fornices holding spermicidal jelly against the cervix. It can be placed an hour before intercourse. Individual fitting is required. If too large a size is used, it can result in urinary retention.
- **Spermicides.** The active ingredient is nonoxynol-9, a surface-active agent that disrupts cell membranes, thus the possible side effect of genital membrane irritation. These can take the form of jellies or foams placed into the vagina.

STEROID CONTRACEPTION

A 44-year-old woman, gravida 4 para 4, presents with questions about oral steroid contraception. She uses a diaphragm but is worried about contraceptive failure. She also expresses concern that her menses have become slightly heavier and more painful. She does not smoke and has no other medical problems.

Mechanisms of Action. These include inhibition of the midcycle luteinizing hormone (LH) surge, thus preventing ovulation; alteration of cervical mucus making it thick and viscid, thus retarding sperm penetration; and alteration of endometrium inhibiting blastocyst implantation.

Table II-9-1. Mechanism of Action of Steroid Contraception

Pituitary	↓ LH surge
Ovary	↓ ovulation
Endometrium	Atrophy
Cervix	Hostile mucus

Estrogen-Mediated Metabolic Effects. These include fluid retention from decreased sodium excretion; accelerated development of cholelithiasis; increase in hepatic protein production (e.g., coagulation factors, carrier proteins, angiotensinogen); healthy lipid profile changes (increase in high-density lipoproteins [HDL]; decrease in low-density lipoproteins [LDL]); and increased venous and arterial thrombosis.

Progestin-Mediated Metabolic Effects. These include mood changes and depression from decreased serotonin levels; androgenic effects (e.g., weight gain, acne); and unhealthy lipid profile changes (decreased HDL, increased LDL).

Absolute Contraindications. These include pregnancy; acute liver disease; history of vascular disease (e.g., thromboembolism, deep venous thrombosis [DVT], cerebrovascular accident [CVA], systemic lupus erythematosus [SLE]); hormonally dependent cancer (e.g., breast); smoker ≥35; uncontrolled hypertension; migraines with aura; diabetes mellitus with vascular disease; and known thrombophilia.

Relative Contraindications. These include migraine headaches, depression, diabetes mellitus, chronic hypertension, and hyperlipidemia.

Noncontraceptive Benefits. These include decreased ovarian and endometrial cancer; decreased dysmenorrhea and dysfunctional uterine bleeding; and decreased PID and ectopic pregnancy.

Table II-9-2. Noncontraceptive Benefits of Steroid Contraception

Mostly Progestin Component
↓ dysmenorrhea
↓ dysfunctional uterine bleeding
↓ pelvic inflammatory disease
↓ ectopic pregnancy

Combination Modalities

Combination OCPs. These contain both an estrogen and a progestin. They are administered most commonly in one of two ways: daily with 21 days on and 7 days off or daily 24 days on and 4 days off. When "off" the hormones, withdrawal bleeding will occur. Of all steroid contraceptives, they are the only one to have regular, predictable menses. Failure rate is 2% with ideal use. A newer combination is with daily hormones for 12 weeks followed by 1 week of placebo.

Oral Contraceptives. A unique combination of OCP (YAZ) reduces severe PMDD symptoms by 50%. It contains ethynyl estradiol and a new progestin, drospirenone. The dosing is 24 days of active pills then 4 days of placebo, rather than the traditional 21 days, followed by 7 days of placebo.

Combination Vaginal Ring. Marketed under the trade name of NuvaRing, this device, inserted into the vagina, contains both an estrogen and a progestin. It is removed after 3 weeks for 1 week to allow for a withdrawal bleed. A major advantage is relatively stable and constant blood levels of hormones. Failure rate is similar to combination OCPs.

Transdermal Skin Patch. Marketed under the trade name of Ortho Evra, this patch contains both an estrogen and a progestin. A patch is replaced every week for 3 weeks then removed for 1 week to allow for a withdrawal bleed. Levels of steroids are 60% higher than combination OCPs.

Progestin-Only Modalities

Progestin-Only OCPs. They contain only progestins and are sometimes called the "minipill." They need to be taken daily and continuously. A frequent side effect is break-through bleeding. Failure rate is 3% with ideal use.

Progestin-Only Injectable. Marketed under the trade name of Depo-Provera, this is an IM injection of depo-medroxyprogesterone acetate (DMPA). The slow release allows administration only every 3 months. A frequent side effect is break-through bleeding. Other side effects are prolonged time for fertility return and decreased bone mineral density. Failure rate is <1%.

Progestin-Only Subcutaneous Implant. Marketed under the trade name of Nexplanon, this uses etonogestrel as the active ingredient. The core contains a small amount of barium, making it visible on x-ray. The continuous release continues for 3 years. A frequent side effect is break-through bleeding. Failure rate is <1%.

"Morning-After" Pill. Marketed under the trade name of "Plan B," it uses levonorgestrel tablets. This postcoital contraception is administered as one tablet, immediately followed by one additional tablet in 12 h. Failure rate is 1%.

General. A recent evaluation of women's views regarding contraceptive health benefits demonstrated that most women are unaware of the protective effects of OCPs against endometrial and ovarian cancer, PID, ectopic pregnancy, benign breast disease, anemia, and dysmenorrhea.

Risks and Benefits. In nonsmoking women age >40, currently available OCPs are extremely safe. Low-dose contraceptive pills do not significantly increase the risk of cancer, heart disease, or thromboembolic events in women with no associated risk factors (hypertension, diabetes, or smoking). The combination estrogen/progestin pill tends to reduce menstrual flow and dysmenorrhea, and it regulates the menses, all of which would be excellent benefits for the patient.

INTRAUTERINE CONTRACEPTION

A 30-year-old woman with Crohn disease who periodically requires steroid therapy seeks advice regarding long-term contraception. She has had 3 pregnancies. A subserosal, fundal fibroid was noted at the time of her previous cesarean section delivery. She states that she is in a mutually monogamous relationship. She was treated for a chlamydia infection 2 months ago but does not like the idea of hormonal contraception and is asking about the risks associated with an IUS.

Intrauterine contraception is a long-acting reversible contraceptive method that involves placement of a small t-shaped object inside the uterus. Failure rate is <1%. Continuation rates at 1 year are almost 80%.

Mechanisms of Action. These include inhibition of sperm transport; increased tubal motility causing failure of implantation of immature zygote; inhibition of implantation secondary to endometrial inflammation; phagocytic destruction of sperm and blastocyst; and alteration of cervical mucus (only progesterone IUSs).

Table II-9-3. Mechanism of Action of Intrauterine System (IUS)

1. ↓ sperm transport
2. ↑ tubal motility
3. ↓ implantation
4. Sperm and blastocyst destroyed
5. Cervical mucus altered (LNG)

Definition of abbreviations: LNG, levonorgestrel.

Absolute Contraindications include a confirmed or suspected pregnancy; known or suspected pelvic malignancy; undiagnosed vaginal bleeding; and known or suspected salpingitis. **Relative Contraindications** include abnormal uterine size or shape; medical condition (e.g., corticosteroid therapy, valvular heart disease, or any instance of immune suppression increasing the risk of infection); nulligravidity; abnormal Pap smears; and history of ectopic pregnancy.

Side Effects. Menstrual bleeding and menstrual pain may be increased with the copper IUS, but not with the progesterone IUSs.

Potential Complications. The popularity of the IUS has varied greatly during the past 2 decades. Despite its excellence as a method of contraception, it has yet to recover from the negative publicity generated by the Dalkon Shield in the late 1970s. The LNG-containing IUS is effective for 5 years, the copper T-380A is effective for 10 years, making it potentially the least expensive contraceptive available.

- **Chlamydia.** This patient's recent chlamydia infection is a significant risk factor for IUS use. Most of the increased risk of infection actually attributable to IUS use is within 20 days after infection; consequently, any vaginal infection should be treated and resolved before insertion of the IUS to prevent introduction of organisms into the upper genital tract. Medical conditions that increase the risk of infection, such as HIV infection and immunosuppressive therapy, are also relative contraindications to IUS use. This patient's periodic need for steroid treatment for Crohn disease is a risk factor.
- **Leiomyomas.** Uterine fibroids could also be a relative contraindication because they alter the shape of the endometrial cavity or cause heavy bleeding. The subserosal fundal fibroids should not interfere with IUS placement.
- **Expulsion** is higher in young, low parity women.
- **Ectopic pregnancy.** The IUS does not increase ectopic pregnancies. However, with pregnancy from failed IUS, the likelihood of it being ectopic is higher because primarily, intrauterine pregnancies are prevented.
- **Septic abortion** occurs in 50% of patients with concurrent pregnancy.
- **Uterine perforation**, although rare, occurs more likely at time of insertion.
- **PID** may occur within the first 2 months after placement if pathogenic organisms are present in the reproductive tract.

IUS Options

- **"Mirena."** A levonorgestrel-impregnated (LNG) IUS that releases the hormone gradually over 5 years. Bleeding and cramping may be decreased. Failure rate is <1%.
- **Skyla**. A smaller (LNG) IUS similar to Mirena but effective for only 3 years. Failure rate is <1%.
- **Copper T-380A IUS.** Marketed under the trade name "Paraguard," this copper-banded IUS releases copper gradually over 10 years. Bleeding and cramping may be increased. Failure rate is <1%.

NATURAL FAMILY PLANNING—PERIODIC ABSTINENCE

This method is based on avoiding sexual intercourse around the time of predicted ovulation. It assumes the egg is fertilizable for 12 to 24 hours and sperm is capable of fertilizing the egg for 24 to 48 hours. Requires high degree of discipline from both sexual partners.

Methods used. Prediction or identification of ovulation may inferred from: menstrual records, basal body temperature charting (temperature rise from thermogenic effect of progesterone), change in cervical mucus from thin and watery to thick and sticky (reflects the change from estrogen dominance preovulation to progesterone dominance postovulation).

Advantages. Inexpensive. Readily available. No steroid hormonal side-effects. May be preferred for religious reasons.

Disadvantages. Inaccurate prediction of ovulation. High failure rate because of human frailities and the passions of the moment.

COITUS INTERRUPTUS

In this practice, also known as **withdrawal** or pull-out method, the man withdraws his penis from the woman's vagina prior to orgasm and ejaculation. It is one of the oldest contraceptive methods described.

Advantages: Readily available. Inexpensive. Free of systemic side effects.

Disadvantages: High failure rates. No protection against STDs. High degree of discipline required. Semen can enter vagina and cervical mucus prior to ejaculation.

VAGINAL DOUCHE

With vaginal douche, plain water, vinegar and other products are used immediately after orgasm to theoretically flush semen out of the vagina. It has a long history of use in the United States.

Advantages: None.

Disadvantages: High failure rates. No protection against STDs. Sperm can enter the cervical mucus within 90 seconds of ejaculation.

LACTATION

With lactation, elevated prolactin levels with exclusive breastfeeding inhibit pulsatile secretion of GnRH from the hypothalamus. Effectiveness is dependent on the frequency (at least every 4-6 hours day & night) and intensity (infant suckling rather than pumping) of milk removal.

Advantages: Enhanced maternal and infant health, bonding, and nutrition. Readily available. Inexpensive. Needs no supplies. Free of systemic side effects. Acceptable to all religious groups.

Disadvantages: High failure rate if not exclusively breastfeeding. Reliable for only up to 6 months. No protection against STDs.

STERILIZATION

A 38-year-old multipara has completed her childbearing and is requesting sterilization. All 3 of her children were delivered vaginally. She has no medical problems and is in good health. General and pelvic examination is unremarkable.

Mechanisms of Action. These are surgical procedures usually involving ligation of either the female oviduct or male vas deferens. After the procedure is performed, there is nothing to forget and nothing to remember. They are to be considered permanent and irreversible.

Tubal Ligation. Destruction or removal of a segment of the oviduct is performed in an operating room through a transabdominal approach usually using a laparoscopy or minilaparotomy. Failure rate is 1 in 200. This is the **most common** modality of pregnancy prevention in the United States. If the procedure fails and pregnancy results, an ectopic pregnancy should be ruled out.

Vasectomy. Destruction or removal of a segment of vas deferens is performed as an outpatient procedure using local anesthesia. Failure rate is 1 in 500. A successful procedure can be confirmed by absence of sperm on a semen specimen obtained 12 ejaculations after the surgery. Sperm antibodies can be found in 50% of vasectomized patients.

Human Sexuality 10

Learning Objectives

- ❑ Take a sexual history
- ❑ Outline the human sexual response cycle
- ❑ List common sexual dysfunctions and their possible causes and treatments
- ❑ Explain the responsibilities of a health professional when examining a sexual assault victim

HUMAN SEXUAL RESPONSE CYCLE

A 31-year-old woman, mother of 4 children, comes to the office stating she has little interest in sexual intercourse with her husband for the past year. She says sex is painful, but she is able to experience orgasm occasionally. She has had no other sexual partners than her husband. These problems are affecting her marriage. She had a tubal sterilization procedure performed after her last delivery 2 years ago. Medications include thyroid replacement and fluoxetine.

Linear Model

Desire. In both women and men the desire for sexual activity is also known as libido. Desire is maintained by a balance between **dopamine** stimulation and **serotonin** inhibition. The threshold of response is determined by androgens, especially **testosterone.** This is true for women as well as men.

Excitement. This phase is also known as **arousal.** It is mediated by **parasympathetic** connections to the pelvic organs and results in vascular **engorgement.** Arousal in women is generally slower, responds more to **touch** and **psychic stimuli**, and is manifested by vaginal lubrication. Arousal in men is generally faster, responds more to **visual** stimuli, and is manifested by penile **erection.**

Plateau. This phase entails progression and intensification of the excitement phase. The length of this phase is variable. The neural pathway and physiologic mechanism is the same as excitement.

Orgasm. This phase is mediated by **sympathetic** connections resulting in reflex tonic-clonic **muscle contractions** of the pelvic floor followed by contractions of the uterus. Women have more individual orgasmic **variability** than men. A unique characteristic of women is the potential for consecutive **multiple orgasms.**

Resolution. This phase is marked by a return to basal physiologic state with reversal of vasocongestion and muscle tension. Resolution tends to be faster for men and slower for women.

Refractory Phase. This is a unique characteristic of men and is the period of inability to be aroused before another orgasm. It frequently varies directly with the age of the man.

Circular Relational Model

Linear biologic model (limitations)

Masters and Johnson's **linear,** 4-stage **biologic** model of sexual response for both men and women assumes that men and women have similar sexual responses. Many women, however, do not move progressively and sequentially through the phases as described. Women may not even experience all of the phases—for example, they may move from sexual arousal to orgasm and satisfaction without experiencing sexual desire, or they can experience desire, arousal, and satisfaction but not orgasm.

- The biologic model may be limited because it does not take into account nonbiologic experiences such as pleasure and satisfaction. It also does not place sexuality into the context of the relationship.
- Much of female sexual desire is actually a reaction to a partner's sexual interest rather than a spontaneous stirring of the woman's own libido. Women have many reasons for engaging in sexual activity other than sexual hunger or drive, as the traditional model suggests.

Circular relationship model (advantages)

The **circular,** variable-stage **relationship** model of female sexual response acknowledges how emotional intimacy, sexual stimuli, and relationship satisfaction affect the female sexual response.

- Female sexual functioning proceeds in a more complex and circuitous manner than does male sexual functioning. Also, female functioning is dramatically and significantly affected by numerous psychosocial issues.
- Many women start from a point of sexual neutrality—where a woman is receptive to being sexual but does not initiate sexual activity—and the desire for intimacy prompts her to seek ways to become sexually aroused via conversation, music, reading or viewing erotic materials, or direct stimulation. Once she is aroused, sexual desire emerges and motivates.
- The goal of sexual activity for women is not necessarily orgasm but rather personal satisfaction, which may be orgasm and/or feelings of intimacy and connection.

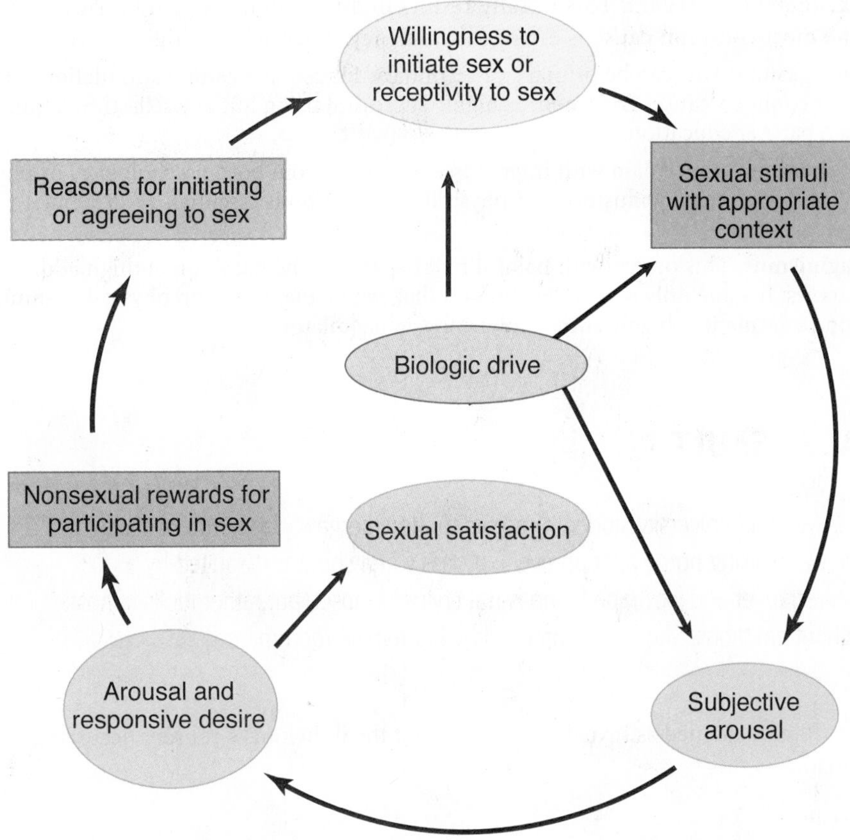

Figure II-10-1. Female Sexual Response Cycle

SEXUAL HISTORY-TAKING

The following questions should be asked of all new patients in developing a medical data base and problem list.

- **Sexual activity.** Start out with the following initial question: Is the patient currently sexually active? If not now, has she been in past?
- **Current history.** If she is currently sexually active, ask the following: Is the relationship with men or women or both? Is the relationship satisfying? Does she have any difficulty lubricating? Does she have pain with intercourse?
- **Previous history.** What was her age at first intercourse? What is the number of lifetime and current sexual partners? Does she have a history of sexual abuse or rape?

SEXUAL DYSFUNCTION

Each phase of the sexual response cycle can be dysfunctional.

- **Desire disorders.** Decreased sexual desire is the most common female sexual complaint. It may be organic (e.g., low androgens), medication related (e.g., selective serotonin reuptake inhibitors [SSRIs]), or psychological (e.g., poor partner relationship). **Treatment** can be difficult if it is relational in etiology.

- **Excitement disorders.** This usually results in difficulty in vaginal lubrication. The most common cause is estrogen deficiency. **Treatment** is highly successful.
- **Anorgasmia.** This can be primary or secondary. Inadequate clitoral stimulation is the most common cause. **Treatment** is highly successful using initially self-stimulation then partner education.
- **Dyspareunia.** Since pain with intercourse may arise from both psychological or physical causes, a thorough history and physical examination is essential. **Treatment** is directed at the specific cause found.
- **Vaginismus.** This occurs with painful reflex spasm of the paravaginal thigh adductor muscles. It is the only sexual dysfunction that can be diagnosed on physical examination. **Treatment** is highly successful using vaginal dilators.

SEXUAL ASSAULT

A 21-year-old university student presents to the emergency department stating she was walking home after an evening class when she was assaulted by a male stranger and was raped. She is not crying or upset, but rather looks almost without emotions. She is accompanied by her female roommate.

Definition. Rape is defined as sexual activity without the individual's consent occurring under coercion.

Management

- **Stabilization.** The first step is to determine the patient's vital signs and take whatever is needed to stabilize them. An informed consent needs to be obtained.
- **History-taking.** Record the events that happened in the patient's own words. Also obtain a reproductive, obstetric, sexual, and contraceptive history.
- **Examination.** A thorough general and pelvic examination should be performed with photographic or drawing documentation of any injuries or trauma.
- **Specimens.** A rape kit should be used to obtain biologic specimens (e.g., vaginal, oral, or anal specimens) for DNA or other evidence for use in potential legal proceedings. These must be appropriately labeled and documented, including signatures of receiving authorities. Also obtain baseline laboratory tests: VDRL, HIV screen, pregnancy test, urine drug screen, and blood alcohol level.
- **Prophylaxis.** Antibiotic therapy should be administered prophylactically for gonorrhea (ceftriaxone 125 mg IM × 1), chlamydia (azithromycin 1 g PO × 1), and trichomoniasis (metronidazole 2 g PO × 1). Antiviral HIV prophylaxis should be administered within 24 hours after exposure, but no medication should be given after 36 hours. Active and passive immunization for hepatitis B is appropriate.
- **Pregnancy prevention.** Administer 2 tablets of high progestin OCPs immediately, repeating two tablets in 12 h. A newly released formulation of levonogesterol tablets (Plan B) are now available specifically for postcoital pregnancy prevention.

Menstrual Abnormalities 11

Learning Objectives

- ❑ Describe the menstrual cycle
- ❑ Give a differential diagnosis and management of disorders of the menstrual cycle, including premenarchal menstrual bleeding, abnormal vaginal bleeding, primary/secondary amenorrhea

MENSTRUAL PHYSIOLOGY

The menstrual cycle is the cyclic pattern of activity of hypothalamus, pituitary, ovary, and uterus that produces a rhythm of bleeding every month for 30 years or more during the active reproductive phase of a woman's life.

Menarche is the first flow that signifies potential reproductivity. Menopause is the termination of the menstrual flow, which signifies diminished ovarian function.

Menstrual cycle occurs with the maturation of the hypothalamic–pituitary–ovarian axis. The hormones produced include gonadotropin-releasing hormone (GnRH) from the hypothalamus, which stimulates follicle-stimulating hormone (FSH) and luteinizing hormone (LH) from the anterior pituitary, which stimulate estrogen and progesterone from the ovarian follicle.

Layers of the Endometrium

Functionalis Zone. This is the superficial layer that undergoes cyclic changes during the menstrual cycle and is sloughed off during menstruation. It contains the spiral arterioles that undergo spasm with progesterone withdrawal.

Basalis Zone. This is the deeper layer that remains relatively unchanged during the menstrual cycle and contains stem cells that function to renew the functionalis. It contains the basal arteries.

Phases of the Endometrium

Menstrual Phase. This is defined as the first 4 days of the menstrual cycle with the first day of menses taken as day 1. It is characterized by disintegration of the endometrial glands and stroma, leukocyte infiltration, and red blood cell (RBC) extravasation. Sloughing of the functionalis and compression of the basalis occurs.

Proliferative Phase. This follows the menstrual phase and is characterized by endometrial growth secondary to estrogen stimulation, including division of stem cells that migrate through the stroma to form new epithelial lining of the endometrium and new endometrial glands. The length of the spiral arteries also increases. **An estrogen-dominant endometrium is unstable** and, in the **presence of prolonged anovulation**, will **undergo hyperplasia with irregular shedding over time**.

Secretory Phase. This follows the proliferative phase and is characterized by glandular secretion of glycogen and mucus stimulated by progesterone from the corpus luteum. Endometrial stroma becomes edematous, and spiral arteries become convoluted. **A progesterone-dominant endometrium is stable** and will **not undergo irregular shedding**. Regression of the corpus luteum occurs by day 23 if there is no pregnancy, causing decreased levels of progesterone and estradiol and endometrial involution. Constriction of the spiral arteries occurs 1 day before menstruation, causing endometrial ischemia and release of prostaglandins, followed by leukocyte infiltration and RBC extravasation. The resulting necrosis leads to painful cramps and menstruation. When a pregnancy occurs, the serum β-human chorionic gonadotropin (β-hCG) becomes positive at day 22–23 of the cycle. The β-hCG becomes positive when the zygote implants into the endometrium, usually 7–8 days after ovulation. Therefore, the serum β-hCG becomes positive before the missed period.

Menstrual Cycle Hormones

FSH stimulates the growth of granulosa cells and induces the **aromatase** enzyme that converts androgens to estrogens. It raises the concentration of its own receptors on the granulosa cells. It stimulates the secretion of inhibin from the granulosa cells and is suppressed by inhibin.

LH stimulates the production of androgens by the theca cells, which then get converted to estrogens in the granulosa cells by the aromatase enzyme (2-cell theory). It raises the concentration of its own receptors in FSH-primed granulosa cells. The LH surge, which is dependent on a rapid rise in estrogen levels, stimulates synthesis of prostaglandins to enhance follicle rupture and ovulation. The LH surge also promotes luteinization of the granulosa cells in the dominant follicle, resulting in progesterone production as early as the 10th day of the cycle.

Estrogen is produced in the granulosa cells in response to even low FSH concentrations, and stimulates proliferative changes in the endometrium. It has a negative feedback to FSH at the hypothalamic–pituitary level, but has a positive feedback to increase GnRH receptor concentrations. At low estrogen levels there is negative inhibitory feedback for LH release, but as the level of estradiol increase is sustained for 50 hours, there is a transition to a positive stimulatory feedback, leading to the LH surge.

Androgens include androstenedione and testosterone. They are precursors of estrogen and are produced in the theca cells. In lower concentrations they stimulate aromatase enzyme activity, whereas at high levels they inhibit it. Androgens inhibit FSH induction of LH receptors.

Progesterone is produced by the corpus luteum and stimulates secretory changes in the endometrium in preparation for blastocyst implantation.

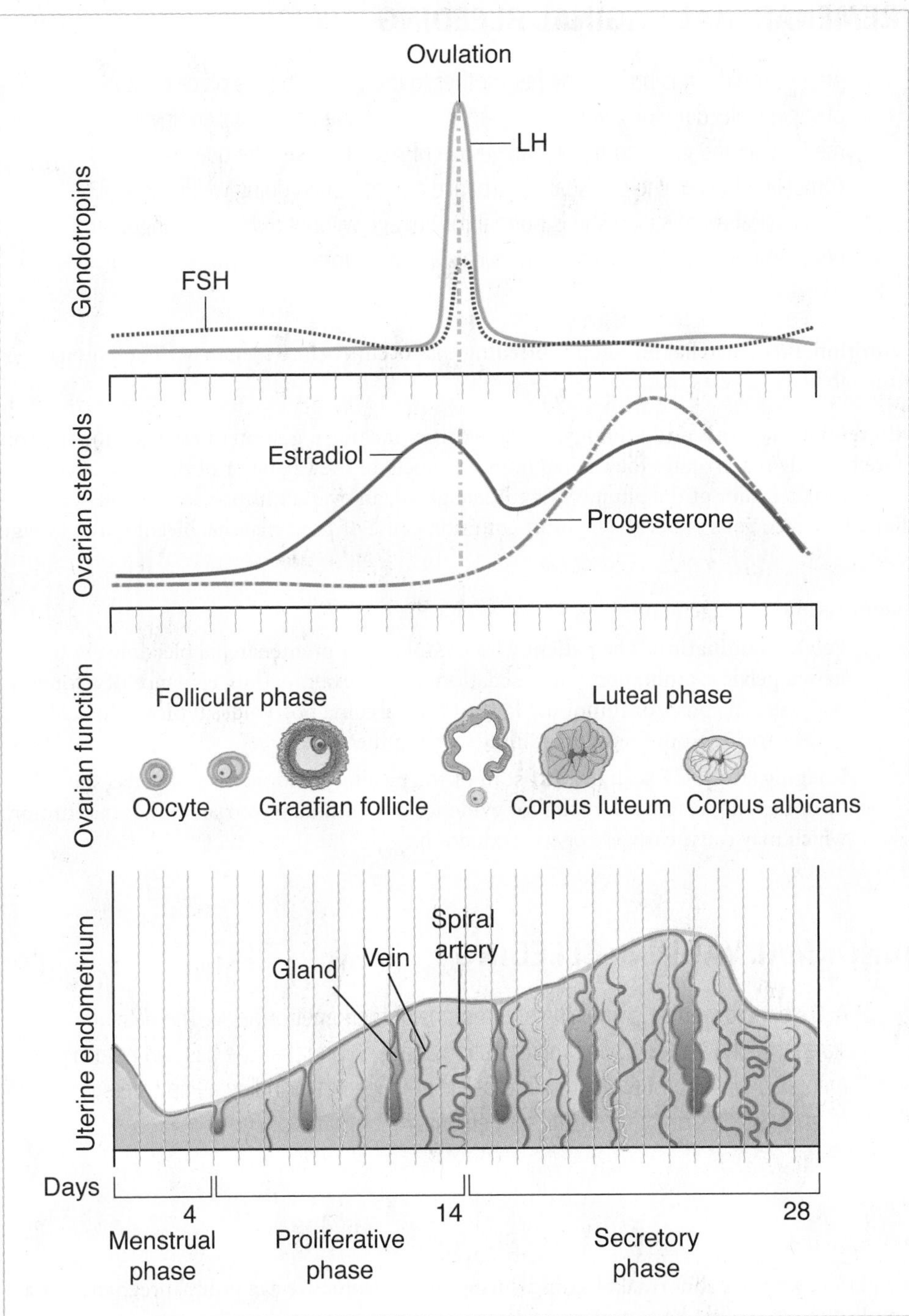

Figure II-11-1. Menstrual Cycle: Pituitary, Ovarian, and Endometrial Correlations

PREMENARCHAL VAGINAL BLEEDING

An 8-year-old girl is brought by her mother to the gynecologist's office because of vaginal bleeding for 2 weeks. The girl states that she has not taken any medication and gives no history suggestive of sexual abuse. She does not complain of headache or visual disturbance and has been doing well in school. On physical examination she is normal for her age without pubertal changes, and pelvic examination under sedation reveals a vaginal foreign body.

Definition. Premenarchal bleeding is bleeding that occurs before menarche. The average age at menarche is 12 years old.

Differential Diagnosis and Etiology. Possible causes include ingestion of estrogen medication, a foreign body that irritates the vaginal lining, a cancer of the vagina or of the cervix (sarcoma botryoides), a tumor of the pituitary or adrenal gland, an ovarian tumor, sexual abuse, or idiopathic precocious puberty. The most common cause of premenarchal bleeding is a foreign body.

Diagnosis and Management

- **Pelvic examination.** The patient who complains of premenarchal bleeding should have a pelvic examination under sedation. In this examination, evidence of a foreign body, sexual abuse, or tumor are looked for. Sarcoma botryoides typically looks like grapes arising from the vaginal lining or from the cervix.
- **Imaging study.** CT scan or MRI scan of the pituitary, abdomen, and pelvis should be done. The scans are looking for evidence of a pituitary, ovarian, or adrenal tumor, which may cause early estrogen production.

ABNORMAL VAGINAL BLEEDING

A 31-year-old woman complains of 6 months of menometrorrhagia. The patient states that she started having menstruation at age 13 and that she has had regular menses until the past 6 months. The pelvic examination including a Pap smear is normal. She has no other significant personal or family history.

Pregnancy

In a patient who has abnormal bleeding during the reproductive age group, pregnancy or a complication must first be considered.

Mechanism. Complications of early pregnancy that are associated with bleeding include incomplete abortion, threatened abortion, ectopic pregnancy, and hydatidiform mole.

Diagnosis. Urine or serum β-hCG test is required to confirm pregnancy. If pregnancy is identified vaginal ultrasound will help sort out which pregnancy complication is operative.

Management. Treatment will vary with the individual diagnosis identified.

Anatomic Lesion

If the pregnancy test is negative, then an anatomic cause of vaginal bleeding should be considered. The classic history is that of unpredictable bleeding (without cramping) occurring between normal, predictable menstrual periods (with cramping).

Mechanism. A variety of lower and upper reproductive tract factors can cause bleeding:

- Vaginal lesions: lacerations, varicosities or tumors
- Cervical lesions: polyps, cervicitis or tumors
- Endometrial lesions: submucous leiomyomas, polyps, hyperplasia or cancer
- Myometrial lesions: adenomyosis

Diagnosis. A number of tests can be used to for anatomic diagnosis.

- Lower genital tract: pelvic and speculum exam
- Upper genital tract: saline sonogram , endometrial biopsy, hysteroscopy

Management. Treatment will vary according to the individual diagnosis identified.

GYN Triad

Endometrial Polyp or Submucosal Leiomyoma

- Predictable vaginal bleeding with intermenstrual bleeding
- 33-year-old woman
- Normal height and weight

Inherited Coagulopathy

Up to 15% of patients with abnormal vaginal bleeding, especially in the adolescent age group, have coagulopathies. Review of systems may be positive for other bleeding symptoms including epistaxis, gingival bleeding and ecchyoses. Von Willebrand disease is the most common hereditary coagulation abnormality. The 3 types can vary in severity.

Mechanism. Coagulopathies can be due to vessel wall disorders, platelet disorders, coagulation disorders and fibrinolytic disorders. Von Willebrand disease arises from a deficiency of von Willebrand factor (vWF), a protein required for platelet adhesion.

Diagnosis. Positive family history and review of systems are helpful for screening. Initial laboratory tests include CBC with platelet count, PT and PTT. The best screening test for Von Willebrand disease is a vWF antigen.

Management. Consultation with hematology specialists is recommended in managing patients with inherited coagulopathies.

Dysfunctional Uterine Bleeding (DUB)

If the pregnancy test is negative, there are no anatomic causes for bleeding and coagulopathy is ruled out, then the diagnosis of hormonal imbalance should be considered. The classic history is that of bleeding that is unpredictable in amount, duration and frequency without cramping occurring.

Mechanism. The most common cause of DUB is anovulation. Anovulation results in unopposed estrogen. With unopposed estrogen, there is continuous stimulation of the endometrium with no secretory phase.

An estrogen dominant endometrium is structurally unstable as it increasingly thickens. With inadequate structural support, it eventually undergoes random, disorderly, and unpredictable breakdown resulting in estrogen breakthrough bleeding.

Diagnosis. Anovulatory cycles can usually be diagnosed from a history of irregular, unpredictable bleeding. Bleeding is usually without cramping since there is no PG release to cause myometrial contractions. Cervical mucus will be clear, thin and watery reflecting the estrogen dominant environment. Basal-body temperature (BBT) chart will not show a midcycle temperature rise due to the absence of the thermogenic effect of progesterone. Endometrial biopsy will show a proliferative endometrium.

GYN Triad

Abnormal Uterine Bleeding

PALM-COEIN Classification (FIGO 2011)

Visualizable by inspection or imaging:

P: Polyps (AUB-P)

A: Adenomyosis (AUB-A)

L: Leiomyoma (AUB-L)

M: Malignancy (AUB-M)

Needs further workup:

C: Coagulopathy (AUB-C)

O: Ovulatory disorders (AUB-O)

E: Endometrial (AUB-E)

I: latrogenic (AU B-1)

N: Not yet classified (AUB-N)

Progesterone trial involves administering progestin to stabilize the endometrium, stop the bleeding and prevent random breakdown. When the progestin is stopped, spiral arteriolar spasm results in PG release, necrosis, and an orderly shedding of the endometrium. A positive progesterone trial confirms a clinical diagnosis of anovulation. A negative progesterone trial rules out anovulation.

Correctable causes of anovulation. Anovulation can be secondary to other medical conditions. It is important to identify and correct a reversible cause of anovulation if present.

- Hypothyroidism is a common cause of anovulation, diagnosed by a high TSH and treated with thyroid replacement.
- Hyperprolactinemia, diagnosed by a serum prolactin test. An elevated prolactin inhibits GnRH by increasing dopamine. Treatment depends on the cause of the elevated prolactin.

Progestin management. Treatment involves replacing the hormone which is lacking (progesterone or progestin). These methods help regulate the menstrual flow and prevent endometrial hyperplasia, but do not reestablish normal ovulation.

- Cyclic MPA. Medroxyprogesterone acetate can be administered for the last 7 to 10 days of each cycle.
- Oral contraceptive pills (OCs). Estrogen-progestin oral contraceptives are often used for convenience. The important ingredient however, is the progestin not the estrogen.
- Progestin intrauterine system (LNG-IUS). The levonorgestrel lUS (Mirena or Skyla) delivers the progestin directly to the endometrium. This treatment can significantly decreasing menstrual blood loss.

Other managements. If progestin management is not successful in controlling blood loss, the following generic methods have been successful:

- **NSAIDs** can decrease dysmenorrheal, improve clotting and reduce menstrual blood loss. They are administered for only 5 days of the cycle and can be used and can be combined with OCs.
- **Tranexamic acid** (Lysteda) works by inhibiting fibrinolysis by plasmin. It is contraindicated with history of DVT, PE or CVA, and not recommended with E+P steroids.
- **Endometrial ablation** procedure destroys the endometrium by heat, cold or microwaves. It leads to a iatrogenic Asherman syndrome and minimal or no menstrual blood loss. Fertility will be affected.
- **Hysterectomy** (removal of the uterus) is a last resort and performed only after all other therapies have been unsuccessful.

PRIMARY AMENORRHEA

A 16-year-old girl presents with her mother, complaining she has never had a menstrual period. All of her friends have menstruated, and the mother is concerned about her daughter's lack of menstruation. On examination she seems to be well-nourished, with adult breast development and pubic hair present. Pelvic examination reveals a rudimentary vagina. No uterus is palpable on rectal examination.

Definition. Amenorrhea means absence of menstrual bleeding. Primary means that menstrual bleeding has never occurred.

Diagnosis. Primary amenorrhea is diagnosed with absence of menses at age 14 **without** secondary sexual development or age 16 **with** secondary sexual development.

Etiology. The origins of primary amenorrhea can be multiple. The two main categories of etiology are anatomic (e.g., vaginal agenesis/septum, imperforate hymen, or Müllerian agenesis) or hormonal (e.g., complete androgen insensitivity, gonadal dysgenesis [Turner syndrome], or hypothalamic-pituitary insufficiency).

Clinical Approach—Preliminary Evaluation

- **Are breasts present or absent?** A physical examination will evaluate secondary sexual characteristics (breast development, axillary and pubic hair, growth). **Breasts are an endogenous assay of estrogen.** Presence of breasts indicates adequate estrogen production. Absence of breasts indicates inadequate estrogen exposure.
- **Is a uterus present or absent?** An ultrasound of the pelvis should be performed to assess presence of a normal uterus.

GYN Triad

Imperforate Hymen

- Primary amenorrhea
- (+) breasts and uterus
- Normal height and weight

Table II-11-1. Müllerian Agenesis versus Androgen Insensitivity

Breasts Present/Uterus Absent	Müllerian Agenesis (46,XX)	Androgen Insensitivity (46,XY)
Uterus absent?	Idiopathic	MIF
Estrogen from?	Ovaries	Testes
Pubic hair?	Present	Absent
Testosterone level?	Female	Male
Treatment	No hormones Create vagina IVF—surrogate	Estrogen Create vagina Remove testes

Definition of abbreviations: MIF, Müllerian inhibitory factor.

Table II-11-2. Gonadal Dysgenesis versus HP Axis Failure

Breasts Absent/Uterus Present	Gonadal Dysgenesis (45,X)	HP Axis Failure (46,XX)
FSH	↑	↓
Why no estrogen?	No ovarian follicles	Follicles not stimulated
Ovaries?	"Streak"	Normal
Treatment pregnancy	E + P Egg donor	E + P Induce ovulation (HMG)
Diagnostic test?	—	CNS imaging

Definition of abbreviations: E + P, estrogen and progestin; HMG, human menopausal gonadotropin.

GYN Triad

Müllerian Agenesis

- Primary amenorrhea
- (+) breasts but (–) uterus
- (+) pubic and axillary hair

GYN Triad

Androgen Insensitivity

- Primary amenorrhea
- (+) breasts but (–) uterus
- **(–) pubic and axillary hair**

GYN Triad

Gonadal Dysgenesis

- Primary amenorrhea
- (–) breasts but (+) uterus
- ↑ FSH levels

GYN Triad

Hypothalamic–Pituitary Failure

- Primary amenorrhea
- (–) breasts but (+) uterus
- ↓ FSH levels

GYN Triad

Kallmann Syndrome

- Primary amenorrhea
- (–) breasts but (+) uterus
- Anosmia

Clinical Approach Based on Findings Regarding Breasts and Uterus

- **Breasts present, uterus present.** Differential diagnosis includes an imperforate hymen, vaginal septum, anorexia nervosa, excessive exercise, and possible pregnancy before first menses.
  - History and physical examination will identify the majority of specific diagnoses.
  - Otherwise the workup should proceed as if for secondary amenorrhea.
- **Breasts present, uterus absent.** Differential diagnosis is Müllerian agenesis (Rokitansky-Kuster-Hauser syndrome) and complete androgen insensitivity (testicular feminization). Testosterone levels and karyotype help make the diagnosis.
  - **Müllerian agenesis.** These are genetically normal females (46,XX) with idiopathic absence of the Müllerian duct derivatives: fallopian tubes, uterus, cervix, and upper vagina; the lower vagina originates from the urogenital sinus.
    - Patients develop secondary sexual characteristics because ovarian function is intact; Müllerian ducts do not give rise to the ovaries.
    - Normal pubic and axillary hair is present. Testosterone levels are normal female.
    - **Management:** surgical elongation of the vagina for satisfactory sexual intercourse
  - **Androgen insensitivity.** In these genetically male (46,XY) individuals with complete lack of androgen receptor function, their bodies do not respond to the high levels of androgens present.
    - Without androgen stimulation, internal Wolffian duct structures atrophy. With testicular Müllerian inhibitory factor present, the Müllerian duct derivatives involute.
    - Without body recognition of dihydrotestosterone, external genitalia differentiate in a female direction. Patients function psychologically and physically as females and are brought up as girls. At puberty, when primary amenorrhea is noted, the diagnosis is made.
    - Female secondary sexual characteristics are present because the testes do secrete estrogens without competition from androgens. No pubic or axillary hair is noted. Testosterone levels are normal male.
    - **Management:** testes removal at age 20 because the higher temperatures associated with the intraabdominal position of the testes may lead to testicular cancer. Estrogen replacement is then needed.
- **Breasts absent, uterus present.** Differential diagnosis is gonadal dysgenesis (Turner syndrome) and hypothalamic–pituitary failure. FSH level and karyotype help make the diagnosis.
  - **Gonadal dysgenesis.** Turner syndrome (45,X) is caused by the lack of one X chromosome, essential for the presence of normal ovarian follicles. Instead of developing ovaries, patients develop streak gonads. FSH is elevated because of lack of estrogen feedback to the hypothalamus and pituitary. No secondary sexual characteristics are noted.
    - **Management:** Estrogen and progesterone replacement for development of the secondary sexual characteristics
  - **Hypothalamic–pituitary failure.** In the patient without secondary sexual characteristic but uterus present by ultrasound, another possibility is the hypothalamic causes of amenorrhea (stress, anxiety, anorexia nervosa, excessive exercise). FSH will be low. Kallman syndrome is the inability of the hypothalamus to produce GnRH and also anosmia. The defect is in the area of the brain that produces GnRH, but it's also close to the olfactory center. CNS imaging will rule out a brain tumor.

– **Management:** These patients should be treated with estrogen and progesterone replacement for development of the secondary sexual characteristics.

SECONDARY AMENORRHEA

A 32-year-old woman states that her last menstrual period was 1 year ago. She started menses at age 12, and was irregular for the first couple of years, but since age 14 or 15 she had menstruated every 28–29 days. She has not been pregnant and is concerned about the amenorrhea. She has not been sexually active and has not used contraception. She has no other significant personal or family history. Physical examination, including a pelvic exam, is normal.

Definition. Amenorrhea means absence of menstrual bleeding. Secondary means that previously menstrual bleeding had occurred.

Diagnosis. Secondary amenorrhea is diagnosed with absence of menses for 3 months if previously regular menses or 6 months if previously irregular menses.

Pathophysiology. There are multiple etiologies for secondary amenorrhea, which can be classified by alterations in FSH and LH levels. They include hypogonadotropic (suggesting hypothalamic or pituitary dysfunction), hypergonadotropic (suggesting ovarian follicular failure), and eugonadotropic (suggesting pregnancy, anovulation, or uterine or outflow tract pathology).

Specific etiology.

- **Pregnancy**. The first step is a β-hCG to diagnose pregnancy. This is the most common cause of secondary amenorrhea.
- **Anovulation**. If no corpus luteum is present to produce progesterone, there can be no progesterone-withdrawal bleeding. Therefore, **anovulation** is associated with unopposed estrogen stimulation of the endometrium. Initially the anovulatory patient will demonstrate amenorrhea, but as endometrial hyperplasia develops, irregular, unpredictable bleeding will occur. The causes of anovulation are multiple, including PCOS, hypothyroidism, pituitary adenoma, elevated prolactin, and medications (e.g., antidepressants).
- **Estrogen Deficiency.** Without adequate estrogen priming the endometrium will be atrophic with no proliferative changes taking place. The causes of hypoestrogenic states are multiple, including absence of functional ovarian follicles or hypothalamic–pituitary insufficiency.
- **Outflow Tract Obstruction.** Even with adequate estrogen stimulation and progesterone withdrawal, menstrual flow will not occur if the endometrial cavity is obliterated or stenosis of the lower reproductive tract is present.

Management

Pregnancy Test. The first step in management of secondary amenorrhea is to obtain a qualitative β-hCG test to rule out pregnancy.

Thyrotropin (TSH) Level. If the β-hCG test is negative, hypothyroidism should be ruled out (TSH level). The elevated thyrotropin-releasing hormone (TRH) in primary hypothyroidism can lead to an elevated prolactin. If hypothyroidism is found, treatment is thyroid replacement with rapid restoration of menstruation.

GYN Triad

Anovulatory Bleeding (Physiologic)

- Irregular, unpredictable vaginal bleeding
- 13-year-old adolescent
- Normal height and weight

GYN Triad

Anovulatory Bleeding (Chronic)

- Irregular, unpredictable vaginal bleeding
- 33-year-old woman
- Obese, hypertensive

Prolactin Level

- **Medications.** An elevated prolactin level may be secondary to antipsychotic medications or antidepressants, which have an anti-dopamine side effect (it is known that the hypothalamic prolactin-inhibiting factor is dopamine).
- **Tumor.** A pituitary tumor should be ruled out with CT scan or MRI of the brain. If a pituitary tumor is found and is <1 cm in its greatest dimension, treat medically with bromocriptine (Parlodel), a dopamine agonist. If >1 cm, treat surgically.
- **Idiopathic.** If the cause of elevated prolactin is idiopathic, treatment is medical with bromocriptine.

Progesterone Challenge Test (PCT). If the β-hCG is negative, and TSH and prolactin levels are normal, administer either a single IM dose of progesterone or 7 days of oral medroxyprogesterone acetate (MPA).

- **Positive PCT.** Any degree of withdrawal bleeding is **diagnostic of anovulation**. Cyclic MPA is required to prevent endometrial hyperplasia. Clomiphene ovulation induction will be required if pregnancy is desired.
- **Negative PCT.** Absence of withdrawal bleeding is caused by either inadequate estrogen priming of the endometrium or outflow tract obstruction.

Estrogen–Progesterone Challenge Test (EPCT). If the PCT is negative, administer 21 days of oral estrogen followed by 7 days of MPA.

- **Positive EPCT.** Any degree of withdrawal bleeding is diagnostic of inadequate estrogen. An FSH level will help identify the etiology.
  - **Elevated FSH suggests ovarian failure.** If this occurs age <25, the cause could be Y chromosome mosaicism associated with malignancy, so order a karyotype. **Savage syndrome** or resistant ovary syndrome is a condition in which follicles are seen in the ovary by sonogram, though they do not respond to gonadotropins.
  - **Low FSH suggests hypothalamic–pituitary insufficiency.** Order a CNS imaging study to rule out a brain tumor. Whatever the result, women with a positive EPCT will need estrogen-replacement therapy to prevent osteoporosis and estrogen-deficiency morbidity. Cyclic progestins are also required to prevent endometrial hyperplasia.
- **Negative EPCT.** Absence of withdrawal bleeding is diagnostic of either an outflow tract obstruction or endometrial scarring (e.g., **Asherman syndrome**). A hysterosalpingogram (HSG) will identify where the lesion is. Asherman is the result of extensive uterine curettage and infection-produced adhesions. It is treated by hysteroscopic adhesion lysis followed by estrogen stimulation of the endometrium. An inflatable stent is then placed into the uterine cavity to prevent re-adhesion of the uterine walls.

Hormonal Disorders 12

Learning Objectives

- ❑ Describe the causes of premenstrual disorders including precocious puberty
- ❑ Describe normal menopause and approaches to treating symptoms
- ❑ Outline the causes of hirsutism
- ❑ Provide epidemiology, diagnosis, and management information about polycystic ovarian syndrome
- ❑ List the steps for diagnosing infertility and treatment options available

PRECOCIOUS PUBERTY

A 6-year-old girl is brought to the office by her mother who has noticed breast budding and pubic hair development on her daughter. She has also experienced menstrual bleeding. Her childhood history is unremarkable until 3 months ago when these changes began.

Diagnosis. Criteria for diagnosis include development of female secondary sexual characteristics and accelerated growth before age 8 in girls and age 9 in boys. Precocious puberty is more common in girls than boys.

Normal Pubertal Landmarks. Complete puberty is characterized by the occurrence of all pubertal changes.

- The **most common** initial change is thelarche (breast development at age 9–10).
- This is followed by **adrenarche** (pubic and axillary hair at age 10–11).
- Maximal growth rate occurs age 11 and 12.
- Finally, the last change is **menarche** (onset of menses at age 12–13).

Table II-12-1. Precocious Puberty

Diagnosis	Female secondary sexual characteristics Accelerated growth <8 years of age in girls	
Normal pubertal landmarks	Thelarche Breast development	9–10 years
	Adrenarche Pubic and axillary hair	10–11 years
	Maximal growth Growth spurt	11–12 years
	Menarche Onset of first menses	12–13 years

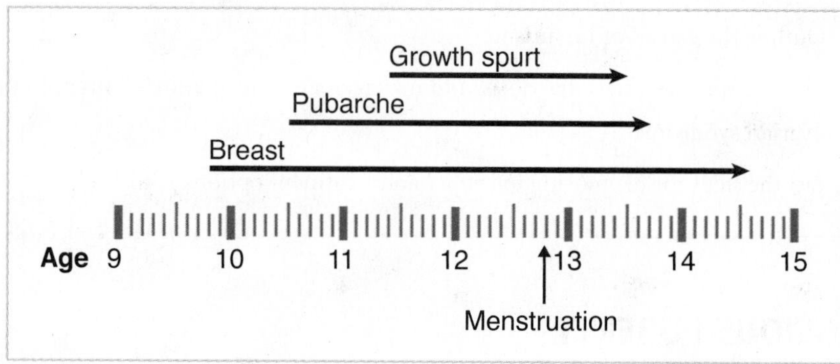

Figure II-12-1. Overview of Puberty

GYN Triad

Idiopathic or Constitutional

- Precocious complete isosexual puberty
- 6-year-old girl
- Normal head MRI

GYN Triad

CNS Lesions

- Precocious complete isosexual puberty
- 4-year-old girl
- Abnormal head MRI

Classification of precocious puberty

Incomplete Isosexual Precocious Puberty. This involves only one change—either thelarche, adrenarche, or menarche. This condition is the result of either transient hormone elevation or unusual end-organ sensitivity. Management is conservative.

Complete Isosexual Precocious Puberty. All changes of puberty are seen including breast development, growth spurt, and menstrual bleeding. The primary concern is premature closure of the distal epiphyses of the long bones, resulting in short stature. Fertility and sexual response are not impaired.

- **Gonadotropin-dependent.** This occurs because of increased secretion of estrogens that are dependent on premature release of gonadotropins from the hypothalamus and pituitary.
  - **Idiopathic.** The **most common** explanation is constitutional without a pathologic process present, accounting for 80% of precocious puberty. The age of the patient is usually 6 or 7 years. The diagnosis is usually one of exclusion after CNS imaging is shown to be normal. **Management** is GnRH agonist suppression (leuprolide or Lupron) of gonadotropins until appropriate maturity or height has been reached.
  - **CNS pathology.** This is a rare cause of precocious puberty. A CNS pathologic process stimulates hypothalamic release of GnRH, which leads to FSH release and ovarian follicle stimulation of estrogen production. This may include hydrocephalus,

von Recklinghausen disease, meningitis, sarcoid, and encephalitis. CNS imaging is abnormal. The age of the patient is usually <6 years. **Management** is directed at the specific pathologic process.

- **Gonadotropin-independent.** This occurs when estrogen production is independent of gonadotropin secretion from the hypothalamus and pituitary.
  - **McCune-Albright syndrome.** Also known as polyostotic fibrous dysplasia, this disorder is characterized by autonomous stimulation of aromatase enzyme production of estrogen by the ovaries. The syndrome includes multiple cystic bone lesions and **café au lait** skin spots. This accounts for 5% of precocious puberty. **Management** is administration of an aromatase enzyme inhibitor.
  - **Granulosa cell tumor.** A rare cause of precocious puberty is a gonadal-stromal cell ovarian tumor that autonomously produces estrogen. A **pelvic mass** will be identified on examination or pelvic imaging. **Management** is surgical removal of the tumor.

Follow-Up. Patients with idiopathic precocious puberty should be maintained with inhibition of the hypothalamic–pituitary–ovarian axis until the chronologic age catches up with the bone age.

Table II-12-2. Management of Precocious Puberty

Idiopathic	GnRH agonist
CNS lesions	Medical or surgical treatment
Ovarian tumor	Surgical excision
McCune-Albright	Aromatase inhibitors

PREMENSTRUAL DISORDERS

Premenstrual Syndrome (PMS)

A 36-year-old patient complains of depression, anxiety, irritability, and breast tenderness, which occur on a monthly basis. On further questioning, the symptoms most commonly occur 2 weeks before her menstruation and disappears with menses.

Definition. PMS includes a wide range of physical and emotional difficulties, as well as the more severe affective changes included in premenstrual dysphoric disorder (PDD).

Diagnosis. The basis for diagnosis is a **symptom diary** the patient keeps throughout 3 menstrual cycles. The specific symptoms are less important than their temporal relationship to the menstrual cycle. All the following must be present about the, symptoms:

- Must be recurrent in at least 3 consecutive cycles
- Must be absent in the preovulatory phase of the menstrual cycle
- Must be present in the 2 postovulatory weeks
- Must interfere with normal functioning
- Must resolve with onset of menses

GYN Triad

McCune-Albright Syndrome

- Precocious complete isosexual puberty
- 6-year-old girl
- Café-au-lait skin lesions

GYN Triad

Granulosa Cell Ovarian Tumor

- Precocious complete isosexual puberty
- 6-year-old girl
- Pelvic mass

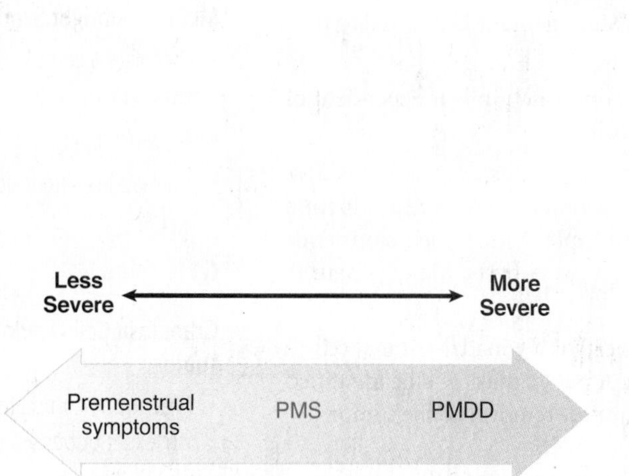

Figure II-12-2. Premenstrual Syndrome Diagnosis by Symptoms

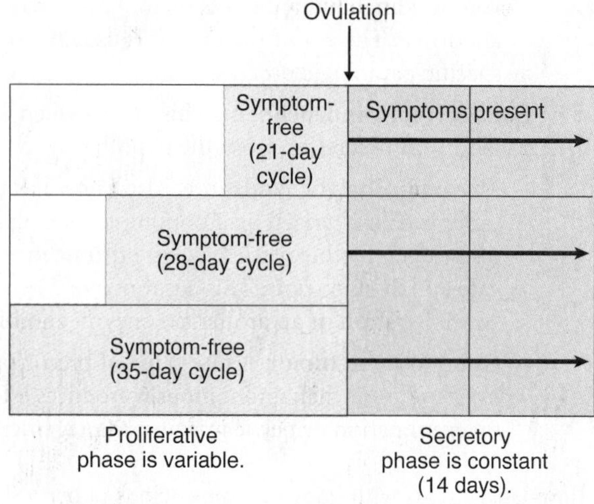

Figure II-12-3. Premenstrual Syndrome Diagnosis by Timing

- **Symptoms.** The symptoms may be of varied descriptions, including fluid retention (bloating, edema, breast tenderness), autonomic changes (insomnia, fatigue, heart pounding), emotional symptoms (crying, anxiety, depression, mood swings), or musculoskeletal complaints (headache, muscle aches, joint aches).

Fluid Retention	Automomic
• Breast tenderness • Extremity edema • Weight gain • Bloating	• Heart pounding • Confusion • Dizziness • Insomnia • Fatigue

Emotional	Musculoskeletal
• Nervous tension • Mood swings • Depression • Irritability • Anxiety, crying	• Muscle aches • Joint aches • Headaches • Cramps

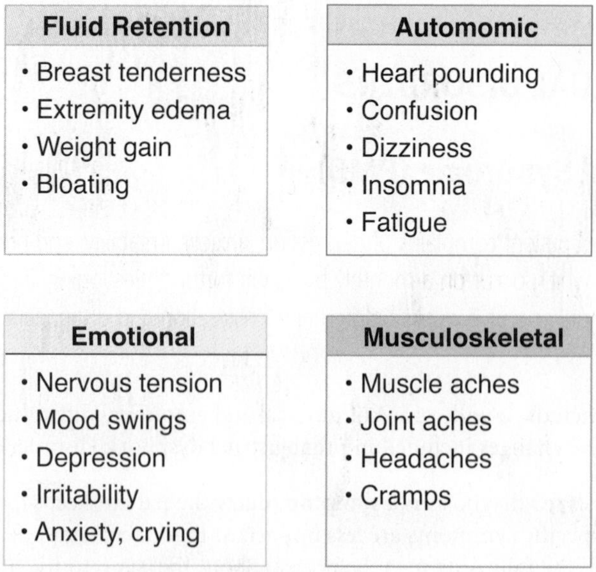

Figure II-12-4. PMS Symptoms

Management of PMS and PMDD

Proven treatments include the following:

- **Selective serotonin reuptake inhibitors (SSRIs).** Fluoxetine hydrochloride (Prozac); natural progesterone vaginal suppositories; MPA (Depo-Provera), spironolactone, and vitamin B_6 (pyridoxine). All of these options have been proposed for the treatment of PMS, but only fluoxetine, alprazolam (Xanax), and GnRH agonists have been shown in controlled, double-blind trials to be superior to placebo for the more severe symptoms of PDD. Recently reported double-blind trials of fluoxetine have shown reductions of 40–75% in troublesome behavioral and emotional symptoms. Similar outcomes have been reported for buspirone hydrochloride (BuSpar) and meclofenamate sodium in descriptive studies. SSRIs are the **treatment of choice** for emotional symptoms of PMS.
- **Yaz (drospirenone/ethinyl estradiol)**, with the unique progestin, drospirinon (DRSP), has been approved by the FDA for the treatment of PMS. Yaz is a low-dose, monophasic combination oral contraceptive with 24 hormone days with only a 4 day hormone-free interval. Studies show that the symptoms of PMS are decreased with a shorter hormone-free time period. DRSP is an analogue of spironolactone which differs from other OCP progestins by exhibiting both antimineralocorticoid and antiandrogenic effects.

Unproven treatments include the following:

- **Progesterone therapy** has a long history in the treatment of PMS, but neither natural progesterone (vaginal suppositories) nor progestin therapy has been shown to be any more effective than placebo. Because of both a lack of efficacy and the possibility of inducing menstrual irregularities, these agents should not be used.
- **Diuretics.** Because of the common complaint of "bloating" voiced by many patients with PMS, diuretics such as spironolactone have been advocated. Spironolactone has been studied in double-blind, randomized trials, and the results have been mixed. Although spironolactone may relieve some symptoms for some patients, the lack of consistent response across the studies in the literature suggests that other therapy is more effective.
- **Pyridoxine.** Vitamin B_6 in doses of 50-200 mg/d has been suggested as a treatment for PMS. A number of randomized, blinded studies have been performed, but no conclusive findings have emerged. Because of the lack of demonstrated efficacy and the possibility of permanent sensory neuropathy associated with high-dose vitamin B_6 consumptions, the use of vitamin B_6 should be discouraged.

Nutritional	Lifestyle
• Balanced diet • ⊠ caffeine • ⊠ sugar • ⊠ salt	• Relaxation techniques • Regular exercise • Support groups

Medications	
• Progesterone • Spironolactone • Pyridoxine (B_6)	**SSRIs** • Fluoxetine **OCPs** • Yaz

Figure II-12-5. PMS Treatment

HIRSUTISM

> A 28-year-old woman complains of increased hair growth on the face and on the chest. She states that this has been going on for the past 10 years; however, she is more conscious of it at the present time. Her menses are irregular and unpredictable. Even though she has been married for 8 years and never used contraception, she has never been pregnant. On pelvic examination the ovaries bilaterally are slightly enlarged, but there are no other abnormalities noted.

Definition. Hirsutism is excessive male-pattern hair growth in a woman on the upper lip, chin, chest, abdomen, back, and proximal extremities. **Virilization** is excessive male-pattern hair growth in a woman **plus other masculinizing signs** such as clitorimegaly, baldness, lowering of voice, increasing muscle mass, and loss of female body contours.

Pathophysiology. Hirsutism involves the conversion of **vellus hair** (fine, nonpigmented hair) to **terminal hair** (coarse, dark hair) within the hair follicle. This conversion is under the influence of androgens. In women, androgens are generally produced in only 3 body locations: the ovaries, the adrenal glands, and within the hair follicle. The workup of hirsutism will seek to identify which of these body locations is producing the androgens that are responsible for the excess terminal hair.

Clinical Approach

- **History.** Is there a positive family history? What was the age of onset? Was onset gradual or abrupt? Have menstrual periods been irregular or regular? Is medication history positive for androgenic steroids?
- **Examination.** What is body-mass index? Location of excess hair? Evidence of virilization (frontal balding, loss of female body contour, clitorimegaly)? Presence of adnexal masses?

Laboratory Tests. The primary purpose of these tests is to identify elevated free androgens.

- **Dehydroepiandrosterone sulfate (DHEAS)** is produced only in the adrenal glands. A markedly elevated DHEAS is consistent with an adrenal tumor.
- **17-OH progesterone** is a precursor in the biosynthesis pathway of cortisol. It is elevated in late-onset congenital adrenal hyperplasia (CAH), with 21-hydroxylase deficiency. It is converted peripherally into androgens.
- **Testosterone** is produced by both the ovary and the adrenal glands. A mildly elevated level is suggestive of PCO syndrome. A markedly elevated level is consistent with an ovarian tumor.

Clinical entities

Adrenal Tumor

- **History.** Typically the onset has been **rapid** without positive family history.
- **Examination.** Physical examination will show evidence of **virilization**. Pelvic examination is unremarkable.
- **Laboratory tests.** DHEAS level is markedly elevated.
- **Imaging.** CT or MRI scan will show an abdominal-flank mass.
- **Management.** Treatment involves surgical removal of tumor.

Ovarian Tumor

- **History.** Typically the onset has been **rapid** without positive family history.
- **Examination.** Physical examination will show evidence of **virilization**. An adnexal mass will be palpated on pelvic examination.
- **Laboratory tests.** Testosterone level is markedly elevated.
- **Imaging.** Pelvic ultrasound will show an adnexal mass.
- **Management.** Surgical removal of the mass, usually either a Sertoli-Leydig cell tumor or hilus cell tumor.

Congenital Adrenal Hyperplasia (21-Hydroxylase Deficiency)

- **History.** Typically the onset has been **gradual** in the second or early third decade of life and is associated with menstrual irregularities and anovulation. Precocious puberty with short stature is common. Family history may be positive. Late-onset CAH is one of the most common autosomal recessive genetic disorders.
- **Examination.** Physical examination will show evidence of **hirsutism** without virilization. Pelvic examination is unremarkable.
- **Laboratory tests.** Serum 17-OH progesterone level is markedly elevated.
- **Management.** Treatment is medical with continuous corticosteroid replacement, which will arrest the signs of androgenicity and restore ovulatory cycles.

GYN Triad

Adrenal Tumor

- Abrupt-onset virilization
- Abdominal/flank mass
- ↑↑ DHEAS levels

GYN Triad

Ovarian Tumor (Sertoli-Leydig)

- Abrupt-onset virilization
- Pelvic mass
- ↑↑ testosterone levels

GYN Triad

Congenital Adrenal Hyperplasia 21-OH Deficiency

- Gradual-onset hirsutism
- Normal exam
- ↑ 17-OH progesterone

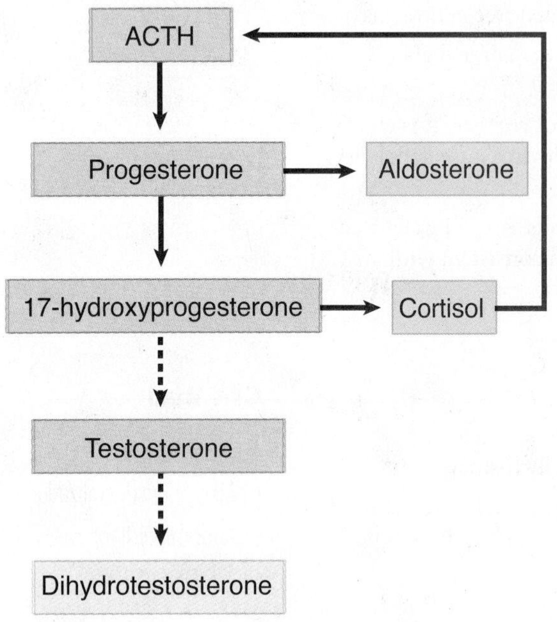

Figure II-12-6. Normal Adrenal Function

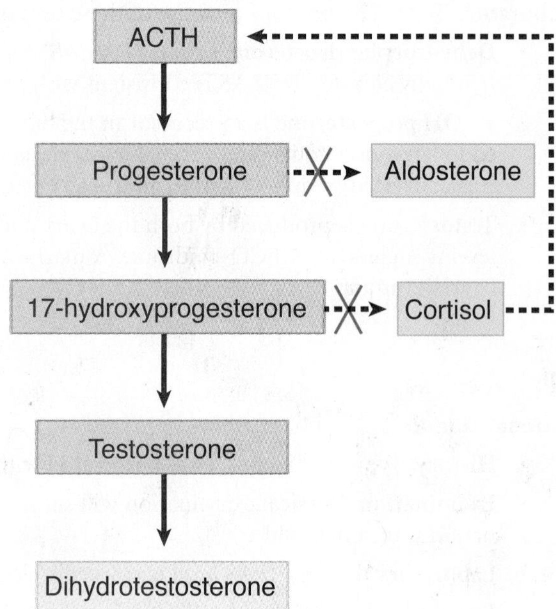

Figure II-12-7. Adrenal Hyperplasia

Polycystic Ovarian Syndrome (PCOS)

- **History.** Typically the onset has been **gradual**, frequently with a positive family history. In addition, the history is positive for irregular bleeding and infertility.
- **Examination.** Physical examination usually reveals **hirsutism** often with obesity and increased acne. Bilaterally enlarged, smooth, mobile ovaries will be palpated on pelvic examination. **Acanthosis nigricans** may be seen.
- **Laboratory tests.** Testosterone level is mildly elevated. LH to FSH ratio is elevated (3:1). Sex hormone binding globulin (SHBG) is decreased.
- **Imaging.** Pelvic ultrasound will show bilaterally enlarged ovaries with multiple subcapsular small follicles and increased stromal echogenicity.
- **Management.** The treatment of choice is combination OCPs. They will lower free testosterone levels in 2 ways. First, OCPs will lower testosterone production by suppressing LH stimulation of the ovarian follicle theca cells. Second, OCPs will also increase SHBG, thus decreasing free testosterone level. Metformin can decrease insulin resistance and lower testosterone levels.

Idiopathic

- **History.** Typically the onset has been **gradual**, frequently with a positive family history. Menses and fertility are normal. This is the **most common** cause of androgen excess in women.
- **Examination.** Physical examination reveals **hirsutism** without virilization. Pelvic examination is normal.
- **Laboratory tests.** Normal levels of testosterone, DHEAS, and 17-OH progesterone are identified.

GYN Triad

Idiopathic (Hair Follicle)
↑ 5-α Reductase Activity

- Gradual-onset hirsutism
- Normal exam
- Normal DHEAS, testosterone, 17-OH progesterone

- **Management.** The treatment of choice is **spironolactone**, a potassium-sparing diuretic. Its mechanism of action as an antiandrogen is twofold. First, it is an androgen-receptor blocker. It also suppresses hair follicle 5-α reductase enzyme conversion of androstenedione and testosterone to the more potent dihydrotestosterone. **Eflornithine** (**Vaniqa**) is the first topical drug for the treatment of unwanted facial and chin hair. It blocks ornithine decarboxylase (ODC), which slows the growth and differentiation of the cells within the hair follicles.

POLYCYSTIC OVARIAN SYNDROME

A 32-year-old woman visits the gynecologist's office complaining of vaginal bleeding, facial hair growth, and obesity. She states that she has noted the facial hair growth for many years and the irregular bleeding has been progressively getting worse during the past 6 months. She has no other significant personal or family history, and on pelvic examination she has slightly enlarged bilateral ovaries. A rectovaginal examination is confirmatory.

Definition. Polycystic ovarian syndrome (PCOS), historically called Stein-Leventhal syndrome, is a condition of chronic anovulation with resultant infertility. The patient presents typically with irregular vaginal bleeding. Other symptoms include obesity and hirsutism.

Pathophysiology

- **Chronic anovulation.** Instead of showing the characteristic hormone fluctuation of the normal menstrual cycle, PCOS gonadotropins and sex steroids are in a steady state, resulting in anovulation and **infertility**. Without ovulation, there is no corpus luteum to produce progesterone. Without progesterone there is unopposed estrogen. Endometrium, which is chronically stimulated by estrogen, without progesterone ripening and cyclic shedding, becomes hyperplastic with **irregular bleeding**. With time **endometrial hyperplasia** can result, which could progress to endometrial cancer.
- **Increased testosterone.** Increased LH levels cause increased ovarian follicular theca cell production of androgens. The increased levels of androstenedione and testosterone suppress hepatic production of SHBG by 50%. The combined effect of increased total testosterone and decreased SHBG leads to mildly elevated levels of free testosterone. This results in **hirsutism**. PCOS is one of the **most common** causes of hirsutism in women.
- **Ovarian enlargement.** On ultrasound the ovaries demonstrate the presence of the necklacelike pattern of multiple peripheral cysts (20–100 cystic follicles in each ovary). The increased androgens prevent normal follicular development, inducing premature follicle atresia. These multiple follicles, in various stages of development and atresia, along with stromal hyperplasia and a thickened ovarian capsule, result in ovaries that are bilaterally enlarged.

Table II-12-3. "HA-IR-AN" Syndrome (Polycystic Ovarian Syndrome)

HA	HyperAndrogenism
IR	Insulin Resistance
AN	Acanthosis Nigricans

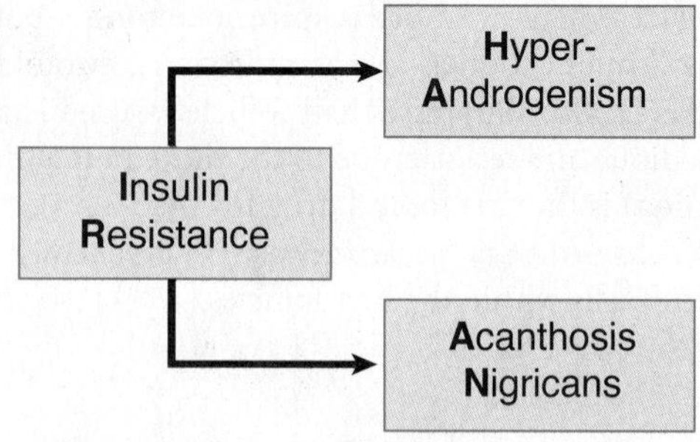

Figure II-12-8. Polycystic Ovarian Syndrome

Diagnosis. Diagnosis is based on the Rotterdam criteria, which requires 2 of the following 3 findings:

1. Oligomenorrhea or menstrual dysfunction
2. Hyperandrogenism, clinically or biochemically
3. Polycystic ovaries on TV sonogram (≥12 peripheral cysts)

Management. Treatment is directed toward the primary problem and the patient's desires.

- **Irregular bleeding.** OCPs will normalize her bleeding. The progestin component will prevent endometrial hyperplasia.
- **Hirsutism.** Excess male-pattern hair growth can be suppressed 2 ways. OCPs will lower testosterone production by suppressing LH stimulation of the ovarian follicle theca cells. OCPs will also increase SHBG, thus decreasing free testosterone levels. Spironolactone suppresses hair follicle 5-α reductase enzyme conversion of androstenedione and testosterone to the more potent dihydrotestosterone.
- **Infertility.** If she desires pregnancy, ovulation induction can be achieved through clomiphene citrate (Clomid) or human menopausal gonadotropin (HMG; Pergonal). Metformin, a hypoglycemic agent that increases insulin sensitivity, can enhance the likelihood of ovulation both with and without clomiphene.

INFERTILITY

A 30-year-old woman comes to the gynecologist's office complaining of infertility for 1 year. She and her husband have been trying to achieve pregnancy for >1 year and have been unsuccessful. There is no previous history of pelvic inflammatory disease and she used oral contraception medication for 6 years. The pelvic examination is normal, and a Pap smear is done.

Definition. Infertility is defined as inability to achieve pregnancy after 12 months of unprotected and frequent intercourse. Both male and female factors have to be evaluated in the patient with infertility. Fifteen percent of American couples suffer infertility.

Fecundability. This is the likelihood of conception occurring with one cycle of appropriately timed midcycle intercourse. With the female partner age of 20 years, the fecundity rate is 20%. By age 35 years, the rate drops to 10%.

Initial Noninvasive Tests

Semen analysis

- **Normal values.** Expected findings are volume >2 ml; pH 7.2–7.8; sperm density >20 million/ml; sperm motility >50%; and sperm morphology >50% normal. If values are abnormal, repeat the semen analysis in 4–6 weeks because semen quality varies with time.
- **Timing.** The first step in the infertility evaluation is a semen analysis, which should be obtained after 2–3 days of abstinence and examined within 2 h.
- **Minimally abnormal.** If sperm density is mild to moderately lower than normal, intrauterine insemination may be used. Washed sperm are directly injected into the uterine cavity. Idiopathic oligozoospermia is the most common male infertility factor.
- **Severely abnormal.** If semen analysis shows severe abnormalities, intracytoplasmic sperm injection may be used in conjunction with in vitro fertilization and embryo transfer.
- **No viable sperm.** With azoospermia or failed ICSI, artificial insemination by donor (AID) may be used.

Anovulation

Of all causes of infertility, treatment of anovulation results in the greatest success.

- **History.** Typically history is irregular, unpredictable menstrual bleeding, most often associated with minimal or no uterine cramping.
- **Objective data.** A basal body temperature (BBT) chart will not show the typical midcycle temperature elevation. A serum progesterone level will be low. An endometrial biopsy shows proliferative histology.
- **Correctible causes.** Hypothyroidism or hyperprolactinemia
- **Ovulation induction.** The agent of choice is **clomiphene** citrate administered orally for 5 days beginning on day 5 of the menstrual cycle. The biochemical structure of clomiphene is very similar to estrogen, and clomiphene fits into the estrogen receptors at the level of the pituitary. The pituitary does not interpret clomiphene as estrogen and perceives a low estrogen state, thus producing high levels of gonadotropins. **HMG** is administered parenterally and is used to induce ovulation if clomiphene fails. Careful monitoring of ovarian size is important because ovarian hyperstimulation is the **most common** major side effect of ovulation induction. When a patient is given clomiphene, her own pituitary is being stimulated to secrete her own gonadotropins, whereas when a patient is administered HMG, the patient is being stimulated by exogenous gonadotropins.

Follow-Up Invasive Tests

Hysterosalpinogram and Laparoscopy

Tubal Disease. Assessment of fallopian tube abnormalities is the next step if the semen analysis is normal and ovulation is confirmed.

- **Hysterosalpingogram (HSG).** In this imaging procedure, a catheter is placed inside the uterine cavity, and contrast material is injected. The contrast material should be seen on x-ray images spilling bilaterally into the peritoneal cavity. It should be scheduled during the week after the end of menses after prophylactic antibiotics to prevent causing a recurrent acute salpingitis. No further testing is performed if the HSG shows normal anatomy. If abnormal findings are seen, the extent and site of the pathology is noted and laparoscopy considered.

- **Chlamydia antibody.** A negative IgG Antibody test for chlamydia virtually rules out infection induced tubal adhesions.
- **Laparoscopy.** If potentially correctible tubal disease is suggested by the HSG, the next step in management is to visualize the oviducts and attempt reconstruction if possible (tuboplasty). If tubal damage is so severe surgical therapy is futile, then IVF should be planned.

Unexplained Infertility

Definition. This diagnosis is reserved for couples in which the semen analysis is normal, ovulation is confirmed, and patent oviducts are noted.

Outcome. Approximately 60% of patients with unexplained infertility will achieve a spontaneous pregnancy within the next 3 years.

Management. Treatment consists of controlled ovarian hyperstimulation (*COH*) with clomiphene, and appropriately timed preovulatory intrauterine insemination (*IUI*). The fecundity rates for 6 months are comparable with IVF with a significantly lower cost and risk.

In Vitro Fertilization. With IVF, eggs are aspirated from the ovarian follicles using a transvaginal approach with the aid of an ultrasound. They are fertilized with sperm in the laboratory, resulting in the formation of embryos. Multiple embryos are transferred into the uterine cavity with a cumulative pregnancy rate of 55% after 4 IVF cycles.

Ovarian Reserve Testing (ORT)

This assessment is mostly reserved for the infertile woman aged 35 or over.

Definition. ORT refers to assessment of the capacity of the ovary to provide eggs that are capable of fertilization.

- It is a function of (1) number of follicles available for recruitment, and (2) the health and quality of the eggs in the ovaries.
- The most significant factor affection ORT is a woman's chronological age with a major decrease around age 35.

Measures of ovarian reserve. These tests help predict whether a woman will respond to ovarian stimulation or whether it would be best to proceed directly to in-vitro fertilization (IVF).

- **Day 3 FSH** is the most commonly used test for ORT. FSH levels are expected to be low due to the feedback of estrogen from the stimulated follicles. An increase in FSH level occurs if there is follicle depletion.
- **Anti-Mullerian hormone** (**AMH**). This glycoprotein is produced exclusively by small antral ovarian follicles and is therefore a direct measure of the follicular pool. As the number of ovarian follicles declines with age, AMH concentrations will decline.
- **Antral follicle count** (**AFC**) is the total number of follicles measuring 2-10 mm in diameter that are observed during an early follicular phase transvaginal sonogram. The number of AF correlates with the size of the remaining follicle pool retrieved by ovarian stimulation. AFC typically declines with age.

MENOPAUSE

A 53-year-old woman visits the gynecologist's office complaining of hot flashes, vaginal dryness, and irritability. She states that her symptoms started 1 year ago and have progressively been getting worse. Her last gynecologic examination was 2 years ago, at which time her mammogram was normal.

Definition. Menopause is a retrospective diagnosis and is defined as 12 months of amenorrhea. This is associated with the elevation of gonadotropins (FSH and LH). The mean age of 51 years is genetically determined and unaffected by pregnancies or use of steroid contraception. Smokers experience menopause up to 2 years earlier.

- **Premature menopause** occurs age 30–40 and is mostly idiopathic, but can also occur after radiation therapy or surgical oophorectomy.
- **Premature ovarian failure** occurs age <30 and may be associated with autoimmune disease or Y chromosome mosaicism.

Diagnosis. The laboratory diagnosis of menopause is made through serial identification of elevated gonadotropins.

Etiology. The etiology of menopausal symptoms is lack of estrogen.

Clinical Findings. The lack of estrogen is responsible for the majority of menopausal symptoms and signs.

- **Amenorrhea.** The **most common** symptom is secondary amenorrhea. Menses typically become anovulatory and decrease during a period of 3–5 years known as perimenopause.
- **Hot flashes.** Unpredictable profuse sweating and sensation of heat is experienced by 75% of menopausal women. This is probably mediated through the hypothalamic thermoregulatory center. Obese women are less likely to undergo hot flashes owing to peripheral conversion of androgens to estrone in their peripheral adipose tissues.
- **Reproductive tract.** Low estrogen leads to decreased vaginal lubrication, increased vaginal pH, and increased vaginal infections.
- **Urinary tract.** Low estrogen leads to increased urgency, frequency, nocturia, and urge incontinence.
- **Psychic.** Low estrogen leads to mood alteration, emotional lability, sleep disorders, and depression.
- **Cardiovascular disease.** This is the **most common** cause of mortality (50%) in postmenopausal women, with prevalence rising rapidly after menopause.
- **Osteoporosis.** This a disorder of decreased bone density leading to pathologic fractures when density falls below the fracture threshold.

GYN Triad

Premature Ovarian Failure r/o Y Chromosome Mosaic

- Hot flashes, sweats
- Age 25 years
- ↑ FSH level

Osteoporosis

Anatomy. The most common bone type of osteoporosis is trabecular bone. The **most common** anatomic site is in the vertebral bodies, leading to crush fractures, kyphosis, and decreased height. Hip and wrist fractures are the next most frequent sites.

Diagnosis. The **most common** method of assessing bone density is with a **DEXA** scan (dual-energy x-ray absorptiometry). The **most common** method of assessing calcium loss is 24-h urine hydroxyproline or NTX (N-telopeptide, a bone breakdown product).

Risk factors. The **most common** risk factor is positive family history in a thin, white female. Other risk factors are steroid use, low calcium intake, sedentary lifestyle, smoking, and alcohol.

Prevention. Maximum bone density is found in the mid-20s. Maintenance of bone density is assisted by both lifestyle and medications.

Table II-12-4. Osteoporosis

Lifestyle	Ca^{2+} and vitamin D intake
	Weight-bearing exercise
	Stop cigarettes and alcohol
Medical	Historic gold standard for comparing therapies: estrogen replacement
	Inhibit osteoclastics: bisphosphonates (alendronate, risedronate)
	Increase bone density: SERMs (raloxifene)

Definition of abbreviations: SERMS, selective estrogen receptor modulators.

- **Lifestyle.** Calcium and vitamin D intake, weight-bearing exercise, and elimination of cigarettes and alcohol.
- **Medications.** Bisphosphates (e.g., alendronate, risedronate) inhibit osteoclastic activity. Selective estrogen receptor modulators (SERMs; e.g., raloxifene) increase bone density. Bisphosphonates and SERMs are the first choices for osteoporosis treatment. Calcitonin and fluoride have also been used. While estrogen is a highly effective therapy, it should not be primarily used to treat osteoporosis because of concerns detailed in the next paragraph.

Hormone Replacement Therapy

Benefits and risks

- Estrogen therapy continues to be the most effective and FDA-approved method for relief of menopausal vasomotor symptoms (hot flashes), as well as genitourinary atrophy and dyspareunia.
- The Women's Health Initiative (WHI) study of the National Institutes of Health (NIH) studied 27,000 postmenopausal women with a mean age of 63 years. These included women with a uterus on hormone therapy (HT), both estrogen and progestin, and hysterectomized women on estrogen therapy (ET) only.

Table II-12-5. Critique of Women's Health Initiative Study

Excludes patients with vasomotor symptoms Primary indication for hormone replacement
Mean patient age was 63 years Missed the 10-year "window of opportunity"
Same dose of hormone for all ages Older women don't need as a high dose as do younger women
Patients were not all healthy Hypertension (40%), ↑ cholesterol (15%), diabetes mellitus (7%), myocardial infarction (3%)

- **Benefits:** Both HT and ET groups in WHI had decreased osteoporotic fractures and lower rates of colorectal cancer.
- **Risks:** Both HT and ET groups in WHI were found to have small increases in deep vein thrombosis (DVT). The HT group also had increased heart attacks and breast cancer, but these were not increased in the ET group.

Table II-12-6. WHI–Benefit and Risk (Mean Age of 63 Years)

	Estrogen and Progestin	Estrogen Only
Vaginal dryness	Benefit	Benefit
Hot flashes	Benefit	Benefit
Vasomotor symptoms	Benefit	Benefit
Osteoporosis	Benefit	Benefit
Breast cancer	Risk	No change
Heart disease	Risk	No change
Stroke	Risk	Risk

Contraindications. Personal history of an estrogen-sensitive cancer (breast or endometrium), active liver disease, active thrombosis, or unexplained vaginal bleeding

Modalities. Estrogen can be administered by oral, transdermal, vaginal, or parenteral routes. All routes will yield the benefits described. Women without a uterus can be given continuous estrogen. All women with a uterus should also be given progestin therapy to prevent endometrial hyperplasia. The **most common** current regimen is oral estrogen and progestin given continuously.

Recommendations. The **Global Consensus Statement on Menopausal Hormonal Therapy (MHT)** by the International Menopause Society (2013) says the following:

Proven Benefits of MHT and Only Indications For Use

- **Vasomotor symptoms.** MHT is the most effective treatment for vasomotor symptoms associated with menopause at any age, but benefits are more likely to outweigh risks for symptomatic women age <60 or within 10 years after menopause.

GYN Triad

Limitations of WHI

- Women with prominent vasomotor symptoms, the most common reason for initiating HT, were excluded from the study.
- The mean age of 63 was 10 years past the age that most women begin HT, thus missing the "window of opportunity" immediately after menopause.
- The same hormone dose was used in both older and younger women.

- **Vaginal dryness.** Local low-dose estrogen therapy is preferred for women whose symptoms are limited to vaginal dryness or associated discomfort with intercourse.
- **Premature menopause.** In women with premature ovarian insufficiency, systemic MHT is recommended at least until the average age of the natural menopause.

Benefits of MHT but Not Indications For Use

- **Osteoporosis.** MHT is effective and appropriate for the prevention of osteoporosis-related fractures in at-risk women age <60 or within 10 years after menopause.
- **Coronary heart disease.** Findings depend on the kind of MHT used.
  - **Estrogen-alone** (ET) may decrease coronary heart disease and all-cause mortality in women age <60 and within 10 years of menopause.
  - **Estrogen plus progestogen** (HT) in this age group shows a similar trend for decreased mortality but no significant increase or decrease in coronary heart disease has been found.

Risks of MHT

- **The risk of venous thromboembolism (VTE) and ischemic stroke** increases with oral MHT but the absolute risk is rare age <60. Observational studies point to a lower risk with transdermaltherapy.
- **The risk of breast cancer** in women age >50 associated with MHT is a complex one. The increased risk of breast cancer is primarily associated with the addition of a progestogen to estrogen therapy (HT) and related to the duration of use. The risk of breast cancer attributable to HT is small and decreases after treatment is stopped. Current safety data do not support the use of MHT in breast cancer survivors.

Administration of Menopausal Hormone Therapy (MHT)

- **Uterus present or absent.** Estrogen as a single systemic agent (ET) is appropriate in women after hysterectomy but additional progestogen (HT) is required in the presence of a uterus.
- **Individualized management.** The option of MHT is an individual decision in terms of quality of life and health priorities as well as personal risk factors such as age, time since menopause and risk of venous thromboembolism, stroke, ischemic heart disease and breast cancer.
- **Dose and duration.** Dose and duration of MHT should be consistent with treatment goals and safety issues, and thus should be individualized.
- **Bioidentical hormones.** The use of custom-compounded bioidentical hormone therapy is not recommended.

Estrogen alternatives

SERMs. In patients with contraindications to estrogen-replacement therapy, SERMs can be used. These are medications with estrogen agonist effects in some tissues, and estrogen antagonist effects on others. Although protective against the heart as well as bone, these medications do not have much effect on hot flashes and sweats.

- **Tamoxifen** (Nolvadex) is an SERM with endometrial and bone agonist effects, but breast antagonist effects.
- **Raloxifene** (Evista) has bone agonist effects, but endometrial antagonist effects.

The Female Breast 13

Learning Objectives

- ❑ Describe normal breast development
- ❑ Differentiate between benign breast disorders and breast cancer, in terms of diagnosis and treatment

NORMAL BREAST DEVELOPMENT

Embryology

Breasts begin developing in the embryo about 7 to 8 weeks after conception, consisting only of a thickening or ridge of tissue.

- From weeks 12 to 16, tiny groupings of cells begin to branch out, laying the foundation for future **ducts** and milk-producing **glands**. Other tissues develop into muscle cells that will form the nipple (the protruding point of the breast) and areola (the darkened tissue surrounding the nipple).
- In the later stages of pregnancy, maternal hormones cause fetal breast cells to organize into branching, tube-like structures, thus forming the milk ducts. In the final 8 weeks, lobules (milk-producing glands) mature and actually begin to secrete a liquid substance called colostrum.
- In both female and male newborns, swellings underneath the nipples and areolae can easily be felt, and a clear liquid discharge (colostrum) can be seen.

Puberty

From infancy to just before puberty, there is no difference between female and male breasts.

- With the beginning of female puberty, however, the release of estrogen—at first alone, and then in combination with progesterone when the ovaries are functionally mature—causes the breasts to undergo dramatic changes that culminate in the fully mature form.
- This process, on average, takes 3 to 4 years and is usually complete by age 16.

Anatomy

> **Note**
>
> Refer to Chapter 1, for a discussion of Tanner Stages.

The breast is made of lobes of glandular tissue with associated ducts for transfer of milk to the exterior and supportive fibrous and fatty tissue. On average, there are 15 to 20 lobes in each breast, arranged roughly in a wheel-spoke pattern emanating from the nipple area. The distribution of the lobes, however, is not even.

- There is a preponderance of glandular tissue in the upper outer portion of the breast. This is responsible for the tenderness in this region that many women experience prior to their menstrual cycle.
- About 80–85% of normal breast tissue is fat during the reproductive years. The 15 to 20 lobes are further divided into lobules containing alveoli (small sac-like features) of secretory cells with smaller ducts that conduct milk to larger ducts and finally to a reservoir that lies just under the nipple. In the nonpregnant, nonlactating breast, the alveoli are small.
- During pregnancy, the alveoli enlarge. During lactation, the cells secrete milk substances (proteins and lipids). With the release of oxytocin, the muscular cells surrounding the alveoli contract to express the milk during lactation.
- Ligaments called **Cooper's ligaments**, which keep the breasts in their characteristic shape and position, support breast tissue. In the elderly or during pregnancy, these ligaments become loose or stretched, respectively, and the breasts sag.
- The lymphatic system drains excess fluid from the tissues of the breast into the axillary nodes. Lymph nodes along the pathway of drainage screen for foreign bodies such as bacteria or viruses.

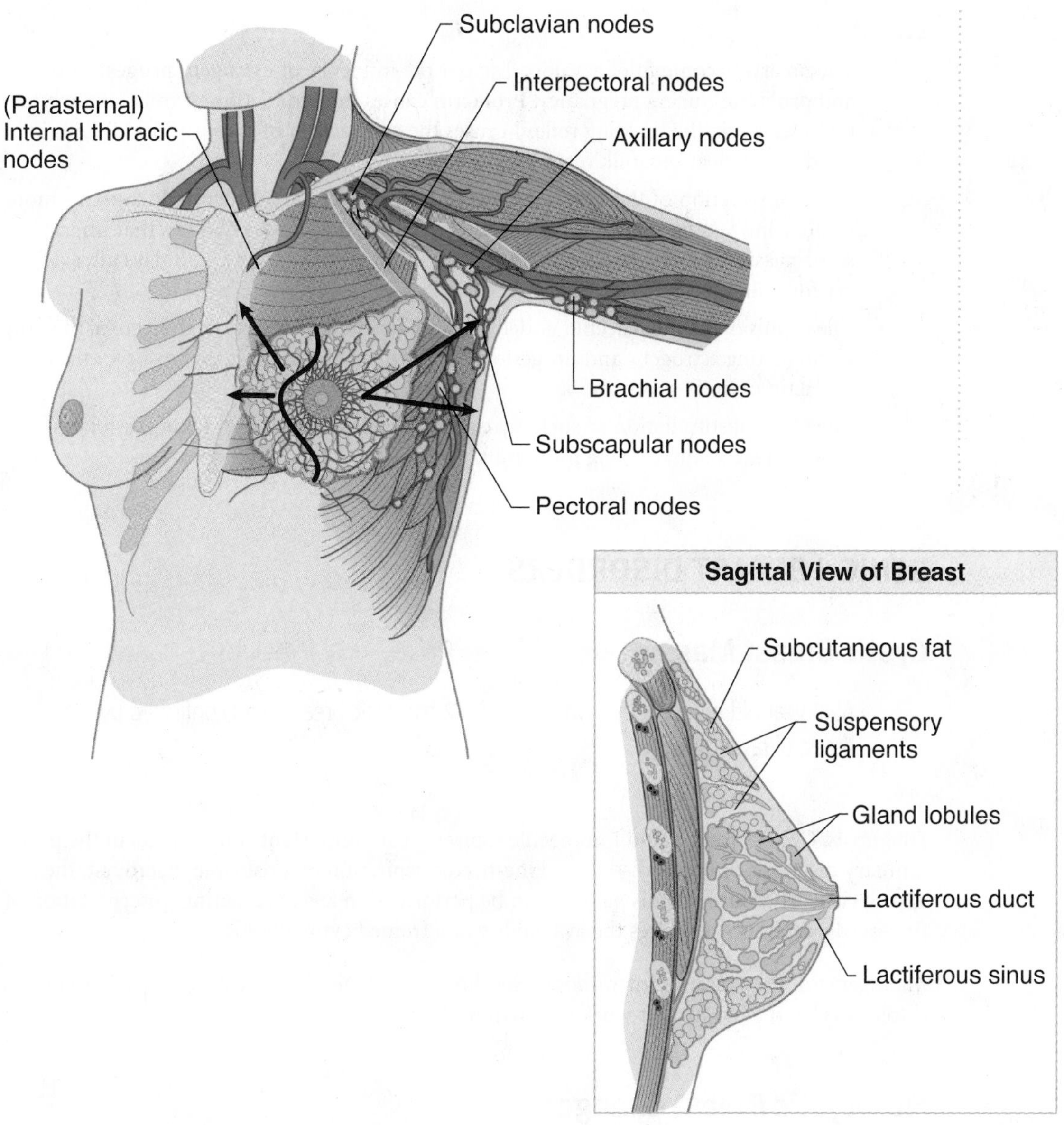

Figure II-13-1. Breast

Hormones

Reproductive hormones are important in the development of the breast in puberty and in lactation.

- **Estrogen**, released from the ovarian follicle, promotes the growth ducts.
- **Progesterone**, released from the corpus luteum, stimulates the development of milk-producing alveolar cells.
- **Prolactin**, released from the anterior pituitary gland, stimulates milk production.
- **Oxytocin**, released from the posterior pituitary in response to suckling, causes milk ejection from the lactating breast.

Lactation

- The breasts become fully developed under the influence of **estrogen**, **progesterone**, and **prolactin** during pregnancy. **Prolactin** causes the production of milk, and **oxytocin** release (via the suckling reflex) causes the contraction of smooth-muscle cells in the ducts to eject the milk from the nipple.
- The first secretion of the mammary gland after delivery is colostrum. It contains more protein and less fat than subsequent milk, and contains IgA antibodies that impart some **passive immunity** to the infant. Most of the time it takes 1 to 3 days after delivery for milk production to reach appreciable levels.
- The expulsion of the placenta at delivery initiates milk production and causes the drop in circulating estrogens and progesterone. **Estrogen** antagonizes the positive effect of prolactin on milk production.
- The physical stimulation of suckling causes the release of oxytocin and stimulates prolactin secretion, causing more milk production.

BENIGN BREAST DISORDERS

Note

Mammograms are discussed in detail in Gynecology, chapter 1.

Cystic Breast Mass

A 40-year-old menstruating woman had a 2-cm cystic breast mass confirmed by breast ultrasonography.

Diagnosis. Cyst aspiration and fine-needle aspiration are important components in the preliminary diagnosis of breast disorders. Fine-needle aspiration of a palpable macrocyst, the appropriate procedure for this patient, can be performed in an office setting. Interpretation of fine-needle aspiration requires the availability of a trained cytopathologist.

Management. Preaspiration mammography should be obtained. If the cyst disappears and the cytology is benign, no further workup is required.

Fibrocystic Breast Changes

A 30-year-old woman experiences bilateral breast enlargement and tenderness, which fluctuates with her menstrual cycle. On physical examination the breast feels lumpy, and the patient indicates a sensitive area with a discrete 1.5-cm nodule, which she says is consistently painful. A fine-needle aspiration is performed, and clear fluid is withdrawn. Clinically the cysts resolved.

Diagnosis. Cyclic premenstrual mastalgia is often associated with fibrocystic changes of the breast; a condition that is no longer considered a disease but a heterogeneous group of disorders. Breast discomfort may be accompanied by a palpable mass. Fine-needle aspiration can easily distinguish whether a mass is solid or cystic. The procedure requires no special skill other than stabilizing the mass so that needle aspiration can be done with precision. The goal of cyst aspiration is complete drainage of the cyst with collapse of the cyst wall.

Management

- **Mass disappears.** If the cyst fluid is clear, it may be discarded. If the cyst fluid is grossly bloody, it should be sent for cytologic examination to rule out the possibility of intracystic carcinoma. After aspiration, the affected area must be palpated to determine whether there is a residual mass. If there is no residual mass, the patient may be reexamined in 4–6 weeks for the reaccumulation of fluid. If fluid reaccumulates, it may be aspirated again.
- **Mass persists.** A mass that persists requires further workup. A persistent accumulation is managed by mammography and excision. Because changes such as hematoma related to aspiration may affect mammographic appearances, it is recommended that mammography not be performed until 2 weeks after aspiration. Definitive evaluation of a persistent mass requires excisional biopsy.
- **Conservative.** Ultrasonography is useful in distinguishing cysts from solid masses. If ultrasonography has been performed before aspiration and had shown a cyst with distinct smooth contours, an alternative management plan would be conservative follow-up with serial ultrasound scans. If the cyst disappears on aspiration and the fluid is clear, no further workup is required.

Breast Fibroadenoma

A 25-year-old woman visits the gynecologist for routine annual examination. During the examination she has a palpable, rubbery breast mass, which has been present and stable for the past 2 years. The pathology report of fine-needle aspiration was consistent with fibroadenoma.

Diagnosis. Fibroadenomas are the **most common** breast tumors found in adolescence and young women. In approximately 15% of patients they occur as multiple lesions. Clinically, fibroadenomas are discrete, smoothly contoured, rubbery, nontender, freely moveable masses. The most distinctive gross feature of fibroadenomas that allows them to be distinguished from other breast lumps is their mobility. Fibroadenomas arise from the epithelium and stroma of the terminal duct lobular unit, most frequently in the upper outer quadrant of the breast. An association of fibroadenomas with the development of breast cancer has not been well established. Any associated increases in breast cancer risk depends on the presence of proliferative changes in the fibroadenoma itself or in the surrounding breast, and on a family history of breast carcinoma.

Although cysts and fibroadenomas may be indistinguishable on palpation, ultrasound examination easily distinguishes cystic from solid lesions. On fine-needle aspiration, cysts typically collapse, whereas samples from a fibroadenoma present a characteristic combination of epithelial and stromal elements.

Management

- **Conservative.** Some clinicians advocate conservative management of fibroadenomas, especially in young women, because they can be diagnosed by ultrasonography and core-needle biopsy or fine-needle aspiration with a high degree of confidence, and in some cases they will resolve. A survey of patient preferences, however, has revealed that many women choose excisional biopsy even when they are assured that the lesion is benign by fine-needle aspiration.

- **Excision.** Typically, the lesion is "shelled out" with a surrounding thin rim of breast tissue to avoid the necessity of reexcision in the rare instances when the tumor proves to be a **phyllodes tumor**. This is a mixed epithelial and stromal tumor that has benign, borderline, and malignant variants. The biology of the phyllodes tumor is determined by its stromal elements; in its fully malignant form, it behaves as a sarcoma.

Mammography Microcalcifications

A 45-year-old woman visits her gynecologist after having her yearly mammogram done. The mammogram reveals a "cluster" of microcalcifications.

Diagnosis. A geographic cluster of microcalcifications is nonpalpable. Although most of these lesions are benign, approximately 15–20% represent early cancer. An occult lesion requires stereotactic needle localization and biopsy under mammographic guidance. The coordinates of the lesion are calculated by the computer according to the basic principles of stereotaxis. The radiologist selects the length of the biopsy needle, and a core biopsy is obtained. The procedure is performed in an outpatient setting.

Management. Treatment is based on the established histologic diagnosis.

Persistent Breast Mass

A 35-year-old woman has a persistent breast mass after a fine-needle aspiration has been performed. The breast mass is confirmed by ultrasonography.

Diagnosis. With the combination of physical examination, fine-needle aspiration or core biopsy, and mammography, open biopsies are being performed less frequently. Excisional biopsy has the advantage of a complete evaluation of the size and histologic characteristics of the tumor before definitive therapy is selected. An excisional biopsy is usually recommended in the following circumstances:

- Cellular bloody cyst fluid on aspiration
- Failure of a suspicious mass to disappear completely upon fluid aspiration
- Bloody nipple discharge, with or without a palpable mass
- Skin edema and erythema suggestive of inflammatory breast carcinoma, and a needle core biopsy cannot be performed

In the past, recurrent or persistent simple breast cysts were routinely excised. Because of improvement in ultrasonographic technology, these cysts may now be followed conservatively. This patient, who has had a fine-needle aspiration before, is a candidate for an excisional biopsy.

Management. Treatment is based on the established histologic diagnosis.

Bloody Nipple Discharge

A 60-year-old woman comes to the gynecologist's office complaining of a left breast bloody nipple discharge.

Diagnosis. A bloody nipple discharge usually results from an intraductal papilloma. The treatment is total excision of the duct and papilloma through a circumareolar incision. Modern ductography does not reliably exclude intraductal pathology and is not a substitute for surgery in patients with pathologic discharge. Its utility is in identifying multiple lesions or lesions in the periphery of the breast.

Management. Treatment is based on the established histologic diagnosis.

BREAST CANCER

Breast Cancer Prognosis

A 65-year-old woman visits the gynecologist with a solid 2-cm mass in the upper outer quadrant of the left breast. A biopsy of the lesion is done, which is consistent with "infiltrating ductal breast cancer."

Epidemiology. Breast cancer continues to be the **most common** cancer diagnosed in women of western industrialized countries. An estimated 182,000 new cases of invasive breast cancer were expected to occur among women in the United States during 2000. After increasing by approximately 4% per year in the 1980s, breast cancer incidence rates in women have leveled off in the 1990s to approximately 110 cases per 100,000 women.

Management. The preferred treatment for most patients with stage I or II breast cancer is considered to be breast-conserving therapy with a wide excision, axillary lymph node dissection or sentinel lymph node biopsy, and radiotherapy. Lymphatic mapping and sentinel lymph node biopsy are new procedures that offer the ability to avoid axillary lymph node dissection and its associated morbidity in patients with small primary tumors who are at low risk of axillary node involvement, while still offering nodal staging information.

Prognostic Factors. Some of the key decisions in the current management of primary breast cancer involve the need for prognostication. Prognostic factors serve to identity those patients who might benefit from adjuvant therapy.

- **Lymph node status.** This is important in determining cancer staging and treatment options. Axillary lymph node status is the most important factor in the prognosis of patients with breast cancer. As the number of positive axillary lymph nodes increases, survival rate decreases and relapse rate increases. An adequate dissection usually contains at least 10 lymph nodes; however, because these tumors in 25–30% of patients with negative nodes eventually recur, other biologic prognostic factors also are needed.
- **Tumor size.** This correlates with the number of histologically involved lymph nodes; however, it is also an independent prognostic factor, particularly in node-negative women. The use of size of the tumor, as the most significant prognostic factor, is problematic because 15% of patients with small tumors have positive nodal involvement.

- **Receptor status.** It is standard practice to determine both estrogen and progesterone receptor status at the time of diagnosis for definitive surgical therapy. Although hormone receptor status correlates with the prognosis, it does so to a lesser degree than nodal status. Hormone receptor determination is, however, of critical importance as a predictive factor. A predictive factor is any measurement associated with response or lack of response of a particular therapy.

> - Estrogen receptor status has clearly shown to be a predictive factor for hormone therapy, either in the adjuvant therapy or the metastatic disease setting. HER-2 (also known as HER-2.neu and c-erbB-2) is an epidermal growth factor receptor on the surface of a cell that transmits growth signals to the cell nucleus.
> - Approximately 25–30% of breast cancers overexpress HER-2, and overexpression of the receptor is associated with poor prognosis. This may be more of a reflection of the biologic correlates of HER-2 overexpression, e.g., rapid tumor cell proliferation, larger tumor size, and loss of hormone receptors, than an independent prognostic indicator.

- **DNA ploidy status.** DNA ploidy status of tumors is determined by flow cytometry. It measures the average DNA per cell. Tumors can be classified as diploid with normal DNA content or aneuploid. Disease-free survival rates are significantly worse in patients with aneuploid tumors than in those with diploid tumors; however, it is unclear whether ploidy has an independent prognostic value.

Infiltrating Ductal Carcinoma

This is the **most common** breast malignancy accounting for 80% of breast cancers. Most are unilateral and start as atypical ductal hyperplasia which may progress to ductal carcinoma in situ (DCIS) which then may break through the basement membrane and progress to invasive ductal carcinoma. Over time the tumor will become a stony hard mass as it increases in size and undergoes a fibrotic response.

Infiltrating Lobular Carcinoma

This is the **second most common** breast malignancy accounting for 10% of breast cancers. Most are unilateral and start as lobular carcinoma in situ (LCIS) which then may break through the basement membrane and progress to invasive lobular carcinoma. The prognosis is better with lobular than with ductal carcinoma.

Inflammatory Breast Cancer

This is an uncommon breast malignancy. Usually, there is no single lump or tumor. It is characterized by rapid growth with early metastasis. As the lymphatics get blocked, the breast becomes erythematous, swollen and warm to examination. The edematous skin of the breast appears pitted, like the skin of an orange, giving the classic **peau d'orange** appearance.

Paget Disease of the Breast/Nipple

This is an uncommon breast malignancy with a generally better prognosis than infiltrating ductal carcinoma. The lesion is pruritic and appears red and scaly often located in the nipple spreading to the areola. The skin appearance can mimic dermatosis like eczema or psoriasis. The nipple may become inverted and discharge may occur. It is almost always associated with DCIS or infiltrating ductal carcinoma.

Breast Cancer Risk Factors

BRCA 1 or 2 gene mutation	RR 15
Ductal or Lobular CIS	RR 15
Atypical hyperplasia	RR 4
Breast irradiation age < 20	RR 3
Positive family history	RR 3

Sentinel Node Biopsy

A sentinel node (SLN) is the first lymph node(s) to which cancer cells are likely to spread from the primary tumor. Cancer cells may appear in the sentinel node before spreading to other lymph nodes. A dye is injected near the tumor to allow flow to the SLN. A biopsy of the dye-stained node is performed to help determine the extent or stage of cancer. Because SLN biopsy involves the removal of fewer lymph nodes than standard lymph node removal procedures, the potential for side effects is lower.

Node-Positive Early Breast Cancer

> A healthy 55-year-old woman had a lumpectomy (negative margins) and axillary node dissection for a 2.5-cm tumor in the upper outer quadrant of the left breast, with three positive lymph nodes. The tumor was positive for both estrogen and progesterone receptors. She comes to the gynecologist's office wanting an opinion about further therapy.

Management. Breast-conserving therapy with a wide excision (lumpectomy), axillary dissection (or sentinel node biopsy), and radiation therapy is considered the preferred treatment for most patients with stage I or II breast cancer.

In patients at moderate or high risk of developing systemic metastasis, it is preferable to give adjuvant therapy, beginning with chemotherapy followed with radiation therapy. This patient has a high risk of recurrence because of the presence of lymph node metastasis, and it would be inappropriate to withhold further therapy.

Another high risk factor that this patient has is that the tumor is larger than 1 cm. Recommended adjuvant treatment for patients with node-positive breast cancer is explained in the table below.

A large number of prospective randomized trials, as well as recent overviews and meta-analysis of adjuvant systemic therapy, have determined that both chemotherapy and tamoxifen therapy reduce the odds of recurrence in breast cancer patients. A few randomized clinical trials and the overview of meta-analysis of randomized clinical trials have suggested that the combination of chemotherapy and tamoxifen is superior to chemotherapy alone or tamoxifen alone in postmenopausal patients with node-positive breast cancer. Women with estrogen receptor-negative breast cancer appear to have no improvement in recurrence or survival from tamoxifen use.

It has been established that combination chemotherapy is superior to single-agent therapy, and that 4 to 6 cycles of combination therapy are as effective as >6 cycles of treatment.

Table II-13-1. Recommended Adjuvant Treatment for Node-Positive Breast Cancer

Patient Group	Treatment
Premenopausal, ER- or PR-positive	Chemotherapy + tamoxifen, Ovarian ablation (or GnRH analog) ± tamoxifen, Chemotherapy ± ovarian ablation (or GnRH analog) ± tamoxifen
Premenopausal, ER- and PR-negative	Chemotherapy
Postmenopausal, ER- or PR-positive	Tamoxifen + chemotherapy
Postmenopausal, ER- and PR-negative	Chemotherapy
Elderly	Tamoxifen, If no ER and PR expression: chemotherapy

Abbreviations: ER, estrogen receptor; PR, progesterone receptor; GnRH, gonadotropin-releasing hormone.

Goldhirsch A, Glick JH, Gelber RD, Senn H-J. Meeting highlights: International Consensus Panel on the Treatment of Primary Breast Cancer. J Natl. Cancer Inst 1998;90:1604. By permission of the National Cancer Institute.

Index

Q

R